AF904353

DYSLEXIA – A COMPREHENSIVE AND INTERNATIONAL APPROACH

Edited by **Taeko N. Wydell** and **Liory Fern-Pollak**

Dyslexia – A Comprehensive and International Approach
Edited by Taeko N. Wydell and Liory Fern-Pollak

Published by InTech
Janeza Trdine 9, 51000 Rijeka, Croatia

Copyright © 2012 InTech
All chapters are distributed under the Creative Commons Attribution 3.0 license, which allows users to download, copy and build upon published articles even for commercial purposes, as long as the author and publisher are properly credited, which ensures maximum dissemination and a wider impact of our publications. After this work has been published by InTech, authors have the right to republish it, in whole or part, in any publication of which they are the author, and to make other personal use of the work. Any republication, referencing or personal use of the work must explicitly identify the original source.

As for readers, this license allows users to download, copy and build upon published chapters even for commercial purposes, as long as the author and publisher are properly credited, which ensures maximum dissemination and a wider impact of our publications.

Notice
Statements and opinions expressed in the chapters are these of the individual contributors and not necessarily those of the editors or publisher. No responsibility is accepted for the accuracy of information contained in the published chapters. The publisher assumes no responsibility for any damage or injury to persons or property arising out of the use of any materials, instructions, methods or ideas contained in the book.

Publishing Process Manager Vana Persen

Technical Editor Teodora Smiljanic

Cover Designer InTech Design Team

Additional hard copies can be obtained from orders@intechopen.com

Dyslexia – A Comprehensive and International Approach, Edited by Taeko N. Wydell and Liory Fern-Pollak
p. cm.
ISBN 978-953-51-0517-6

We are IntechOpen, the world's leading publisher of Open Access books

Built by scientists, for scientists

3,750+
Open access books available

115,000+
International authors and editors

119M+
Downloads

151
Countries delivered to

Our authors are among the
Top 1%
most cited scientists

12.2%
Contributors from top 500 universities

WEB OF SCIENCE™

Selection of our books indexed in the Book Citation Index
in Web of Science™ Core Collection (BKCI)

Interested in publishing with us?
Contact book.department@intechopen.com

Numbers displayed above are based on latest data collected.
For more information visit www.intechopen.com

For EU product safety concerns:
IN TECH d.o.o., Prolaz Marije Krucifikse Kozulić 3, 51000 Rijeka, Croatia,
info@intechopen.com or visit our website at intechopen.com.

Meet the editors

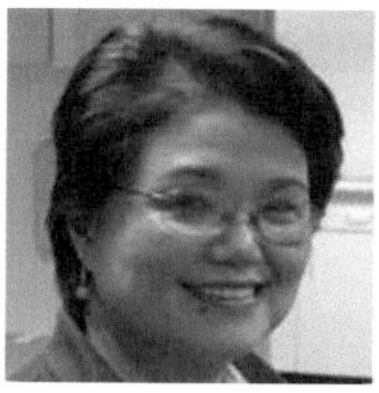

Professor Taeko N. Wydell is a professor in cognitive neuroscience/neuropsychology, and Co-Director of the Centre for Cognition and Neuroimaging (CCNI) at Brunel University, UK. Her research interests include: cognitive and neural processes involved in language, in particular, reading using behavioural and brain imaging (EEG, MEG, & fMRI) techniques; normal and impaired language/reading processes including developmental dyslexia, acquired dyslexia (with neurological patients), and SLI (Specific Language impairment) in different languages (e.g., Chinese, English, Finnish, & Japanese) and bilingual's language/reading processes. Professor Wydell is an internationally recognised researcher who has established several international collaborations in Europe and Asia-Pacific. She has many publications in prestigious journals such as Cognition, Cortex, JEP:LMC, J. of Cognitive Neuroscience, and Reading & Writing.

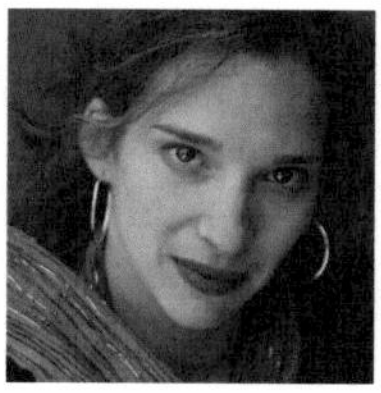

Dr Liory Fern-Pollak (BSc, MSc, PhD) is a cognitive neuroscientist at the Centre for Cognition and Neuroimaging (CCNI) of Brunel University, West London, investigating the neural correlates of multilingual language processing, reading and dyslexia in adults and children. Dr Fern-Pollak teaches biopsychology and statistics at Birkbeck, the Institute of Education, University of London and Kingston University.

Contents

Preface

This book covers all aspects of developmental dyslexia from the underlying aetiology to currently available, routinely used diagnostic tests and intervention strategies, and also addresses important social, cultural and quality of life issues of those with developmental dyslexia.

The ability to read and write is a remarkable trait of humanity. This trait enables us to convey spoken language through the conversion of symbols composed of lines, dashes, circles and dots, into words, phrases and sentences. This ability seems to have emerged around 3,500 years ago; in terms of evolution, this is a relatively recent phenomenon in human history, which dates back some 200,000 years! Unlike spoken language, learning to read and write does not happen through mere exposure during infancy, but requires systematic instruction and applied study, which normally begins in early childhood. While most children are able to reach a skilled level of reading and writing within 5-6 years, some struggle to acquire the skill and may be subsequently diagnosed as having Developmental Dyslexia. This term stands in contrast to Acquired Dyslexia, which is associated with brain damage in individuals who prior to the incident which caused the condition had adequate reading skills.

Developmental Dyslexia is characterised primarily by reading difficulty in the absence of any profound sensory, neurological and intellectual disorders or socio-cultural factors. However, it may co-occur with other developmental disorders such as attention deficit hyperactivity disorder (ADHD), dyscalculia, or dyspraxia, and may therefore manifest as delayed language production, spelling difficulties, and/or difficulties associating sounds and meanings with written words. The precise incidence of Developmental Dyslexia is not known, although it is thought that up to 12% of school children in some countries may face reading difficulties, with higher incidence in boys than girls.

Although now widely regarded as a neurobiological disorder with genetic origin, Developmental Dyslexia may be caused by deficits in auditory processing or visual processing skills, or visual attentional skills as well as a deficit in visual or verbal short-term memory, which can affect its manifestation in isolation or in conjunction. Moreover, different languages exert different cognitive demands on the process of reading. For example, reading in Spanish or Italian, where a close relationship exists between letters and their corresponding sounds, words can be pronounced correctly by assigning to each written consonant the sound of the vowel that follows. In contrast, reading in English often requires prior knowledge of the correct pronunciation, since the phonology of a large proportion of words is not consistent with their spelling (e.g., *pint* vs. hint, lint, mint, tint; *bread, head* vs. *bead; mead* vs. *steak; bough* vs. *cough* vs. *dough* vs. *through* vs. *thorough; colonel; gauge; yacht*). In logographic writing-systems such as Chinese and Japanese Kanji, phonemes do not form part of written text since these languages use intricate characters to directly convey meaning. Reading in these languages therefore requires rote memorization and a complete understanding of the combination of strokes included in each character. Dyslexia may therefore manifest itself differently for speakers of different languages.

Diagnosis of Developmental Dyslexia is a complex process, which requires intellectual, educational, speech and language, medical, and psychological evaluations, as well as a careful consideration of the properties of the particular language. Treatment is typically provided through educational support, which can help dyslexics to complete everyday reading and writing tasks through compensatory strategies, but cannot 'cure' or eliminate the underlying cause. Importantly, beyond the cognitive symptoms and the ensuing difficulty with reading and writing, Dyslexic children may suffer social exclusion, which can lead to behavioural and affective problems. Current research on Developmental Dyslexia therefore comprises various strands; some focusing on the aetiology, some on diagnosis and intervention, and others on psychological and behavioural aspects. All strands aim to provide new insight in order to facilitate early detection, efficient intervention and management of this challenging condition.

In nine chapters written by researchers from different parts of the world, this book brings together leading international research from all strands.

The first three chapters discuss the manifestation of Dyslexia in very different languages; Japanese, Chinese and Spanish, respectively, thus highlighting the effects of the orthographic properties of different languages on differential manifestation of reading difficulty.

The following three chapters explore specific cognitive and biological factors which affect the observed symptoms of Dyslexia among French speakers; namely degraded phonological representations, maturation of the oculomotor system and visual attention span. The eighth chapter provides a comprehensive review of different intervention programs used in UK schools, highlights individual differences in dyslexic children, and the difficulties they face in light of the available diagnostic tools and provision. It further proposes that beyond reading, focus must be shifted towards writing and spelling both for early screening and diagnosis tools and for successful intervention.

The final two chapters touch upon the affective aspect of living with dyslexia among French children in Switzerland and among British adults, respectively.

Professor Taeko N. Wydell and Dr. Liory Fern-Pollak
Centre for Cognition and Neuroimaging (CCNI)
School of Social Sciences
Brunel University
Middlesex
UK

1

Cross-Cultural/Linguistic Differences in the Prevalence of Developmental Dyslexia and the Hypothesis of Granularity and Transparency

Taeko N. Wydell
Centre for Cognition and NeuroImaging, Brunel University, Middlesex, UK

1. Introduction

In this chapter, cross-cultural and cross-linguistic differences in the prevalence of developmental dyslexia will be discussed. In order to account for the differences, the Hypothesis of Granularity and Transparency postulated by Wydell and Butterworth (1999) will be revisited.

Developmental dyslexia is defined as a failure to acquire reading skills, despite adequate intelligence, education and sociocultural opportunity (Chrichey, 1975), and it is generally accepted that it is a neurobiological disorder with a genetic origin (e.g., Eden & Moat, 2002; Fisher & DeFries, 2002). It has been reported that up to 10 – 12% of children in the English speaking world suffer from developmental dyslexia (e.g., Shaywitz, Shaywitz, Fletcher, & Escobar, 1990; Snowling, 2000). Extensive research has been conducted in order to ascertain the causes of dyslexia (and subsequently to develop intervention programmes), since dyslexia sufferers form a large minority group, and yet there seems to be no consensus amongst the researchers as to what causes developmental dyslexia.

Ramus (2003) reviewed recent empirical studies in relation to major theories accounting for the causes of developmental dyslexia, such as for example, *the auditory processing* (in particular, *rapid or temporal processing) deficit hypothesis* (e.g., Tallal, 1980; Share, Jorm, MacLean, & Matthews, 2002); *the visual processing deficit hypothesis including magnocellular dysfunction hypothesis* (e.g., Hansen, Stein, Orde, Winter and Talcott, 2001; Stein, 2001; 2003); *the motor control deficit hypothesis* (e.g., Wolf, 2002) including *the cerebellar dysfunction hypothesis* (e.g., Nicholson, Fawcett, & Dean, 2001); *the general sensorimotor processing deficit hypothesis* (e.g., Laasonen, Service, & Virsu, 2001; 2002) and the *phonological processing deficit hypothesis* (e.g., Ramus, 2001; Snowling, 2000). In his succinctly written review, Ramus pointed out that behavioural genetic studies revealed that phonological deficits are highly heritable, whereas auditory and visual deficits are not (e.g., Davis, Gayan, Knopik, Smith, Cardon, Pennington, Olson, & DeFries, 2001; Olson & Datta, 2002), and concluded that "although the phonological deficit is still in need of a complete cognitive and neurological characterisation, the case for its causal role in the aetiology of the reading and writing disability of the great majority of dyslexic children is overwhelming" (p.216).

Indeed, many behavioural studies in English have found core phonological deficits in children with developmental dyslexia (e.g., Stanovich, 1988; Stanovich & Siegel, 1994;

Snowling 2000). The phonological deficits tend to interfere with the acquisition of appropriate grapheme-to-phoneme conversion skills. Moreover, adults with childhood diagnoses of dyslexia also revealed persistent phonological deficits (e.g., Bruck, 1992). For example, Felton, Naylor, and Wood (1990) found that adults with developmental dyslexia were impaired compared with normal controls using Rapid-Automatized-Naming (RAN), phonological awareness skills and non-word reading tests. Similarly, Paulesu, Frith, Snowling, Gallagher, Morton, Frackowiak and Frith (1996) found that even well-compensated dyslexic adults showed residual phonological deficits on phoneme deletions and Spoonerizing (exchange the initial phonemes of a pair of words, e.g., /car/ /park/ -> /par/ /cark/) tests.

2. Dyslexia and poor phonological recoders

More recently, Wydell in Shapiro, Hurry, Masterson, Wydell and Doctor (2009) tested 158 male and female students aged 14–15 in a state-funded selective and highly academic secondary school in the UK, and identified a subset students with phonological deficits.

The following five phonological tests (in written format) were administered to all the participating students: Rhyme-Judgements in words (e.g., YES to 'head–bed'), Rhyme-Judgement in nonwords (e.g., YES to 'kape-bap'), Homophone-Judgements in words (e.g., YES to 'their-there'), Homophone-Judgements in nonwords (e.g., YES to 'kane-kain'), Phonological-Lexical Decisions (e.g., YES to 'brane').

Wydell identified 16 students out of this cohort (*approximately just over 10%*), whose scores on any of these tests fell more than 1.5 standard deviations (SD) below the mean of the group, as *poor phonological recoder (PPR) readers* (i.e., those with phonological deficits).

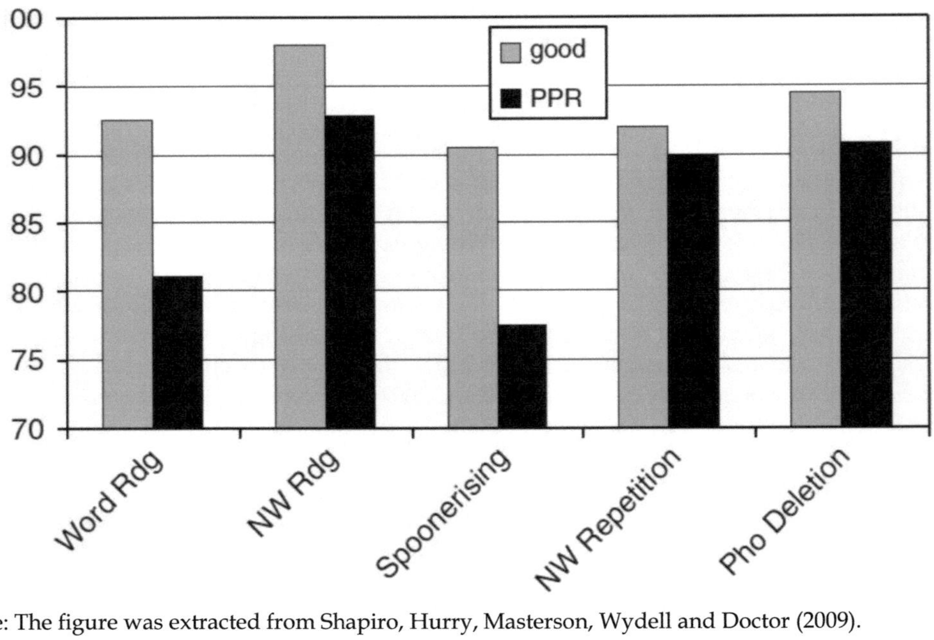

Note: The figure was extracted from Shapiro, Hurry, Masterson, Wydell and Doctor (2009).

Fig. 1. Proportion correct for reading and phonological tasks of PPR-Readers compared with that of the controls.

Those PPR-readers and 16 randomly selected normal readers were further tested for their skills in Word Reading, Nonword Reading, Spoonerizing, Phoneme Deletions, and Non-word Repetition. As illustrated in *Figure 1*, the results revealed that PPR-readers were significantly worse than the controls on all the tests (p>.01 – p>.0001) except for Phoneme Deletions (p=.08) and Non-word repetition (p>1). Note that Gathercole and Baddeley's (1996) Non-word Repetition test is known to be one of the most effective diagnostic tools to identify developmental dyslexia in young children. Yet, this test did not show any difference between the PPR-readers and the normal controls. This might be because the test was developed primarily to assess young children's phonological skills, and that the test might not be sensitive enough for these adolescent individuals.

Furthermore, Wydell compared these PPR-readers' performance on SATs[1] in English, Science and Mathematics individually, with that of the normal controls using z-scores[2].

The results revealed that 60% of PPR-readers' SAT-English scores, and 70% of their SAT-Science scores were significantly lower than those of normal controls (both at p<.001). In SAT-Maths scores, however, none of the PPR-readers were significantly worse than the controls, indicating that cognitive processes involved in reading may be different from those involved in mathematical operations (a similar pattern of data can be seen in the case study reported by Wydell & Butterworth, 1999).

Wydell thus identified a subset of students aged 14-15 with phonological deficits even in a selective and competitive academic environment, where all students appeared to be performing well against the national average. Yet, these PPR-readers can still be considered as academic underachievers, as Hannell (2004) suggested.

3. Dyslexia and the hypothesis of granularity and transparency

Wydell and Butterworth (1999) reported the case of an adolescent English-Japanese bilingual male, AS, whose reading and writing difficulties are confined to English only. Extensive investigations into his reading/writing difficulties in English revealed that he has typical phonological processing deficits (Wydell & Butterworth, 1999; Wydell & Kondo, 2003). *Figure 2* illustrates his performance in reading and phonological processing tests in English together with those of age-matched English and Japanese monolingual controls, which clearly indicate his phonological processing deficits.

However his ability to read Japanese was equivalent and often better than that of his Japanese peers, as illustrated in *Table 1*.

Note that the Japanese writing system consists of two qualitatively different scripts: logographic, morphographic Kanji, derived from Chinese characters, and two forms of syllabic Kana, Hiragana and Katakana which are derived from Kanji characters (see Wydell, Patterson, & Humphreys, 1993 for more details). These three scripts are used to write different classes of words. Kanji characters are used for nouns and for the root morphemes

---

[1] SATs - Standard Assessment Tests: national achievement tests given to all the children across the UK at the end of Year-2 (aged seven), Year-6 (aged 11) and Year-9 (aged 14).

[2] This is because it has been reported that there are marked individual differences among children with developmental dyslexia both in terms of the extent of the severity and the nature of difficulties/impairments (e.g., Snowling & Griffiths, 2005).

of inflected verbs, adjectives and adverbs. Hiragana characters are used mainly for function words and the inflections of verbs, adjectives and adverbs, and for some nouns with uncommon Kanji representations. Katakana characters are used for the large number of foreign loan words (e.g. テレビ/terebi/TV) in contemporary Japanese.

Both forms of Kana have an almost perfect one-to-one relationship between character and pronunciation. That is, one character always represents one particular syllable or mora (syllable like unit) of the Japanese language and its sound value does not change whether the character appears in the first position, the middle position or at the end of a multi-syllable word. This is different from English, where orthographic units not only map onto sub-syllabic phonological units, but the mapping will also depend on context, i.e. the location within the word.

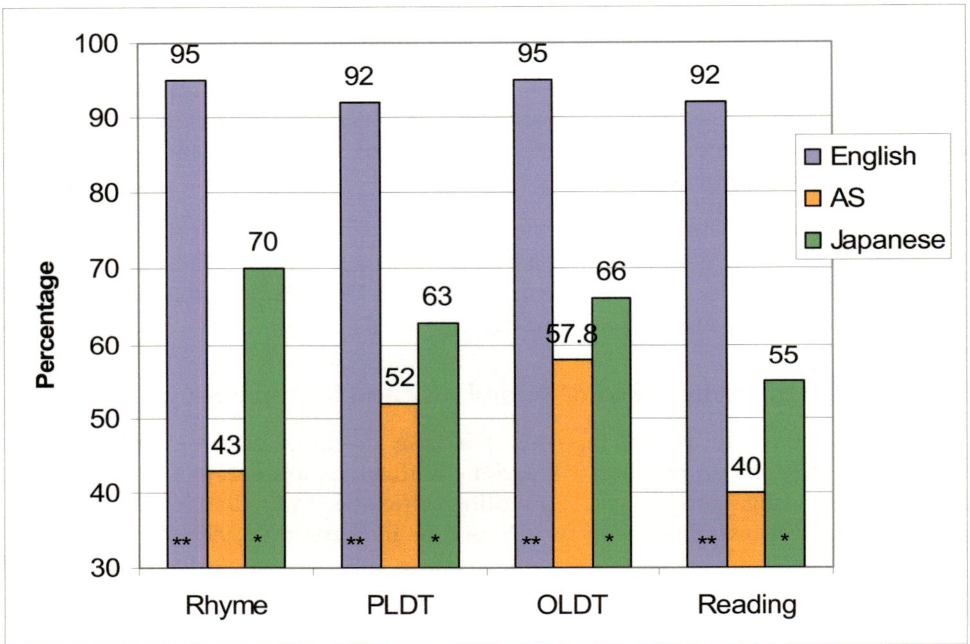

Note: These tests are in written format: Rhyme = Rhyme judgements; PLDT = Phonological lexical decision task (YES to psudohomophones, e.g., brane); PLDT = Orthographic lexical decision task (i.e., spell checking); Reading = reading aloud. ** = p<.01; * = p<.05.
The data were extracted from Wydell and Kondo (2003).

Fig. 2. A comparison of AS's performance with that of Japanese and English monolingual controls for reading and phonological tests

Words in Kanji have 1–5 characters with two being the modal number, and 2.4 the mean.

The relationship between character and pronunciation in Kanji is very opaque. This is because each Kanji character is a morphographic element that cannot phonetically be decomposed in the way that an alphabetic word can be. There are no separate components of a character that correspond to the individual phonemes (see Wydell, Patterson & Butterworth, 1995 for a further discussion). Also, most Kanji characters have one or more ON-readings, (pronunciations that were imported from spoken Chinese along with their corresponding characters) as well as a KUN-reading from the original Japanese spoken language. Some characters have no KUN-reading, but for those which have, the KUN-reading is almost always the correct reading when this character constitutes a word on its own (e.g., 花/hana/ in KUN-reading, meaning 'flower' which represents a single-character word; 花束/hana-taba/ in KUN-reading, meaning 'bouquet' vs. 花瓶/ka-bin/ in ON-reading, meaning 'vase').

Word type	AS	(Control)		AS	(Control)	
	High frequency (n = 40)			Low frequency (n = 40)		
		S.7	S.14		S.7	S.14
Consistent	95%	(99.2%)		95%	(97.9%)	
RT (ms)	880	*814*	*924*	800	*786*	*776*
Inc-ON	100%	(98.7%)		90%	(89.2%)	
RT (ms)	883	*813*	*812*	802	*760*	*810*
Inc-KUN	100%	(97.9%)		80%	(87.2%)	
RT (ms)	965	*919*	*1377*	838	*791*	*916*
Jukujikun	85%	(89.2%)		60%*	(81.7%)	
RT (ms)	1070	*1119*	*1215*	843	*960*	*1052*

*Outside of the range of normal adults (aged between 20 and 54 years, mean age 31 years). The control data are the adult data from Wydell et al. (1997).

Note: Consistent = each character in a two-character Kanji word has one invariant ON (or occasionally KUN)-reading; Inc-ON (Inconsistent ON-reading) = each character takes ON-reading in a two-character word, but each character has a KUN-reading and/or another ON-reading; Inc-KUN (Inconsistent KUN) = each character takes KUN-reading in a two-character word, but each character has at least one ON-reading; Jukujikun = truly exception words, neither character in a two-character Kanji word takes typical ON or KUN-reading, e.g., 雪崩/nadare/ meaning 'avalanche' however the first character means 'snow', and it is /yuki/ in KUN-reading, while it is /setsu/ in ON-reading; the second character means 'collapse', and it is /kuzu/ in KUN-reading, while it is /hou/ in ON-reading.
The table was extracted from Wydell & Butterworth (1999).

Table 1. AS's Performance for two-character Kanji word naming

Table 1 shows that his accuracy in reading two-character Kanji words is equivalent to Japanese undergraduate level except for low familiar Jukujikun (z = -3.63, P , 0.0009). Wydell and Butterworth stated that the latter may be due to the fact that he had not had enough exposure to low familiar Jukujikun. When AS was tested with these words, he was 16 years old, while the youngest participant who took part in the experiment of Wydell, Butterworth, Shibahara and Zorzi (1997) was 20 years old (mean age was 31 years old). Kanji learning is essentially a life-long continuous learning process. If he were continuously educated within the Japanese educational system, he would most probably be able to read these low familiar Jukujikun by the time he graduated from a Japanese university.

In order to account for the dissociation between his ability to read in English and Japanese, Wydell and Butterworth (1999) put forward the Hypothesis of Granularity[3] and

[3] In their review paper, Ziegler and Goswami (2005) also pointed out the importance of 'granularity' in order to explain developmental dyslexia across different languages, and postulated the "Psycholinguistic grain size theory", which, however, "does not predict that orthographic consistency

Transparency as illustrated in *Figure 3*. The hypothesis maintains that orthographies can be described in these two dimensions - (1) any orthography, where the print-to-sound translation is one-to-one or transparent *would not produce a high incidence of phonological dyslexia* (i.e., dyslexia due to phonological deficits) regardless of the level of translation, i.e. phoneme, syllable, character, etc. This is the 'transparency' dimension, and (2) even when this relationship is opaque and not one-to-one, any orthography whose smallest orthographic unit representing sound is coarse, i.e. a whole character or whole word, *would not produce a high incidence of phonological dyslexia*. This is the 'granularity' dimension. Any orthography used in any language can be placed in the transparency-granularity orthogonal dimension described by this hypothesis.

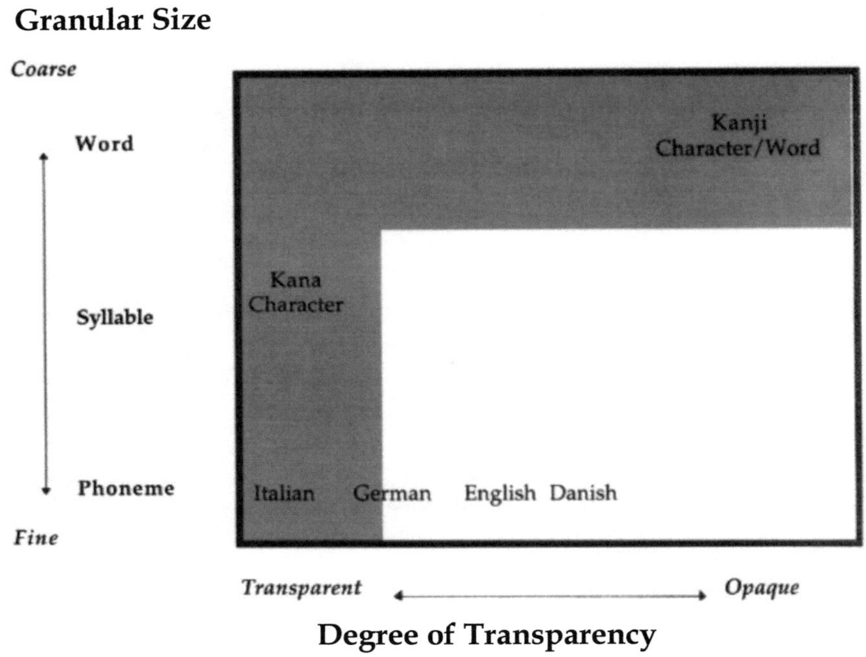

Fig. 3. Hypothesis of Granularity and Transparency and orthography-to-phonology correspondence.

For example, the granularity of the smallest orthographic unit representing phonology for *Japanese Kana* is finer than the whole word, but coarser than the grapheme, and its orthography-to-phonology mapping is at the level of syllables and one-to-one. In contrast, for *Japanese Kanji*, the unit of granularity is much coarser, i.e. a character or a whole word,

(i.e., transparency) reduced developmental dyslexia" (p.20). They further argued that had Wydell and Butterworth included nonword reading tasks in terms of "timed performance", he (AS) would have "displayed clear deficits in reading" in both languages (p.20). However, Zigler and Goswami did not include Wydell and Kondo (2003)'s follow-up study in their review paper. Wydell and Kondo stated that "AS's reading was never laborious and slow" (p.40). Although they did not measure RT for each stimulus word or nonword in milliseconds, they measured AS's reading latencies for stimulus lists (in minutes/seconds), which included nonwords in English and Japanese Kana. AS's reading latencies were comparable to those of the English controls, and were shorter than those of the Japanese controls.

and the orthography -to-phonology mapping is very opaque, hence Kanji can be placed in the shaded area. By this hypothesis, therefore, either of the two scripts used in Japanese should *not lead to a high incidence of phonological dyslexia.*

Now with this categorisation, English can be placed outside of the shaded area, since the granularity for English is small/finer, however, the orthography-to-phonology mapping is not always one-to-one and not transparent. By this hypothesis, English orthography *may lead to a high incidence of phonological dyslexia.* Given the differences between the two orthographies used in Japanese and English, therefore, the hypothesis of granularity and transparency argues that it might be possible for an English-Japanese bilingual individual to be dyslexic in English but not in Japanese.

4. Prevalence of dyslexia and the hypothesis of granularity and transparency

Indeed, researchers have argued that the difference in the prevalence of developmental dyslexia in the different languages might be primarily due to the differences inherent in the characteristics of each orthography, in particular, the way in which phonology is computed from orthography (e.g., de Luca, Burani, Paizi, Spinelli, Zoccolotti, 2010; Landerl, Wimmer, Frith, 1997; Wydell & Butterworth, 1999; Zoccolotti, de Luca, de Pace, Gasperini, Judica, Spinelli, 2005). Earlier it was mentioned that in English up to 10 - 12% of children are reported to suffer from developmental dyslexia (e.g., Shaywitz, et al., 1990; Snowling, 2000). In Danish, as many as 12% of adults in Denmark have difficulties in reading, which was revealed in the study conducted by Elbro, Moller, and Nielsen (1995). In these languages, orthography-to-phonology correspondence (which means grapheme-to-phoneme correspondence in alphabetic languages) is not consistent, i.e., not always one-to-one or transparent (e.g., hint, lint, tint vs. pint; bread, head vs. bead, mead; colonel; yacht; bough vs. dough vs. through vs. thorough). However, in alphabetical languages whereby the grapheme-to-phoneme correspondence is consistent or transparent, such as for example, Dutch, German, or Italian, the prevalence of developmental dyslexia is much lower (e.g., de Luca, et al., 2010; Zoccolotti et al., 2005 for Italian; Landerl, et al., 1997 for the comparison between German and English speakers; Paulesu, De´monet, Fazio, McCrory, Chanoine, Brunswick, Cappa, Cossu, Habib, Frith, C.D., & Frith U., 2001 for the comparison between English, French and Italian speakers).

For example, Landerl et al. (1997) examined the reading and phonological processing skills of English and German dyslexic children against their normal chronological and reading age-matched controls, and found that although the same underlying phonological processing deficit might exist in both German and English dyslexic children, there were differences in the severity of the reading impairment. English dyslexic children showed a marked adverse effect in the acquisition of reading skills compared to German dyslexic children. These differences were also seen between the normal German and English control children in their reading performance. Landerl et al. suggested that these differences were due to differences in orthographic 'consistency'. That is, different orthographies have different mapping rules, and there is a wide range in the degree of consistency with which alphabets represent phonemes by graphemes. 'Consistency' here is interchangeable with 'transparency'. For orthographies such as German, Italian or Spanish, the grapheme-to-phoneme mapping is, in general, one-to-one, and consistent/transparent. For other orthographies such as English or Danish, the grapheme-to-phoneme mapping is often one-to-many (e.g., food vs. hood vs. flood or blood), and less consistent/transparent (e.g. Seidenberg, Waters, Barnes, & Tanenhaus, 1984). Thus it was assumed that orthographic consistency/transparency affects both the nature and degree of reading difficulties (de Luca, et al., 2010; Zoccolotti et al., 2005).

Landerl et al. further argued that phonological recoding itself may not necessarily be a demanding task. When grapheme-to-phoneme mapping is consistent/transparent, children can easily acquire the grapheme-phoneme correspondence rules, and use these to assemble pronunciations for novel letter strings (as seen with Italian or Spanish children for example). Therefore, the phonological recoding may become a demanding task, only when the grapheme-phoneme correspondence in an orthography is not consistent/transparent, such as for example, English (Snowling, 2000) or Danish (Elbo et al., 1995). Therefore, if the grapheme-phoneme correspondence is consistent, even children with phonological deficits may be able to learn to map print onto sound thus without showing a delay in reading acquisition. Similarly, the 'hypothesis of granularity and transparency' in particular, the transparency dimension predicts that *developmental phonological dyslexia* should not manifest itself in a writing system where the print-to-sound correspondence is transparent regardless of the size unit of granularity.

Moreover, the granularity dimension of the hypothesis predicts that developmental phonological dyslexia should not manifest itself in a writing system where the unit of granularity is coarse at a whole character or whole word level. It should therefore be possible to find a bilingual individual with monolingual dyslexia, especially between two orthographies such as English and Japanese.

Further evidence which lends support to the Hypothesis can be seen in a recent cross sectional study conducted in Japanese by Uno, Wydell, Haruhara, Kaneko and Shinya (2009). In their study, 495 Japanese primary school children (from 2nd Grade aged eight to 6th Grade aged 12) in Japan were tested for their reading, writing and other cognitive skills including phonological awareness (STRAW, 2006). The results showed that percentages of children who had reading difficulties (defined as those whose reading/writing/phonological tests' scores fell below -1.5SD) in syllabic Hiragana, syllabic Katakana, and logographic Kanji were 0.2%, 1.4%, and 6.9% respectively – these figures were significantly lower than those reported in the studies in English (Shaywitz et al., 1997; Snowling, 2000) or Danish (Elbo et al., 1995). Yet there was no significant difference in the IQ scores between the normal group and reading/writing disabled (RWD) group (measured by Ravens Coloured Progressive Matrices, 1976).

The study also suggested that different reading strategies might be adopted when reading in Kana and Kanji. For Kana, where the character-to-sound-mapping is transparent, a simple on-line phonological processing (i.e., sublexical analytical reading) strategy might be used (Wydell & Butterworth, 1999; Rastle, Havelka, Wydell, Coltheart, Besner 2009), just like other consistent orthographies such as Italian (de Luca, et al., 2010; Zoccolotti et al., 2005) or German (Landerl et al., 1997). In contrast, for Kanji, because the character-to-sound-relationship is opaque, and the correct pronunciation is determined at the whole-word level, a lexical whole-word reading strategy might be used (e.g., Morton, Sasanuma, Patterson & Sakuma, 1992; Wydell, 1998; Wydell & Butterworth, 1999; Wydell, et al., 1993; Wydell, Butterworth & Patterson, 1995; however also see Fushimi, Ijuin, Patterson & Tatsumi, 1999 for counter argument).

Thus the results of Uno et al.'s (2009) study further lend support to the Hypothesis of Granularity and Transparency. Wydell and Butterworth (1999) argued that English orthography would require a fine tuning of the orthography-to-phonology mapping, because English orthography is not completely transparent at the subsyllabic level (i.e. smaller grain-unit than syllables). In contrast, the grain size for Kana is at the whole character level (i.e., greater grain-unit than graphemes), and its orthography-to-phonology mapping is transparent (one-to-one). Hence Japanese children in general find it easier to master reading in Kana. This is because, as Landerl et al. (1997) argued for German, the phonological recoding of Kana is not a demanding task. Moreover, although the grain size for Kanji is either at whole character or whole word level, its orthography-to-phonology mapping is opaque (one-to-many). Consequently learning to read in Kanji for Japanese children is harder than that in Kana. The results thus indicate that reading Kanji may require different reading strategies or different cognitive skills to those required for reading Kana. If so, reading English may yet require different reading strategies to those required for Kanji or Kana.

Wydell and Butterworth (1999) thus speculated that it is therefore possible to be a Danish or English-Japanese bilingual with monolingual dyslexia in Danish or English.

5. Dyslexia and cross-cultural and cross-linguistic differences

Interestingly, in Japan rather than group studies, single case studies of children with reading disorders have started to emerge (e.g., Kaneko, Uno, Kaga, Matsuda, Inagaki, & Haruhara, 1997; 1998; Uno, Kaneko, Haruhara, Matsuda, Kato, & Kasahara, 2002). The majority of these children in Japan tend to have both reading and writing difficulties, and often the writing impairment is more severe than the reading impairment[4]. Significantly, in Japan there are very few reported cases of children with reading impairments only. The Japanese researchers usually attribute these reading and writing impairments among children to 'visual' or 'visuospatial' processing problems (e.g., Kaneko et al., 1998) rather than phonological processing problems.

Unlike alphabetic orthographies but similar to Japanese KANJI, the Chinese language uses a logographic writing system whereby the basic orthographic units, the Chinese characters, correspond directly to morphemic meanings and to syllables in the spoken language. The pronunciations of Chinese characters are represented at the monosyllabic level, and no phonemes are represented in a character. That is, reading a Chinese character does not allow the segmental analysis (i.e., grapheme-to-phoneme conversion), which is fundamental in alphabetic orthographies (Wanga, Bi, Gao, &Wydell, 2010). Therefore Chinese is often referred as a morphosyllabic writing system (Shu & Anderson, 1997). Further, Meng, Sai, Wang X., Wang, J., Sha, and Zhou (2005) pointed out that there is only limited systematic correspondence between orthography and phonology. Moreover, Mandarin Chinese has a large number of homophonic morphemes and homophonic characters. Therefore it is often stated that the use of phonological information may not be as critical in reading Chinese as it is in reading alphabetic languages (Ho, Chan, Lee, Tsang, & Luan, 2004; Ho, Chan, Tsang, & Lee, 2002; Shu, McBride-Chang,Wu, & Liu, 2006). If this were the case, then a high incidence

[4] In English, it is often the case that when reading is impaired, writing is also impaired, and therefore dyslexia is assumed to mean both reading and writing impairments.

of phonological dyslexia in Chinese should not be seen (*cf* the Hypothesis of Granularity and Transparency (Wydell & Butterworth, 1999)).

Similar to Uno et al.'s (2009) study in Japanese, Li, Shu, McBride-Chang, Liu and Peng (in press) investigated the acquisition of reading in Chinese, and tested 184 kindergarten children and 273 primary school children from Beijing, Mainland China for their skills in (a) Chinese character recognition, (b) visual-spatial relationships and visual memory, (c) orthographic judgement, (d) phonological awareness including (d1) Rime deletion, (d2) Syllable deletion, (d3) Phoneme deletion and (d4) Rapid number naming, (e) Morphological awareness including (e1) Homophone judgements, (e2) Morphological construction, and (e3) Morpheme production.

The results showed that especially for the primary school children, a unique and relatively strong relationship between (c) orthographic knowledge (and not (b) visual skills) and reading was found. In addition, (d) phonological and (e) morphological awareness "appear to be somewhat important for reading throughout the very beginning and intermediate periods of character acquisition" (p.15). However, (d3) phoneme deletion was not uniquely associated with reading particularly for the primary school children. Li et al. thus argued that "phoneme awareness by itself is relatively unimportant for reading Chinese because the phoneme is not explicitly represented in the Chinese orthography" (p.16). Li et al. further argued that unlike most alphabetic writing systems where there is a strong relationship between phoneme awareness and reading skills, in Chinese larger unit size such as syllable or rime may be a better predictor variable for reading Chinese characters.

Indeed, recent research has revealed that the major cause of developmental dyslexia in Chinese is a deficit in orthographic processing skills, rather than in phonological processing skills (e.g., Chan, Ho, Tsang, Lee, & Chung, 2006; Ho et al., 2004; Shu et al., 2006), though some studies did show that Chinese dyslexic children had phonological deficits (e.g., deficits in rapid naming (e.g., Ho, Law, & Ng, 2000) and auditory processing (e.g., Meng et al., 2005).

In order to ascertain neurophysiologically a cause of developmental dyslexia in Chinese, Wang, Bi, Gao, and Wydell (2010) conducted an ERP (Event Related Potential) study with Chinese dyslexic and chronological-age-matched, and reading-level-matched non-dyslexic children from Beijing, Mainland China, employing a psychophysical experiment, i.e., the motion-onset paradigm. A similar psychophysical paradigm was first employed by Rogers-Ramachandran and Ramachandran (1998) with English-speakers as their participants, whereby two distinct visual systems/pathways in human vision were identified, namely, "a fast, sign-invariant system concerned with extracting controls" (p.71) which is the magnocellular visual system, and "a shallower, sign-sensitive system concerned with assigning surface colour" (p.71), which is the parvocellular visual system. Subsequent similar psychophysics studies with English-speaking children as participants showed that the performance of the participating children significantly correlated with the measures of orthographic skills in the Magnocellular Condition (e.g., Sperling, Lu, Manis, and Seidenberg, 2003; Talcott, Witton, McLean, Hansen, Rees, & Green, 2000).

Wang et al.'s ERP study revealed that the Chinese dyslexic children's orthographic processing skills were significantly compromised, when compared to their Chinese chronological and reading age-matched control children, which in turn, Wang et al. argued, is linked to a deficit in the visual magnocelluar system.

Other brain imaging studies using fMRI (functional Magnetic Resonance Imaging) in Chinese such as Siok, Niu, Jin, Perfetti, and Tan (2008) or Siok, Perfetti, Jin, & Tan (2004) revealed functional and structural abnormalities in the left middle frontal gyrus of Chinese dyslexic children, but not in the left temporoparietal and occipitotemporal regions that are important for reading in alphabetic languages (e.g., Paulesu, McCrory, et al., 2000; Wydell, Vuorinen, Helenius & Salmelin, 2003), and are typically compromised in dyslexic children in alphabetic languages (e.g., Horwitz, Rumsey, & Donohue, 1998; Temple, Poldrack, Salidis, Deutsch, Tallall, Merzenich, & Gabriel, 2001). These researchers therefore argued that reading Chinese characters might require firstly greater cognitive demand for visual processing than reading in alphabetic languages such as English, and secondly a greater inter-activity between orthography and phonology. This is because, like Japanese Kanji, reading Chinese characters requires retrieving phonology as a whole rather than addressing phonology in piece-meal fashion (see Wang et al., 2010 for more details). Therefore Siok and his colleagues also suggested that the neural abnormality found in impaired readers is dependent on culture (see also Paulesu, Frith, et al., 2001 for a similar argument).

Thus in this Chapter, having reviewed recent empirical studies in alphabetical as well as non-alphabetic languages such as Chinese and Japanese, the chapter has shown significant cross-cultural/linguistic differences in the prevalence of developmental dyslexia in different languages.

6. References

Bruck, M. (1992). Persistence of dyslexics' phonological awareness deficits. *Developmental Psychology, 28*, 874–886.

Chan, D.W., Ho, C.S.H., Tsang, S.M., Lee, S.H., & Chung, K.K.H. (2006). Exploring the reading–writing connection in Chinese children with dyslexia in Hong Kong. *Reading and Writing, 19*(6), 543–561.

Chrichey, M. (1975). Specific developmental dyslexia. In: Lenneberg, E.H., Lenneberg, E. (Eds.), *Foundations of Language Development*, Vol. 2. Academic Press, New York.

Davis, C.J., Gayan, J., Knopik, V.S., Smith, S.D., Cardon, L.R., Pennington, B.F., Olson, R.K., & DeFries, J.C. (2001). Etiology of reading difficulties and rapid naming: the Coloradotwin study of reading disability. *Behavioral Genetics, 31*:625-635.

de Luca M, Burani C, Paizi D, Spinelli D, Zoccolotti P. (2010). Letter and letter-string processing in developmental dyslexia. *Cortex 46,* 1272–83.

Eden, G., & Moats, L. (2002). The role of neuroscience in the remediation of students with dyslexia. *Nature Neuroscience, 5,* 1080–1084.

Elbo, C., Moller, S., & Nielsen, E.M., (1995). Functional reading difficulties in Denmark: a study of adult reading of common text. *Reading and Writing 7,* 257–276.

Felton, R. H., Naylor, C. E., & Wood, F. B. (1990). Neuropsychological profile of adult dyslexia. *Brain and Language, 39,* 485–497.

Fisher, S. E., & DeFries, J. (2002). Developmental dyslexia: genetic dissection of a complex cognitive trait. *Nature Reviews Neuroscience, 3,* 767–780.

Fushimi, T., Ijuin, M., Patterson, K., & Tatsumi, I. (1999). Consistency, frequency, and lexicality effects in naming Japanese Kanji. *Journal of Experimental Psychology: Human Perception and Performance, 25,* 382–407.

Gathercole, S.E., & Baddeley, A.D. (1996). The Children's Test of Nonword Repetition. London: The Psychological Corporation.

Hannell, G. (2004). *Dyslexia: Action plans for successful learning*. Great Britain: David Fulton Publishers.

Hansen, P.C., Stein, J.F., Orde, S.R., Winter, J.L., & Talcott, J.B. (2001). Are dyslexics' visual deficits limited to measures of dorsal stream function? *NeuroReport, 12*:1527-1530.

Ho, C. S. H., Chan, D. W. O., Lee, S. H., Tsang, S. M., & Luan, V. V. H. (2004). Cognitive profiling and preliminary subtyping in Chinese developmental dyslexia. *Cognition, 91*(1), 43–75.

Ho, C. S. H., Chan, D. W. O., Tsang, S. M., & Lee, S. H. (2002). The cognitive profile and multiple-deficit hypothesis in Chinese developmental dyslexia. *Developmental Psychology, 38*(4), 543–553.

Ho, C. S. H., Law, T. P. S., & Ng, P. M. (2000). The phonological deficit hypothesis in Chinese developmental dyslexia. *Reading and Writing, 13*(1–2), 57–79.

Horwitz, B., Rumsey, J. M. & Donohue, B. C. (1998). Functional connectivity of the angular gyrus in normal reading and dyslexia. *Proceeding of the National Academy of Sciences, USA, 95*, 8939–8944 (1998).

Kaneko, M., Uno, A., Kaga, M., Matsuda, H., Inagaki, M., Haruhara, N. (1997). Developmental dyslexia and dysgraphia: a case report (in Japanese). *NO TO HATTATSU (Brain and Child Development) 29*, 249–253.

Kaneko, M., Uno, A., Kaga, M., Matsuda, H., Inagaki, M., Haruhara, N. (1998). Cognitive Neuropsycho-logical and Regional Cerebral Blood Flow Study of a Developmentally Dyslexic Japanese Child. *Journal of Child Neurology Brief Communications 13*, 9.

Laasonen, M., Service, E., & Virsu, V. (2001). Temporal order and processing acuity of visual, auditory, and tactile perception in developmental dyslexic young adults. *Cogn Affect Behav Neurosi, 1*; 394-410.

Laasonen, M., Service, E., & Virsu, V. (2002). Crossmodal temporal order and processing acuity in developmental dyslexic young adults. *Brain & Language, 80*, 340-354.

Landerl, K., Wimmer, H., & Frith, U. (1997). The impact of orthographic consistency on dyslexia: a German-English comparison. *Cognition 63*, 315–334.

Li, H., Shu, H., McBride-Chang, C., Liu, H., & Peng, H. (in press). Chinese children's character recognition: Visuo-orthographic, phonological processing and morphological skills. Journal of Research in Reading. *DOI: 10.1111/j.1467-9817.2010.01460.x*

Meng, X. Z., Sai, X. G., Wang, C. X., Wang, J., Sha, S. Y., & Zhou, X. L. (2005). Auditory and speech processing and reading development in Chinese school children: Behavioural and ERP evidence. *Dyslexia, 11*(4), 292–310.

Morton, J., Sasanuma, S., Patterson, K., & Sakuma, N. (1992). The organisation of lexicon in Japanese: Single and compound Kanji. *British Journal of Psychology 83*, 517–531.

Nicolson, R.I., Fawcett, A.J., & Dean, P. (2001). Dyslexia, development and the cerebellum. *Trends in Neuroscience, 24*:515-516.

Olson. R., & Datta, H. (2002). Visual-temporal processing in readingdisabled and normal twins. *Reading and Writing15*:127-149.

Paulesu, E., Frith, U., Snowling, M., Gallagher, A., Morton, R.S.J., Frackowiak, R., & Frith, C.D. (1996). Is developmental dyslexia a disconnection syndrome? Evidence from PET scanning. *Brain 119*, 143–157.

Paulesu, E., De´monet, J-F., Fazio, F., McCrory, E., Chanoine, V., Brunswick, N., Cappa, S.F., Cossu, G., Habib, M., Frith, C.D., & Frith U. (2001). Dyslexia: cultural diversity and biological unity. *Science, 291*:2165-2167.

Paulesu, E., Frith, U., Snowling, M., Gallagher, A., Morton, R.S.J., Frackowiak, R., & Frith, C.D. (1996). Is developmental dyslexia a disconnection syndrome? Evidence from PET scanning. *Brain 119*, 143–157.

Paulesu, E., McCrory, E., Fazio, F., Menoncello, L., Brunswick, N., Cappa, S., Cotelli, M., Cossu, G., Corte, F., Lorusso, M., Pesenti, S., Gallagher, A., Perani, D., Price, C., Frith, C., &Frith, U. (2000). A cultural effect on brain function. *Nature Neuroscience, 3*, 91–96.

Ramus, F. (2001). Outstanding questions about phonological processing in dyslexia. *Dyslexia, 7*; 125-149.

Ramus, F. (2003). Developmental dyslexia: specific phonological deficit or general sensorimotor dysfunction? *Current Opinion in Neurobiology, 13*, 212-218.

Rastle K, Havelka J, Wydell T, Coltheart M, & Besner D. (2009). The cross-script length effect: Further evidence challenging PDP models of reading aloud. *Journal of Experimental Psychology: Learning, Memory and Cognition 35*, 238–46.

RCPM (*Ravens Coloured Progressive Matrices)* by Ravens (1976).

Rogers-Ramachandran, D. C., & Ramachandran, V. S. (1998). Psychophysical evidence for boundary and surface systems in human vision. *Vision Research, 38*(1), 71–77.

Seidenberg, M.S., Waters, G.S., Barnes, M.A., & Tanenhaus, M.K. (1984). When does irregular spelling or pronunciation incluence word recognition? *Journal of Verbal Learning and Verbal Behavior, 23*, 383-404.

Shapiro, L.R., Hurry, J., Masterson, J., Wydell, T.N., & Doctor, E. (2009). Classroom implications of recent research into literacy development: from predictors to assessment. *Dyslexia, 15 (1)*, 1-22.

Share, D.L., Jorm, A.F., MacLean, R., & Matthews, R. (2002). Temporal processing and reading disability. *Reading and Writing, 15*:151-178.

Shaywitz, S. E., Shaywitz, B. A., Fletcher, J. M., & Escobar, M. D. (1990). Reading disability in boys and girls. *Journal of the American Medical Association, 264*, 998–1002.

Shu, H. & Anderson, R.C. (1997). Role of radical awareness in the characters and word acquisition of Chinese children. *Reading Research Quarterly, 32(1)*, 78-89.

Shu, H., McBride-Chang, C., Wu, S., & Liu, H. Y. (2006). Understanding Chinese developmental dyslexia: Morphological awareness as a core cognitive construct. *Journal of Educational Psychology, 98(1)*, 122–133.

Snowling, M.J. (2000). *Dyslexia.* 2nd Edn. Oxford: Blackwell.

Siok, W. T., Niu, Z. D., Jin, Z., Perfetti, C. A., & Tan, L. H. (2008). A structural-functional basis for dyslexia in the cortex of Chinese readers. *Proceedings of the National Academy of Sciences of the USA, 105(14)*, 5561–5566.

Siok, W. T., Perfetti, C. A., Jin, Z., &Tan, L. H. (2004). Biological abnormality of impaired reading is constrained by culture. *Nature, 431*(7004), 71–76.

Snowling, M. J., & Griffiths, Y. M. (2005). Individual differences in dyslexia. In T. Nune & P. E. Bryant (Eds.). *Handbook of Literacy*. Dordrecht: Kluwer Press.

Stanovich, K.E. (1988). Explaining the differences between the dyslexic and the garden-variety poor reader: the phonological-core variable-difference model. *Journal of Learning Disability, 21*, 590-604.

Stanovich, K. E., & Siegel, L. S. (1994). Phenotypic performance profile of children with reading disabilities: A regression-based test of the phonological-core variable-difference model. *Journal of Educational Psychology, 86*, 24–53.

Stein, J. (2001). The magnocellular theory of developmental dyslexia. *Dyslexia, 7*(1), 12–36.

Stein, J. (2003). Visual motion sensitivity and reading. *Neuropsychologia, 41*(13), 1785–1793.

STRAW (*The Screening Test for Reading and Writing for Japanese Primary School Children*) by Uno, Haruhara, Kaneko, & Wydell (2006)

Tallal, P. (1980). Auditory temporal perception, phonics, and reading disabilities in children. *Brain and Language, 9*(2), 182–198.

Talcott, J. B., Witton, C., McLean, M. F., Hansen, P. C., Rees, A., & Green, G. G. R. (2000). Dynamic sensory sensitivity and children's word decoding skills. *Proceedings of the National Academy of Sciences of the USA, 97*(6), 2952–2957.

Temple, E., Poldrack, R.A., Salidis, J., Deutsch, G.K., Tallal, P., Merzenich, M.M., Gabriel, J.D.(2001). Disrupted neural responses to phonological and orthographic processing in dyslexic children: an fMRI study. *Neuroreport, 12*, 299-307.

Uno A, Kaneko M, Haruhara N, Matsuda H, Kato M, Kasahara, M. (2002) Developmental dyslexia: neuropsychological and cognitive- neuropsychological analysis (in Japanese). *Shitsugoshoukenkyu 22*, 130–6.

Uno, A., Wydell, T.N., Haruhara, N., Kaneko, M., & Shinya, N. (2009). Relationship between reading/writing skills and cognitive abilities among Japanese primary-school children: normal readers versus poor readers (dyslexics). *Reading & Writing 22*, 755-789. *DOI 10.1007/s 11145-008-9128-8*

Uno, A., Wydell, T.N., Kato, M., Itoh, K., & Yoshino, F. (2009) Cognitive neuropsychological and regional cerebral blood flow study of a Japanese–English bilingual girl with specific language impairment (SLI). *Cortex, 45:2*, 154-163.

Wang, J-J., Bi, H-Y., Gao, L-Q., & Wydell, T.N. (2010). The visual magnocellular pathway in Chinese-speaking children with developmental dyslexia. *Neuropsychologia, 48*; 3627-3633

Wolf, P.H. (2002). Timing precision and rhythm in developmental dyslexia. *Reading and Writing, 15*:179-206.

Wydell, T.N., & Butterworth, B. (1999). An English-Japanese bilingual with monolingual dyslexia. *Cognition, 70*, 273-305

Wydell, T.N., Butterworth, B., Shibahara, N., Zorzi, M. (1997). The irregularity of regularity effects in reading: the case of Japanese Kanji. Paper presented at the meeting of the Experimental Psychology Society, Cardiff, UK.

Wydell, T. N., & Kondo, T. (2003). Phonological deficit and the reliance on orthographic approximation for reading: A follow up study on an English–Japanese bilingual with monolingual dyslexia. *Journal of Research in Reading, 26*, 33–48.

Wydell, T.N., Butterworth, B.L., & Patterson, K.E. (1995). The inconsistency of consistency effects in reading: Are there consistency effects in Kanji? *Journal of Experimental Psychology: Language. Memory and Cognition, 21*: 1156–1168.

Wydell, T.N., Patterson, K., & Humphreys, G.W. (1993). Phonologically mediated access to meaning for KANJI: Is a ROWS still a ROSE in Japanese KANJI? *Journal of Experimental Psychology: Learning, Memory and Cognition 19*, 491–514.

Wydell, T.N., Vuorinen, T., Helenius, P., & Salmeline, R. (2003). Neural Correlates of Letter-String Length and Lexicality during reading in a regular orthography. *Journal of Cognitive Neuroscience, 15:7*, 1052-1062.

Ziegler, J.C. & Goswami, U. (2005). Reading acquisition, developmental dyslexia, and skilled reading across languages: A psycholinguistic grain size theory. *Psychological Bulletin, 131*(1), 3–29

Zoccolotti, P., de Luca, M., de Pace, E., Gasperini, F., Judica, A., & Spinelli, D. (2005). Word length effect in early reading and in develop-mental dyslexia. *Brain & Language 93*, 369–73.

2

Typical and Dyslexic Development in Learning to Read Chinese

Hua Shu and Hong Li
Beijing Normal University, China

1. Introduction

Compared with research on alphabetic languages, research on reading acquisition and impairment in Chinese has a relatively short history. However, this field has attracted more and more attention, and increasing number of findings have been reported in recent years. In the present chapter, we will firstly describe some important features of the Chinese language, and how these features influence reading acquisition of normal Chinese children. Then, we will summarize a series of studies of dyslexic development in learning to read Chinese, in which the critical deficits for Chinese dyslexic children were identified. Finally, several longitudinal studies will be reviewed, in which the early predictors and developmental trajectories of reading acquisition and impairment in Chinese children were explored.

2. Properties of the Chinese language and the cognitive correlates in reading acquisition of Chinese children

It has long been recognized that phonological skills are highly correlated with reading ability in alphabetic languages (Bradley & Bryant, 1983; Wagner & Torgesen, 1987; Ziegler & Goswami, 2005). In recent years, increasing research evidence has been reported that the contribution of the cognitive skills on reading acquisition is also related to the nature of the orthographies. For example, naming speed (Wimmer et al., 2000) and letter knowledge (Gallagher, Frith, & Snowling, 2000) have been identified to be also the important cognitive correlates of reading acquisition in transparent orthographies.

Chinese is a logographic writing system. The basic units of written Chinese are characters. More than 80% of modern Chinese characters are phonetic compound characters and consist of sub-character components or radicals arranged under the orthographic rules. For example, a compound character (e.g., 盯, /ding1/, *stare*) consists of two parts: one component is called semantic radical (e.g., 目, *eye*), which carries the meaning information of a character, and another component called phonetic radical (丁, /ding1/), which provides the information about pronunciation of a character. The corpus study by Shu, Chen, Anderson, Wu, and Xuan (2003) showed that, in all of the characters taught in elementary schools, about 88% of the compound characters are semantic transparent (e.g. the character妈 (*mother*) is with a female radical "女") or semi-transparent (e.g. the character猎

(*hunting*) is with an animal radical "犭"). However, only about 39% of the compound characters are regular in pronunciation (e.g., the character 逗 /dou4/ is with the phonetic radical "豆" /dou4/).

The semantic and phonetic radicals may be further divided into about 600 subcomponents (e.g. 十, 口) which have fixed internal structures. The components or subcomponents are combined to form thousands of characters. Many of the radicals or components have their legal positions within the characters, although others can occur on flexible positions. For example, some components can appear only on the left (e.g. 扌), on the right (e.g. 刂), on the top (艹) or on the bottom (灬) of characters. Awareness of inter-structure and position of components within characters are important in character recognition and it makes relatively greater demands on basic visual or orthographic analysis in Chinese reading. Previous studies have demonstrated that visual skill and orthographic awareness (e.g. Huang & Hanley, 1995; Ho & Bryant, 1997; Ho, Chan, Lee, Tsang, & Luan, 2004; Li, Peng, & Shu, 2006; Li, Shu, McBride-Chang, Liu, & Peng, in press) play significant roles in Chinese reading development. The brain mechanism of orthographic processing in Chinese reading were also reported in the fMRI studies (Liu, Zhang, Tang, Mai, Chen, Tardif & Luo, 2008; Tan, Liu, Perfetti, Spinks, Fox, & Gao, 2001; Wang, Yang, Shu & Zevin, 2011)

The unit of interface between the written word and spoken language in Chinese is *morpheme*. A character corresponds with one syllable and usually represents one morpheme. It makes morphological awareness potentially important in Chinese reading. Morphological awareness in Chinese is suggested to consist of three types of knowledge related to reading (Wu, Packard, & Shu, 2009). First, the fact that there are about 7,000 morphemes but only 1,200 syllables in Mandarin Chinese suggesting that more than five morphemes or characters share one syllable. Therefore the knowledge of homophones becomes important when reading Chinese, in which a reader is required to distinguish the homophone characters which share the same syllable (e.g. /yi4/) but with different morphemes (e.g. 义 *'meaning'*, 易 *'easy'*, 亿 *'a hundred million'*, 宜 *'appropriate'*, 益 *'benefit'*, 艺 *'art'*, 议 *'discuss'*, and so on. The second is knowledge of homographs which requires a reader to be aware that a single written character (e.g. 草) may represent different morphemes ('grass' or 'careless'). The different morphemes contribute to the word's meaning when they are in different compound words (e.g. *'grass'* in 草地 *'lawn'* or *'careless'* in 草率 *'cursory'*). The third is knowledge of the morphemic structure of compound words which requires the awareness of the contribution of the individual morphemes (e.g. 飞 *'fly'* and 机 *'machine'*) to the meaning of the whole word (e.g. 飞机, *'airplane'*) . Because of the central role played by the morpheme in Chinese orthography, sensitivity to morphological knowledge is especially important in the development of oral and written vocabulary in Chinese. Morphological awareness is critically important for children learning to read and write, and emerges early and develops with age in preschool children (Chen, Hao, Geva, Zhu, & Shu, 2009; McBride-Chang, Shu, Zhou, Wat, & Wagner, 2003).

Chinese has a relatively simple syllable structure: a syllable consists of an onset and a rime and the combination is regular in spelling; mapping from spelling to sound is syllable-based. However, numerous studies on Chinese children's reading development and impairment have demonstrated that phonological skills, including syllable awareness, onset awareness and rime awareness, are associated with Chinese character recognition (e.g.

Chow, McBride-Chang, & Burgess, 2005; Siok & Fletcher, 2001; Ho, Law, & Ng, 2000). Lexical tone is a fundamental feature of Chinese spoken language in which four tones are used to distinguish meanings that are not differentiated by segmental information. Studies showed that different levels of phonological awareness in Chinese emerge as the results of age or experience. Syllable and rhyme awareness appear to develop naturally with age in preschool children. However, onset and tone awareness appear to depend upon school instruction (Shu, Peng, & McBride-Chang, 2008).

Rapid Automatized Naming (RAN) refers to tasks that require readers to name a list of familiar stimuli as rapidly as possible. RAN tasks were suggested to predict reading better in transparent orthographies than in opaque orthographies. However, recent studies have suggested RAN to be a consistent predictor of Chinese reading development, in which linking printed information with a given phonological representation arbitrarily is important. It predicts reading fluency and accuracy in both typically developing children and dyslexics (Ho & Lai, 1999; Ho et al., 2000; Shu, McBride-Chang, Wu, & Liu, 2006; Lei, Pan, Liu, McBride-Chang, Li, Zhang, Chen, Tardif, Liang, Zhang, & Shu, 2011; Pan, McBride-Chang, Shu, Liu, Zhang, & Li. in press).

To summarize, studies have reported a strong link between phonological awareness and character recognition in Chinese children (e.g., Siok & Fletcher, 2001; Shu et al., 2008). The role of morphological awareness, visual-orthographic skills, and rapid automatized naming in reading acquisition and impairment has also been demonstrated (e.g., Ho et al., 2004; Shu et al., 2006). What assessments can best examine those cognitive skills and are most sensitive to differences in reading ability at different stages of development? Li et al., (in press) administered 184 kindergarten children at age 5 to 6, and 273 primary school children at age 7 to 9 from Beijing with a comprehensive battery of tasks, including those for visual-orthographic, phonological, morphological skills, rapid automatized naming abilities, and Chinese character recognition skills, in order to explore the cognitive correlates which can better predict Chinese reading acquisition across preschool and early grade levels. Visual Spatial Relationships and Visual Memory subtests were administered to test children's visual skills. An orthographic judgment task was created to measure orthographic awareness of Chinese children, in which children were asked to judge 4 types of critical items, including black and white line drawings (e.g. ), ill-formed structure with radicals in the illegal positions (e.g. ) , ill-formed components (e.g. 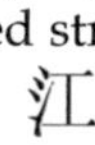), and well-formed structure pseudo-characters items (e.g. 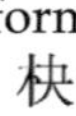). Phonological awareness contained syllable deletion, rime detection, and phoneme deletion. Three tasks were designed for measurement of morphological awareness, specifically for knowledge of compound words, knowledge of homophones, and knowledge of homographs. The morphological construction task aims to test if children are able to decompose a compound word (大红花, *big red flower*) into morphemes (大 *big*, 红 *red*, 花*flower*) and construct a new compound word based on the new morphemes (e.g. "If a big flower that is red in color is called "大红花, *big red flower*", what should we call the big flower that is blue?" The correct answer is "大蓝花, *big blue flower*"). The homophone judgment task aims to test if children can distinguish the morphemes with the same sound but different meanings based on the compound word context. For example, the second syllable of the words "蛋(*egg*)糕(*cake*), /dan4-gao1/, *cake*" and "跳(jump)高(high), /tiao4-gao1/, *high jump*" share the same sound /gao1/ but with different meanings "糕, *cake*" and "高, *high*". Children were asked to judge "If the compound words 蛋糕 */dan4 gao1/* and 跳高 */tiao4 gao1/* share the same morpheme /gao1/?" The correct answer is "No". Morpheme production task aimed to test if children can distinguish homographs, that is, the morphemes with same character and same sound, but with different meanings based on the compound word context. For example, the morpheme "明"in word "明(next)天(day), */ming2 tian1/, tomorrow*" and"明(bright)亮(light), */ming2 liang4/, brighten*" share the same character and same sound, but with the different meanings 'next' and *'bright'*. In the task, the experimenter spoke a word (e.g. "明(next)天(day), */ming2 tian1/, tomorrow'*) to children. Children were asked to produce two compound words containing the same character and sound but with different morphemes (homograph). The possible correct words are 明(next)年(year) */ming2 nian2/'next year'* with the morpheme *'next'* and 明(bright)亮(light) */ming2 liang4/, 'brightness'* with the morpheme *'bright'*).

Regression analyses indicated that only syllable deletion, morphological construction, and speed number-naming were unique correlates of Chinese character recognition in kindergarten children. Among primary school children, the independent correlates of character recognition were rime detection, homophone judgment, morpheme production, orthographic knowledge, and speed number-naming. Results confirmed that phonological awareness, morphological awareness and speed naming are important in explaining character recognition for both kindergarten and lower grade primary school children. Orthographic awareness becomes significant to character recognition of school children as they learn to read. It is important to choose tasks which are suitable for the age of children that are being tested, since some tasks are sensitive to a wide range of ages, while others are more age-specific.

3. Chinese children with dyslexia and its early prediction

3.1 The characteristics and core deficits of Chinese children with dyslexia

About 5%-10% of school-aged children, in any language, have a persistent difficulty in learning to read that could not be explained by sensory deficits, low general intelligence, poor educational opportunity, or lack of motivation (Fisher, DeFries, 2002; Shaywitz, Shaywitz, Fletcher, Escobar, 1990). However, for a long time developmental dyslexia was believed to be a problem that exists only in western languages, since the strong assumption that phonological awareness has a major impact on the acquisition of literacy only in alphabetic languages. Since Stevenson, Stigler, Lucker, Lee, Hsu, and Kitamura (1982) first found that the prevalence of dyslexia among American, Japanese and Chinese children is comparable, a great number of studies in Hong Kong, Taiwan and Mainland China have congruously reported that between 5% and 10% of school-aged children in Chinese were dyslexic in the past years (Zhang, Zhang, Yin, Zhou, & Chang, 1996; Yin and Weekes, 2003). Research has revealed that, just like in alphabetic languages, dyslexic children in Chinese mainly suffered from the accuracy and speed of word reading and spelling, so that reading measures widely used in distinguishing dyslexic from normal children are single character or word recognition measures ((Ho, et. al, 2002, 2004; Meng, Shu & Zhou, 1999; Shu, Wu, McBride-Chang, 2006).

According to the dual-route model of reading, mapping from print to sound is achieved through at least two pathways, a lexical semantic route and a nonsematic GPC route (Coltheart, Rastle, Perry, Langdon & Ziegler, 2001). Yin and Weekes (2003) proposed a framework for understanding acquired and developmental dyslexia in Chinese derived from a cognitive neuropsychological account of reading and writing Chinese. Their model assumes that normal oral reading in Chinese depends on a division of labor between the lexical semantic pathway and a nonsemantic pathway. Impairment to the lexical semantic pathway will result in acquired surface dyslexia, while impairment to the nonsemantic pathway results in deep dyslexia. In a case study, Shu, Meng, Chen, Luan, and Cao, (2005) reported two types of dyslexic children, surface and deep, who showed the impairment in different pathways. Two dyslexic children, Child-L and Child-J, were tested by a word recognition task, in which they were asked to name a character and then to compose a compound word based on the target character. It was found that Child-L, identified as 'surface dyslexic', could correctly pronounce many of regular characters but made many regularization errors in irregular character naming. And Child-L also made many homophone errors when he composed a compound word based on the target character. According to Hillis and Caramazza (1995), the information from semantic-lexical and OPC routes integrate to provide the constraint for the selection of word pronunciation. For a Chinese reader, a compound character 拦 /lan2/*'obstruct'*may active a set of homophone characters /lan2/, and also active the characters with the meaning related with *'obstruct'*. The correct pronunciation and meaning of the character will be accessed with the two pathways. However, Child-L could correctly pronounce a target character (e.g. 拦 /lan2/) based on its phonetic cue (e.g. 兰 /lan2/), but he could not access the semantic information of the character. Then he composed a wrong compound word 篮子 /lan2 zi/, *'basket'* with a homophone character 篮 /lan2/, as illustrated in Figure 1. It suggests that as a surface dyslexic, Child-L normally developed the nonsemantic or sublexical route so that he could utilize phonetic radical information in character naming. But his semantic pathway was developmentally delayed or deficient.

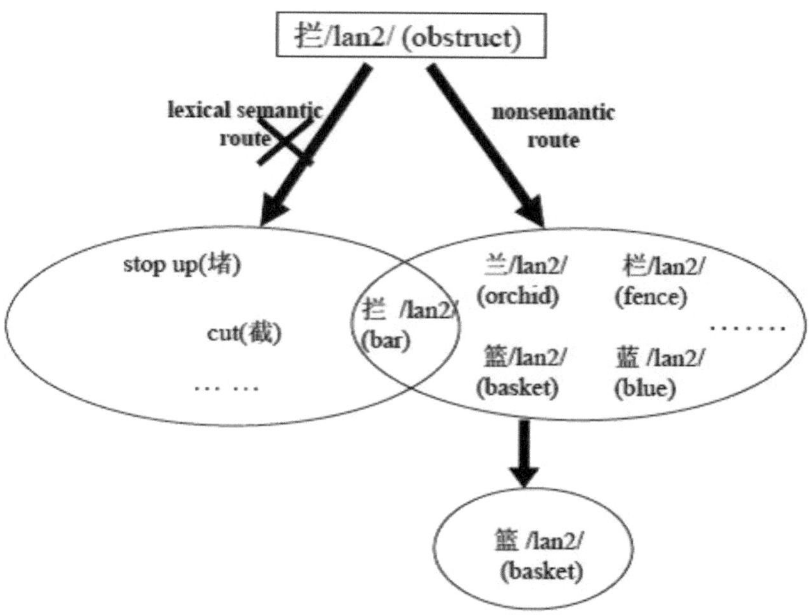

Fig. 1. An example of reading model for surface dyslexic Child L

In contrast, Child-J, identified as 'deep dyslexic', made a relatively large percentage of semantic related errors (26%) in pronunciation. For example, he named the character 煎 /jian1/ *'fry'*, which is with the phonetic 前 /qan2/, as 炖 /dun4/ *'braise'*, a character which is semantically related with the target character煎*'fry'*, but with the phonetic 屯 /tun2/. He composed a compound word炖肉 /dun4-rou4/ *'stew'*, (see Figure 2). It is clear that he ignored the phonological information provided by the phonetic 前 /qan2/ of the target character煎 /jian1/, but accessed the meaning of the target 煎*'fry'* and also the characters with the meanings related with *'fry'* were activated. Child-J's performance showed the characteristics of deep dyslexia. That is, his nonsemantic pathway was developmentally delayed or deficient, but his semantic pathway was relatively normal.

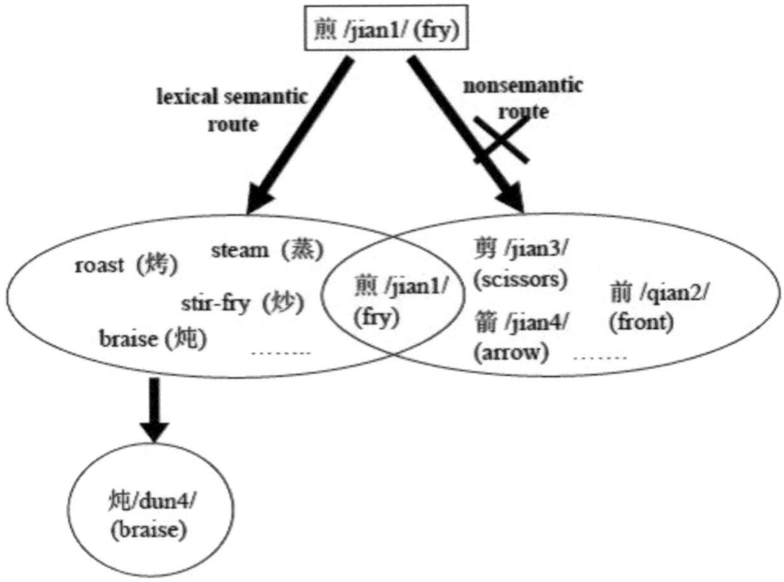

Fig. 2. An example of reading model for deep dyslexic Child J

The resulting patterns of the two children support the framework proposed by Yin and Weekes (2003) that surface dyslexia (Child-L) may be explained by developmental delay or deficit in the *semantic* pathway and deep dyslexia (Child J) can be explained by delay or deficit in the *nonsemantic* pathway in reading acquisition. The impairment in different pathways could explain the fact that child L could not distinguish the target from homophone characters, and child J could not utilize sublexical phonetic information in pronunciation. The response patterns of the dyslexic children were simulated and confirmed by the results from a triangle model in Chinese (Yang, McCandliss, Shu, & Zevin, 2008).

Phonological deficit has been treated as the main cause of developmental dyslexia and sufficient to explain poor reading performance in alphabetic languages (Bradley & Bryant, 1983; Ramus, 2003; Snowling, 2000; Ziegler, Bertrand, Tórth, Csépe, Reis, Faísca, Saine, Lyytinen, Vaessen, & Blomert, 2010). However, the important links of cognitive skills with reading success and failure vary across orthographies (Ziegler & Goswami, 2005; Lyytinen, Erskine, Tolvanen, Torppa, Poikkeus, & Lyytinen, 2006). What are the core deficits for dyslexic children in Chinese?

Research has revealed that phonological, naming-speed and orthographic deficits are important features in Chinese dyslexic children. Testing 147 Hong Kong children with dyslexia on a number of literacy and cognitive tasks, Ho, et al. (2004) found that rapid naming deficit (57%) and orthographic deficit (42%) were the most dominant types of cognitive deficits in Chinese developmental dyslexia, while the relatively small proportion of dyslexic children has phonological deficits (29%) and visual deficits (27%).

Shu, et al. (2006) specifically examined the role of morphological skills in Chinese dyslexia besides other cognitive skills. Comparing 75 dyslexic with 77 normal children from primary schools in Beijing, the study systematically examined their literacy skills (character naming, reading comprehension, and dictation), linguistic and nonlinguistic cognitive skills with morphological awareness, rapid naming, phonological awareness, verbal short-term memory, lexical vocabulary, visual spatial test, articulatory rate, visual attention and nonverbal short-term memory tasks. In the logistic regression analysis, dyslexic children were found to be best distinguished from age-matched controls with tasks of morphological awareness, speeded number naming and vocabulary skills, while performance on tasks of visual skills and phonological awareness failed to distinguish the two groups. Path analysis revealed that phonological awareness, morphological awareness and rapid naming were all uniquely associated with the three literacy tasks: character recognition, reading comprehension and dictation. Based on the same data, Wu (2004) further found that, compared with phonological (53%) and speed (45%) problems, the largest proportion (96%) of dyslexic children had morphological problems. Figure 3 shows all the children with dyslexia grouped by their deviant performance on the different tasks.

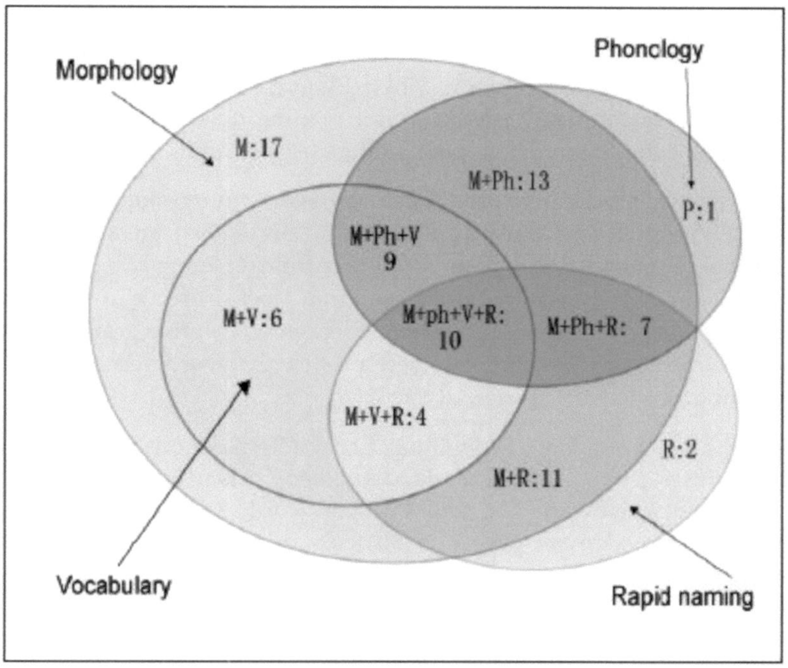

Fig. 3. Classification of dyslexic outliers by morphology, phonology, vocabulary and rapid naming. (from Wu, 2004).

The significance of morphological awareness was supported in a following study in which children with and without dyslexia were tested on the tasks including paired associative learning (visual-visual and visual-verbal PAL), phonological awareness, morphological awareness, rapid naming, verbal short-term memory and character recognition. The logistic regression demonstrated that morphological awareness, rapid naming and visual-verbal PAL uniquely distinguished children with and without dyslexia, even with other metalinguistic skills controlled (Li et al., 2009).

Researchers found that Chinese children with dyslexia tend to possess more than one kind of cognitive deficits. Ho, et al. (2002) reported that 20% of the dyslexic children have only one deficit and about 50% of dyslexic children possess more than two deficits. In Wu, et al. (2009) study, the results further confirmed that 24% of the dyslexic children were found to have only one deficit and about 80% of dyslexic children possessed more than one deficit.

3.2 Early prediction of reading acquisition and impairment

Dyslexia has been defined as a developmental disorder starting at childhood. Many factors interact to shape children's language and reading development before they start school. However, dyslexic children usually are diagnosed after they failed in learning to read at school. Could children with reading difficulties at school be identified at an earlier stage? Longitudinal research provides the best way to understand early prediction of reading acquisition and impairment. Longitudinal studies in alphabetic languages have revealed that slow vocabulary development, language grammatical skills, phonological awareness, rapid naming, and letter knowledge begin to differ between children with and without risk for dyslexia around 3 or 4 years old (Lyytinen et al., 2006). Research even reported that ERP response to speech sound at 6 month discriminated infants with familial risk for reading disorder at age 8 (Leppänen, Richardson, Pihko, Eklund, Guttorm, Aro, & Lyytinen,, 2002). What are the most effective early predictors for reading development and impairment in Chinese? Are we able to identify latent poor readers from early indicators?

In recent years, several studies explored those questions through longitudinal studies. Liu, McBride-Chang, Wong, Tardif, Stokes, Fletcher, and Shu (2009) investigated the extent to which language skills at ages 2 to 4 years could discriminate Hong Kong Chinese poor from adequate readers at age 7. It was found that children's performance at age 2 in vocabulary knowledge, at age 3 in Cantonese articulation, and age 4 receptive grammar skill, sentence imitation, and story comprehension can best predict the word recognition performance between the poor and adequate readers at age 7.

McBride-Chang, Lam, Lam, Doo, Wong, and Chow (2008) found that the group of Hong Kong children with a genetic risk for dyslexia showed particular difficulties in lexical tone detection, morphological awareness, and Chinese word reading, whereas the language delayed group performed more poorly in all tasks administered. Their follow-up study (McBridge-Chang, et al., 2011) further reported that 62% of the children with an early language delay subsequently manifested dyslexia and 50% of those with familial risk become dyslexic at school. The deficits which best distinguish dyslexic from nondyslexic children at age 7 were morphological awareness, rapid automatized naming, and word reading at age 5, suggesting that rapid automatized naming and morphological awareness are relatively strong correlates of developmental dyslexia in Chinese.

Lei et al. (2011) reported a 10-year longitudinal study in Beijing which revealed the dynamic change of reading disabled children and their heterogeneous characteristics in development. 261 children were followed from 3 to 8 years old. They were administered 7 language and cognitive skills (Compound awareness, Grammatical skill, Nonword repetition, Syllable deletion, Morphological construction, Rapid automatized naming, Vocabulary definition) between ages three and six, and then literacy skills (Character recognition, and Reading fluency) were tested at age eight. Individual differences in developmental profiles across tasks were estimated using growth mixture modeling which identified not only the important early predictors but also different subgroups with different developmental trajectories. The results showed that there were four developmental trajectories from ages three to six years and two of them were identified as poor readers (see Figure 4).

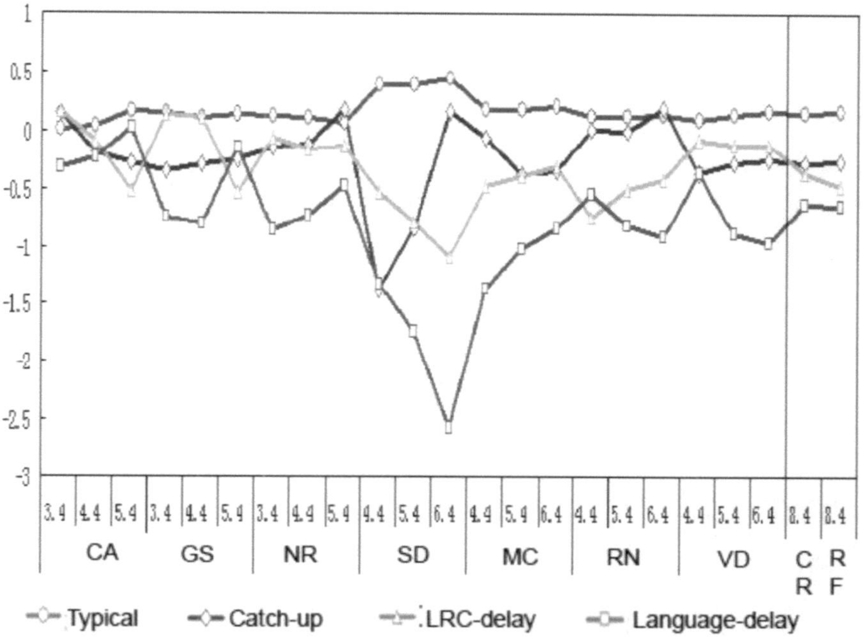

Note: CA-Compound awareness, GS-Grammatical skill, NR-Nonword repetition, SD-Syllable deletion, MC-Morphological construction, RN-Rapid automatized naming, VD-Vocabulary definition, CR-Character recognition, and RF-Reading fluency (from Lei, 2008).

Fig. 4. Subgroup members' average performance in the seven skills and in reading.

The initial level and subsequent growth on three deficits together (phonological awareness, morphological awareness and rapid naming) from age three to six were best to predict their reading difficulties at age eight. Early language deficits in addition to a combination of deficits in phonological awareness, morphological awareness, and rapid naming might lead to more severe reading problems for Chinese children. The results from the longitudinal study support those from dyslexic and control group comparison studies (e.g., Shu et al., 2006), suggesting that phonological awareness, morphological awareness, and rapid naming should be simultaneously considered in Chinese, given the use of broad skills required to learn to read this orthography.

4. Conclusions

In summary, the research confirmed some universal aspects of reading acquisition in alphabetic languages and in Chinese. Just like in alphabetic languages, Chinese children with dyslexia have mainly deficits in the accuracy and speed of character or word recognition. Mastery of a writing system depends upon acquiring an adequate phonological knowledge of the language, especially in early age. Phonological awareness and naming-speed are the two deficits shared by both dyslexic children in Chinese and in alphabetic languages. The specific aspects of reading acquisition in Chinese are related with the characteristic of Chinese language and orthography. It makes morphological and orthographic awareness particularly important to consider in understanding Chinese reading development and dyslexia. Furthermore, most of Chinese children with dyslexia tend to have more than one kind of cognitive deficits. The longitudinal studies reveal that it is possible to identify the school-age poor readers from early stage. The effective predictors include phonological awareness, morphological awareness, rapid naming and oral vocabulary.

In the future, more basic research is needed in order to understand further the cognitive causes of reading failures of Chinese children and the underlying brain mechanism.

Although it has not been discussed in this chapter, systematic work is also needed to explore the role of family and education environment on children's reading acquisition and dyslexia; With family's support and better education environment, more effective assessments could be developed, and early predictors for which children with dyslexia or children at risk for dyslexia could be identified; and in turn better intervention programmes for both preschool and school children could be developed, which could improve dyslexic children's reading ability and reduce the risk of the reading failures.

5. Acknowledgment

The research work was supported by a grant from the Natural Science Foundation of China (30870758), by a grant from Fundamental Research Fund for the Central Universities. It also was a part of a project of Beijing Key Lab of Applied Experimental Psychology supported by the Beijing Educational Committee and Beijing Science and Technology Committee.

6. References

Bradley, L., Bryant, P. E. (1983). Categorizing sounds and learning to read: A Causal connection. *Nature, 30*, 419-421.

Chen, X., Hao, M., Geva, E., Zhu, J. & Shu, H. (2009). The role of compound awareness in Chinese children's vocabulary acquisition and character reading. *Reading and Writing*, 22, 615-631.

Coltheart, M., Rastle, K., Perry, C., Langdon R. & Ziegler, J. (2001). DRC: A dual route cascaded model of visual word recognition and reading aloud. *Psychological Review, 108(1)*, 204-256.

Chow, Y.-W., McBride-Chang, C., & Burgess, S. (2005). Phonological Processing Skills and Early Reading Abilities in Hong Kong Chinese Kindergarteners Learning to Read English as an L2. *Journal of Educational Psychology*, 97, 81-87.

Fisher, S., DeFries, J. (2002). Developmental dyslexia: genetic dissection of a complex cognitive trait. *Nature Reviews Neuroscience*, 3, 767-780.

Gallagher, A., Frith, U., & Snowling, M.J. (2000). Precursors of literacy delay among children at genetic risk of dyslexia. *Journal of Child Psychology and Psychiatry*, 41, 203–213.

Harm, M. W., & Seidenberg, M. S. (2004). Computing the Meanings of Words in Reading: Cooperative Division of Labor Between Visual and Phonological Processes. *Psychological Review, 111*(3), 662-720.

Hillis, A.E. & Caramazza, A. (1995). Converging evidence for the interaction of semantic and sublexical phonological information in accessing lexical representations for spoken output, *Cognitive Neuropsychology*, 12, 187-227.

Ho, C. S., & Bryant, P. (1997). Phonological skills are important in learning to read Chinese. *Developmental Psychology*, 33, 946-951.

Ho, C. S.-H., Chan, D. W., Chung, K. K. H., Lee, S.-H., Tsang, S.-M. (2007). In search of subtypes of Chinese developmental dyslexia. *Journal of Experimental Child Psychology*, 97, 61-83.

Ho, C. S.-H., Chan, D. W.-O., Lee, S.-H., Tsang, S.-M., & Luan, V. H. (2004). Cognitive profiling and preliminary subtyping in Chinese developmental dyslexia. *Cognition, 91*, 43-75.

Ho, C.S.-H., Chan, D.W.-O., Tsang, S. M., & Lee, S.-H. (2002). The cognitive profile and multiple-deficit hypothesis in Chinese developmental dyslexia. *Developmental Psychology, 38*, 543-553.

Ho, C. S.-H., & Lai, D. N.-C. (1999). Naming-speed deficits and phonological memory deficits in Chinese developmental dyslexia. *Learning and Individual Differences*, 11, 173–186.

Ho, C. S.-H., Law, T. P. S., & Ng, P. M. (2000). The phonological deficit hypothesis in Chinese developmental dyslexia. *Reading and Writing: An Interdisciplinary Journal, 13*, 57-79.

Huang, H. S., & Hanley, J. R. (1995). Phonological awareness and visual skills in learning to read Chinese and English, *Cognition*, 54, 73-98.

Lei, L. Developmental trajectories and early predictors of poor readers in Chinese. Unpublished Master degree thesis of Beijing Normal University, 2008.

Lei, L., Pan, J., Liu, H., McBride-Chang, C., Li, H., Zhang, Y., Chen, L., Tardif, T., Liang, W., Zhang, Z., & Shu, H. (2011). Developmental trajectories of reading development and impairment from ages 3 to 8 years in Chinese children. *Journal of Child Psychology and Psychiatry, 52*, 212-220.

Leppänen, P. H. T., Richardson, U., Pihko, E., Eklund, K.M., Guttorm, T.K., Aro, M., & Lyytinen, H. (2002). Brain responses to changes in speech sound durations differ between infants with and without familial risk for dyslexia. Developmental Neuropsychology, 22(1), 407-422.

Li, H., Peng, H., & Shu, H. (2006). A study on the emergence and development of Chinese orthographic awareness in preschool and school children. *Psychological Development and Education*. 18(1), 35-38. (In Chinese)

Li, H., Shu, H., McBride-Chang, C., Liu, H., & Peng, H. (In press). Chinese Children's Character Recognition: Visuo-orthographic, Phonological Processing, and Morphological Skills. *Journal of Research in Reading*.

Li, H., Shu, H., McBride-Chang, C., Liu, H. & Xue, J. (2009). Paired associate learning in Chinese children with dyslexia. *Journal of Experimental Child Psychology, 103*, 135-151.

Liu, C., Zhang, W.T., Tang, Y.Y., Mai, X.Q., Chen, H.C., Tardif, T. & Luo, Y.J. (2008). The visual word form area: Evidence from a fMRI study of implicit processing of Chinese characters, *Neuroimage*, 40, 1350-1361.

Liu, P. D., McBride-Chang, C., Wong, A. M.-Y., Tardif, T., Stokes, S., Fletcher, P., & Shu, H. (2009). Early language markers of poor reading performance in Hong Kong Chinese children. *Journal of Learning Disabilities, 43*, 322-331.

Lyytinen, H., Erskine, J., Tolvanen, A., Torppa, M., Poikkeus, A. M., & Lyytinen, P. (2006). Trajectories of reading development: A follow-up from birth to school age of children with and without risk for dyslexia. *Merrill-Palmer Quarterly, 52*, 514-546.

McBride-Chang, C., Lam, F., Lam, C., Chan, B., Fong, C., Wong, T., Wong, S. (2011). Early predictors of dyslexia in Chinese children: familial history of dyslexia, language delay, and cognitive profiles, *Journal of Child Psychology and Psychiatry, 52*, 204-211.

McBride-Chang, C., Lam, F., Lam, C., Doo, S., Wong, S. W. L., & Chow, Y. Y. Y. (2008). Word recognition and cognitive profiles of Chinese pre-school children at risk for dyslexia through language delay or familiar history of dyslexia. *Journal of Child Psychology and Psychiatry*. *49*, 211-218.

McBride-Chang, C., Shu, H., Zhou, A., Wat, C. P., & Wagner, R. K. (2003). Morphological awareness uniquely predicts young children's Chinese character recognition. *Journal of Educational Psychology*, 95(4), 743-751.

Pan, J., McBride-Chang, C., Shu, H., Liu, H., Zhang, & Li, H. (in press). What is in the naming? A 5-year longitudinal study of early rapid naming and phonological sensitivity in relation to subsequent reading skills in both native Chinese and English as a second language. *Journal of Educational Psychology*.

Ramus F. (2003). Developmental dyslexia: Specific phonological deficit or general sensorimotor dysfunction? *Current Opinion in Neurobiology*, *13*, 212-218.

Shaywitz, S.E., Shaywitz, B.A., Fletcher, J.M., & Escobar, M.D. (1990). Prevalence of reading disability in boys and girls. *Journal of the American Medical Association*, 264, 998-1002.

Shu, H., Chen, X., Anderson, R. C., Wu, N., & Xuan, Y. (2003). Properties of school Chinese: Implications for learning to read. *Child Development*, *74*, 27-47.

Shu, H., McBride-Chang, C., Wu, S., & Liu, H. (2006). Understanding Chinese Developmental Dyslexia: Morphological Awareness as a Core Cognitive Construct. *Journal of Educational Psychology, 98,* 122-133.

Shu, H., Meng, X., Chen, X, Luan, H., & Cao, F. (2005). The subtypes of developmental dyslexia in Chinese: Evidence from three cases. *Dyslexia, 11,* 311-329.

Shu, H., Meng, X., & Lai, A. (2003). The lexical representation and processing in Chinese-speaking poor readers. In H.-C. Chen (Ed.) *Reading development in Chinese children* (pp.199-214). New Haven: Greenwood Press.

Shu, H., Peng, H., & McBride-Chang, C. (2008). Phonological awareness in young Chinese children. *Developmental Science, 11,* 171-181.

Snowling, M. J. (2000). *Dyslexia.* Malden: Blackwell Publishing.

Siok, W.T., & Fletcher, P. (2001). The role of phonological awareness and visual-orthographic skills in Chinese reading acquisition. *Developmental Psychology, 37,* 886-899.

Stevenson, H.W., Stigler, J.W., Lucker, G.W., Lee, S.Y., Hsu, C.C., & Kitamura, S. (1982). Reading disabilities: The case of Chinese, Japanese and English. *Child Development, 53,* 1164-1181.

Tan, L. H., Liu, H.-L., Perfetti C. A., Spinks, J. A., Fox, P. T., & Gao, J.-H. (2001). The neural system underlying Chinese logograph reading. *NeuroImage,* 13(5), 836-846.

Wang,X., Yang,J., Shu,H. & Zevin, J. (2011). Left fusiform BOLD responses are inversely related to word-likeness in a one-back task, *Neuroimage,*2011, 55(3), 1346-1356.

Wagner, R. K., & Torgesen, J. (1987). The nature of phonological processing and its causal role in the acquisition of reading skills. *Psychological Bulletin,* 101, 192-212.

Wu, S., Morphological deficit and dyslexia subtypes in Chinese children, Unpublished PhD dissertation of Beijing Normal University, 2004.

Wu, S., Packard, J., & Shu, H. (2009), Morphological deficit and dyslexia subtypes in Chinese (pp.199-214). In S.-P. Law, B. S. Weekes, & A. M.-Y. Wong (Eds.) *Language disorders in speakers of Chinese* (pp. 112-137). Bristol: Multilingual Matters.

Wimmer, H., Mayringer, H., & Landerl, K. (2000). The double-deficit hypothesis and difficulties in learning to read a regular orthography. *Journal of Educational Psychology, 92,* 668–680.

Yang, J., McCandliss, B., Shu, H. & Zevin, J. (2008) Division of labor between semantics and phonology in normal and disordered reading development across languages. In B. C. Love, K. McRae, & V. M. Sloutsky (Eds.), Proceedings of the 30th Annual Conference of the Cognitive Science Society (pp. 445-450). Austin, TX: Cognitive Science Society.

Yin, W. & Weekes, B. (2003). Dyslexia in Chinese: Clues from cognitive neuropsychology. *Annals of Dyslexia, 53,* 255-279.

Zhang, C., Zhang, J., Yin, R., Zhou, J., & Chang, S. (1996). Experimental research on reading disability of Chinese students. *Psychological Science,* 19, 222-256.

Ziegler, J. C., Bertrand, D., Tórth, D., Csépe, V., Reis, A., Faísca, L., Saine, N., Lyytinen, H., Vaessen, A., & Blomert, L. (2010). Orthographic depth and its impact on universal predictors of reading: A cross-language investigation. *Psychological Science,* 21, 551-559.

Ziegler, J. C., & Goswami, U. (2005). Reading acquisition, developmental dyslexia, and skilled reading across languages: A psycholinguistic grain size theory. *Psychological Bulletin, 131,* 3-29.

3

The Role of Phonological Processing in Dyslexia in the Spanish Language

Juan E. Jiménez
University of La Laguna, The Canary Islands, Spain

1. Introduction

This chapter presents theoretical arguments and empirical evidence to support the idea that the phonological deficit in dyslexia in a language with a transparent orthography such as Spanish is at the phoneme level in the phonological awareness continuum, suggesting that a phonemic deficit is curtailing the development of phonological decoding. Results of two studies are presented to demonstrate the role of phonological processing in dyslexia in the Spanish language. The first study examines the dyslexic subtypes within the context of a reading-level match in a transparent orthography. In this research we explored whether developmental dyslexics form a homogeneous population, with a unique underlying impairment, or whether they form distinct subgroups. The second study examines the effects of a computer-assisted intervention designed to improve the visual word recognition of Spanish-speaking children identified with a learning disability (LD).

The classical phonological explanation ascribes dyslexics' reading deficit to a specific cognitive deficiency in phonological processing, primarily, in phonemic awareness and in phonological short-term memory.

Nevertheless, other current non-phonological explanations according to which dyslexics' phonological deficit is secondary to more basic sensori-motor impairment: a deficiency in either rapid auditory processing, or in the visual magnocellular pathway, or in motor skills (see for a review, Sprenger-Charolles, Colé, & Serniclaes, 2006).

Deficits in phonological awareness have been identified as the critical factor underlying the severe word decoding problems displayed by individuals with reading difficulties in languages with an opaque orthography such as English (Goswami & Bryant, 1990). Studies in English have found phonemic deficits in dyslexic children compared to children matched by chronological age (CA) or by reading level (RL) (Olson, 1994). In addition, dyslexic children appear to have more difficulty reading nonwords than nondisabled readers matched in age or in reading level supporting the deficit model in phonological processing (Rack, Snowling, & Olson, 1992). However, Goswami (2002, p. 150) suggests that "the consistency of the phoneme-grapheme correspondences in languages with a transparent orthography such as Spanish should facilitate the further development of both phonemic awareness and grapheme-phoneme recoding skills. These skills would, therefore, be expected to develop more slowly in dyslexic children learning to read in such consistent orthographies, but they would not be expected to be massively disrupted".

However, empirical evidence in Spanish indicates that dyslexic children exhibit the same difficulties in phonemic segmentation exhibited by older English dyslexic children (Jiménez, 1997). For example, Jiménez (1997) analyzed phoneme awareness within the context of a reading-level match design, demonstrating a deficit in the Spanish reading disabled (RD) children in phonemic tasks, but not in intrasyllabic tasks. In another study, Jiménez et al. (2005) examined the effects of linguistic complexity (e.g., complexity in the syllable structure) and task differences without taking into account verbal working memory. The assumption was that if students, identified as dyslexic, performed worse in a phonemic task compared to RL and CA matched children, the hypothesis of a phonemic deficit in explaining dyslexia in a transparent orthography would be confirmed. Results indicated that the complexity of the syllable structure had no particularly marked effect on the dyslexic children. Rather, the isolation task revealed the phonological deficit across all syllable structures.

Jiménez, García and Venegas (2008) examined whether phonological processes are the same or different in low literacy adults and children with or without reading disabilities in a transparent orthography. They selected a sample of 150 subjects organized into four different groups: (1) 53 low literacy adults, (2) 29 reading disabled children, (3) 27 younger normal readers at the same reading level as those with reading disabilities and low literacy adults, and (4) 41 normal readers matched in age with the reading disabled group. Phonological awareness tasks that included different complexities of the syllable structure (e.g., words with CV and CCV structure) were administered. Results indicated that the complexity of the syllable structure did not have a significant effect on low literacy adults. These adults appear to experience more difficulty in deleting phonemes irrespective of the complexity of the syllable structure.

Moreover, findings from studies that looked at whether phonological processes or lexical processes differentiated Spanish readers with and without reading difficulties indicated that the cause of the reading difficulties appeared to reside in the grapheme-phoneme decomposition procedure than in the lexical processes (Domínguez & Cuetos, 1992; Jiménez & Hernández-Valle, 2000; Rodrigo & Jiménez, 1999). This finding reinforces the hypothesis that the basis of reading problems is a difficulty in phonological processing, indicating that a lack of phonemic awareness is curtailing the acquisition of word recognition skill.

A major question posed by researchers relates to whether a major variable affecting the level of difficulty in learning to read also depends on the transparency/opacity of the writing system (e.g., Wydell & Butterworth, 1999). Specifically, the question relates to whether the effect of the transparency/opacity of the writing system is not only quantitative, but also qualitative. For instance, research indicated that English-speaking children perform reading tasks worse than do children who speak Spanish, French or German. A plausible reason is because the dissociation between sublexical and lexical procedures is greater for English-speaking children than for children who speak other languages. Sprenger-Charolles et al. (2006) reviewed cross-linguistic studies and longitudinal studies that examined the stability of dyslexic performance patterns across languages, and over time as reading develops. Group studies, single case studies, and multiple case studies conducted in various languages to evaluate the reliability and prevalence of the dyslexic performance pattern were included in the review. Assessments to determine the lexical and sublexical routes used both high frequency irregular word reading, and pseudoword reading. However, not all studies included a standard measure of lexical processing (i.e., irregular word reading) because it is impossible to find enough irregular words in some of the languages (e.g., Spanish) included in the review. Findings indicated a higher incidence rate of phonological dyslexia in English in comparison to other languages (e.g., Wydell & Butterworth, 1999; Wydell & Kondo 2003) where researchers found a higher incidence of surface dyslexia. Note that surface dyslexia is characterized by impaired orthographic skills and fairly well-preserved phonological skills (Stanovich, et al., 1997b), while a phonological dyslexia is characterized by impaired phonological skills and fairly well-preserved orthographic skills (Castles & Coltheart, 1993; Manis, Seidenberg, Doi, McBridge-Chang & Petersen, 1996; Stanovich, Siegel & Gottardo, 1997b).

Thus, studies that indicate the extent to which the dual-route hypothesis (i.e., differences between phonological and surface dyslexia (e.g., Manis, et al, 1996; Stanovich, et al, 1997b) is also applicable to languages with a transparent orthography, are still necessary. Moreover, studies designed to demonstrate that the consistency of mappings from graphemes to phonemes in different languages has a marked effect on the development of phonemic awareness and of grapheme-phoneme recoding strategies in dyslexic children are necessary. Two Spanish studies of dyslexic subtypes and computer-assisted practice on visual word recognition are presented here to provide empirical evidence in favor of the deficit model in phonological processing in a transparent orthography. Next we report results of the two studies.

2. Study 1: Identifying dyslexic subtypes in a transparent orthography

A question posed by reading researchers is whether readers with developmental dyslexia form a homogeneous group with a unique underlying impairment, or whether this group actually consists of distinct subgroups. In English, research indicates the existence of two distinct profiles of developmental dyslexia. In our own review of studies of dyslexic performance patterns, we have found the opposite pattern when we reviewed studies conducted in orthographies less opaque than English (e.g., Swedish: Wolff, 2009). These discrepancies between the Spanish versus the anglophone or francophone studies may be due to (a) linguistic factors, (b) the measures used, and (c) differences in the dyslexics' chronological age. Given that grapheme-phoneme correspondences are more regular in Spanish than in English and in French, Spanish-speaking dyslexics may manage to use the sublexical reading route with less difficulty than English-speaking or French speaking dyslexics. This could explain why fewer phonological dyslexics were found in languages that are less opaque than English. A similar trend was observed when time measures were used in Spanish or in French (Genard et al., 1998) suggesting that the phonological deficit of Spanish-speaking dyslexics manifests itself as slow processing more than in accuracy.

The study presented here was first published by Jiménez and Ramirez (2002) and replicated later by Jiménez, Rodríguez, and Ramírez (2009). It employed the same procedure used by Castles and Coltheart (1993) for identifying dyslexic subtypes based on pseudoword and irregular word reading. Given that Spanish does not have any irregular words, we compared the reaction times (RTs) of students reading high frequency words and pseudowords between the group of dyslexic children and the group of children similar in chronological-age, and reading-level (RL).

Some difficulties have been encountered in research using traditional research designs. So, for example, when reading-disabled subjects are matched in age with normal readers, differences between the groups on non-reading measures have been presumed to reflect deficits causally related to the reading failure of the reading-disabled group (Backman, Mamem, & Ferguson, 1984). When two groups that have different reading levels are compared, any differences found between them could be interpreted as a product rather than as a cause of such differences (Bryant & Goswami, 1986). However, if the children are at the same reading level, any differences between them cannot be attributed to one group being more successful readers than the other group. However, as has been suggested by Bryant and Goswami (1986) the studies that analyze correlates of reading disability should involve a combination of reading level and chronological age matched groups. In the three-group design, there are two control groups in addition to the target group, one for reading level and one for chronological age. Thus, the paradigm allows not only comparison of children of different chronological ages with the same reading level as in the two-group approach, but also comparison within chronological age across reading levels. The addition of the third group, i.e., chronological age controls, allows examination of differing performance levels across two chronological age levels in normal children, as well as relative performance within chronological age and reading level-matched groups (Backman et al, 1984). As several authors have pointed out (Backman et al, 1984; Bryant & Goswami, 1986) positive results (a difference between reading disabled children and normal controls) in experiments that use a reading level match allows us to conclude that the measure under consideration is probably causally related to the reading disabilities. As has been suggested by Manis et al. (1996), "the developmental forms result in patterns that are not observed in normal readers at any age or level of reading acquisition - a *deviant* developmental pattern. Another possibility is that a subgroup might lag in a broad spectrum of reading skills and hence resemble younger normal readers - a *developmental delay* pattern" (p. 162).

Therefore, we conducted further exploration of the validity and reliability of the subgroup assignments by examining the performance on phonological awareness tasks. We predicted that if the subgrouping was valid, phonological dyslexics (Ph-Dys) should perform relatively poorly on the phonological awareness tasks compared to younger normal readers, supporting a specific deficit in phonological processing, whereas there should not be differences on the phonological awareness tasks between surface dyslexics (S-Dys) and younger normal readers.

2.1 Method

Participants. In the initial sample, teachers selected children who they believed were normally achieving readers or were reading-disabled. We assessed these children with different subtests of the Standardized Literacy Skills Test T.A.L.E. (Test de Análisis de Lectoescritura; Toro & Cervera, 1980). The study employed a reading-level-match design including three groups: (1) The reading-disabled sample consisted of 89 third-grade children who achieved a performance below the grade 3 norms (i.e., two years) on each of the subtests of TALE individually; (2) A control group of 37 normal readers matched in age with the reading-disabled group; (3) A control group of 39 younger children at the same reading level as the reading-disabled group. Both reading disabled and younger normal readers were matched on each of the subtests of TALE individually (i.e., letter, syllable, and word reading) based on grade 1 norms. Normal readers matched in age achieved a performance according to grade 3 norms.

Measures. We used three different phonological awareness tests (i.e., odd-word-out task, phoneme segmentation and phoneme reversal). The *Odd-word-out task* was designed to test the awareness of intrasyllabic units and was based on a similar measure by Bowey and Francis (1991). The difference between the Bowey and Francis measure and ours was that we used pictures. In the *Phoneme segmentation test*, children counted the phonemes of words presented orally. Children were aloud to use aids such as rods to count the phonemes they heard in words. In the *Phoneme reversal test* the children counted the phonemes of words by reversing the order of segments in each word.

Procedure. We used the same regression-based procedure introduced by Castles and Coltheart (1993) and used the same-aged normal readers' performance to identify subtypes of dyslexics. We used RTs to high frequency words and pseudowords, controlling for the number of letters. That is, the RT for each stimulus (word and pseudoword) was divided by the number of letters. We hypothesized that children who have greater RTs for familiar word reading compared to RTs for pseudoword reading would have difficulties using a lexical procedure to read words. On the other hand, children who would show longer latencies for pseudoword reading as compared to familiar word reading would have more difficulties in using a phonological route. To conduct this experiment, the program UNICEN was designed and used together with a device that detected the sounds within the broad band of the human voice but was not affected by the fairly high percentage of background noise. High-frequency words used in the experiment were selected on the basis of ratings generated from a normative study conducted by Guzmán and Jiménez (2001), who employed a sample of 3,000 words obtained from different texts of children's literature. Word familiarity was measured using these authors' procedure of frequency estimation, which involved the separation of the 3,000 words into different sets. Each set was printed and then different groups of 30 children rated each word on a 5-point scale, ranging from *least frequent* (1) to *most frequent* (5). The estimated frequency was calculated for each word by averaging the rating across all 30 judges. On the basis of these ratings, high-frequency words were selected. Pseudowords were extracted from research by de Vega, Carreiras, Gutiérrez, and Alonso-Quecuty (1990). The order of presentation of words and pseudowords was counterbalanced. Items were presented in random order within each set. In total, there were 32 words and 48 pseudowords.

Results. We carried out two different analyses: (1) a comparison of dyslexic subgroups to the CA control group, and (2) a comparison of dyslexic subgroups to the RL control group. The first analysis allows us to know how the performance of the dyslexic children differs from normal readers of the same age (Manis, et al., 1996). The soft subtypes were defined by running a regression line with 90% confidence intervals through the Word RTs x Pseudoword RTs plot for the CA and RL control children. This regression line and confidence intervals were then superimposed on the scatterplot of the performance of the dyslexic sample. A surface dyslexic is a child who is an outlier when word RTs are plotted against pseudowords RTs, but is within the normal range when pseudowords RTs are plotted against words RTs. Ph-Dys are defined conversely.

If we compare our results with the English and French studies, the percentage of dyslexic subtypes were quite different. Table 1 shows the proportion of Ph-Dys and S-Dys identified in our study and the proportion in other studies. Castles and Coltheart (1993) found 55% Ph-Dys, Manis, et al. (1996) found 33.3% Ph-Dys, and Stanovich, et al. (1997b) found 25% Ph-Dys in their samples. In our study, we found 18% Ph-Dys and 53% of S-Dys, a greater proportion of S-Dys in comparison to Castles and Coltheart (30%), Manis, et al. (29%) and Stanovich, et al. (22%). Similarly, Genard, et al. (1998) found 56% of S-Dys, and only 4% of Ph-Dys. In general, controlling for CA, there were more Ph-Dys than S-Dys. Similarly, compared to RL controls, there were more Ph-Dys readers than S-Dys; however, the S-Dys profile almost disappeared.

On the other hand, in the Chinese orthography, Ho (2001) found that the incidence of S-Dys and Ph_Dys differs. In general more Chinese dyslexic children have a surface dyslexia (26%) than Ph-Dys (13%), ascertaining our assumption that phonological dyslexia appears to be less common in Chinese than in English.

Studies	PD*	SD.*	D.D*.	ND.*	Variables
Castles & Coltheart. (1993)	55%	30%	6%	9%	Accuracy
Manis et al. (1996)	33%	29%	10%	28%	Accuracy
Stanovich et al. (1997)	25%	22%	28%	25%	Accuracy
Genard et al. (1998)	4%	56%	3%	37%	Accuracy
Sprenger et al. (2000)	52%	32%	3%	13%	Reaction Times
Jiménez & Ramírez. (2002)	18%	53%	3%	26%	Reaction Times/number of letters

*(PD:phonological dyslexics, SD:surface dyslexics, DD: double deficits ND: non-deficit)

Table 1. Classification of dyslexics based on regression method on CA control group

The second analysis focused on whether the performance of dyslexics resembled the performance of younger children learning to read at a normal rate (Manis, et al., 1996). RTs of the dyslexics were plotted so as to identify phonological dyslexics (children with high pseudoword RTs relative to word RTs). The Pseudoword RTs were plotted against the Word RTs. The regression line and confidence intervals are based on the data from the 39 RL controls. Overall, nineteen of the 48 surface dyslexics identified in the regression analysis for the CA group fell below the confidence limit for the RL control group. In contrast, the same 20 phonological dyslexics were identical to those identified from the CA regression lines.

With regard to the validity of subtypes, three separate analyses of variance (ANOVAs) for one factor (younger normal readers vs. phonological dyslexics vs. surface dyslexics) were conducted using the number of correct responses on each of the three phonological awareness tests as dependent variables. Bonferroni's correction was used to determine the acceptable alpha level for rejecting the null hypothesis.The ANOVA on the odd-word-out task was significant [$F (2, 104) = 9.48$; $p < .001$]. A multiple comparison test indicated that younger normal readers scored significantly higher than the phonological dyslexics ($t = 4.50$;

$p < .001$) and surface dyslexics ($t = 2.19$; $p < .05$). The ANOVA on the phoneme segmentation task revealed significant differences [$F (2, 105) = 3.26$; $p < .05$], and the test indicated that the younger normal readers performed significantly better than the phonological dyslexics ($t = 2.56$; $p < .01$) and surface dyslexics ($t = 3.80$; $p < .001$). The ANOVA on the phoneme reversal revealed similar results [$F (2, 105) = 5.95$; $p < .05$] indicating again that younger normal readers scored significantly higher than surface dyslexics ($t = 3, 84$; $p < .001$) and phonological dyslexics ($t = 3.72$; $p < .001$).

2.1.1 Discussion

Studies in English have presented a consistent picture of developmental deviancy and developmental lag that appears to characterize the phonological and surface subtypes (e.g., Manis, et al., 1996; Stanovich et al., 1997b). Phonological dyslexia reflected true developmental deviancy. In contrast, surface dyslexia resembled a form of developmental delay. In the Spanish studies (Jiménez, et al., 2002; Jiménez, et al., 2009) surface and phonological subtypes both represent deviations from normal development. However, the results of the phonological awareness tasks did not validate the division of the dyslexic sample into these two subgroups. Both dyslexic subtypes exhibited significant discrepancies between pseudoword and familiar word reading but they shared the same phonological problems, because both performed more poorly than the younger children in analyzing the phonemic structure of spoken words.

In another study, Jiménez et al. (2009) examined the prevalence, cognitive profile, and home literacy experiences of dyslexic children with different subtypes in Spain. Just like in the other study, we examined the response of three groups (a) a chronological-age-matched group, (b) a reading-level control group, and (c) a dyslexic group. Using regression-based procedures, the author identified 8 phonological and 16 surface dyslexics from a sample of 35 dyslexic 4th-grade children by comparing them to chronological-age-matched controls on RTs for high frequency word and pseudoword reading. However, when the dyslexic subtypes were defined by reference to reading-level controls, 12 phonological dyslexics were defined but only 5 surface dyslexics were identified. Both dyslexic subtypes showed a deficit in phonological awareness, but children with surface dyslexia also showed a deficit in orthographical processing assessed by a homophone comprehension task. This deficit was associated with poor home literacy experiences because the group of parents with children matched in reading age, in comparison to parents with children with surface dyslexia, reported more literacy home experiences.

Sprenger-Charolles, et al. (2000) found that the phonological impairment of the two dyslexic groups was quite severe, since it emerged even relative to younger average readers. Therefore, they suggested that these results are more in line with the hypothesis that a phonological deficit is at the core of developmental dyslexia than with Castles and Coltheart's idea that a "clear double dissociation exists between surface and phonological reading patterns" (1993, p. 174).

Recently, Sprenger-Charrolles, Siegel, Jiménez, and Ziegler (2011) carried out a review of studies conducted in languages varying in the transparency of their orthography. They also concluded that the regression-based method appears to result in less reliable subtypes within and between languages.

In sum, we concluded that in a transparent orthography developmental dyslexics do form a homogeneous population with a unique underlying phonological impairment.

3. Study 2: Computer speech-based remediation for reading disabilities in Spanish dyslexics

An increasing number of researchers have used computers in experiments on the remediation of reading disabilities (e.g., Jones, Torgesen & Sexton, 1987; Olofsson, 1992; Olson & Wise, 1992; Torgesen & Barker, 1995; Van Daal & Reitsma, 1993; Van der Leij, 1994). It has been demonstrated that reading on the computer with speech feedback significantly improved disabled reader's phonological decoding and word recognition. With regard to the best instructional intervention for remediating reading disabilities, Swanson (1999) tested in his study whether certain models of instruction (e.g., direct instruction, strategy instruction, etc.) have broad effects across word-recognition and comprehension measures. He found that effect sizes were higher for word recognition when studies included direct instruction. Moreover, studies of computer-aided remediation for reading-disabled children demonstrated that word recognition skill improved when different forms of orthographic units were manipulated (Olson & Wise, 1992). The study presented here was first published by Jiménez et al. (2003). We had predicted that reading on the computer with speech feedback can provide a helpful remedial tool for children with RD in a transparent orthography.

3.1 Method

Participants. A sample of 73 Spanish children was obtained ranging between 7 years 1 month and 10 years 6 months of age. Using the standard-score discrepancy method, the children with reading difficulties were classified into two groups based on the difference, or lack thereof, between their scores on the IQ test and their standard scores on the Pseudoword subtest of the PROLEC (Cuetos, Rodríguez, & Ruano, 1996). Children were classified as having dyslexia if their pseudoword standard score was more than 15 points lower than their IQ score (N=14), and if their score on an IQ test was >80. Children were considered poor readers if their pseudoword score was less than 15 points lower than their IQ score (N=31), and if their score on an IQ test was >80. The overall sample was classified into three different groups: (1) an experimental group of 14 dyslexics (8 male, 6 female) who received computer-based reading practice; (2) an experimental group of 31 garden variety poor readers (GV) (17 male, 14 female) who also received the same type of practice, and (3) a control group of 28 reading-disabled children (20 male, 8 female) who did not receive computer-assisted practice.

Measures. We used the Standardized Reading Skills Test PROLEC. This test includes different reading subtests. We only administered the following subtests: (1) word reading, (2) pseudoword reading, and (3) text comprehension. Word and Pseudoword reading subtests required correct identification of ordinary words and pseudowords. Both subtests are based on the accuracy of the responses. The comprehension subtest includes a short story and questions which were given to the children after reading. We used the same phonological awareness tests as in Study 1 (i.e., odd-word-out task, phoneme segmentation and phoneme reversal).

Procedure. All the tests were administered by psychologists in a random order, to avoid any effect of the presentation of the material. Once the computer equipment was installed in the schools, the children were randomly assigned to the experimental and control conditions. We first carried out a general trial session, in which the children were trained in all of the TEDIS (Tratamiento Experimental de la Dislexia = Experimental Treatment of Dyslexia) program requirements. Once the treatment sessions started, the examiners were present just to guarantee the optimal technical functioning of the program. The children came to the computer room for 40 minutes per day during language arts time, to keep equivalent the reading instruction time for experimental subjects and for matched untrained controls in the same class. A core technical component in the TEDIS remedial program is the "talking" computer, which gives support and feedback through digitized speech. The TEDIS program provided feedback segmented into sub-word units (i.e., phonemes, syllables, onset-rime segments) which were sequentially highlighted and spoken by the computer. All children received orthographic and speech feedback that was presented in syllable or sub-syllable units. In each session the words were presented on the center of the screen. These words were pronounced by a professional speech trainer and recorded on tape in a studio.

First of all, the computer segmented the word into sub-word units whereas a woman's voice was pronouncing them. Children were asked to attempt to pronounce each segment before clicking the mouse again to hear the speech support. Then, the subject had two options to choose, clicking with the mouse: (1) to repeat the same task with the same sub-word units, or (2) to pronounce the whole word. When the subject was able to pronounce the word correctly, the subjects had to press the keyboard to obtain the next word. When speech feedback was requested, the sub-word sound was immediately delivered through the headphones. When the subject asked for speech feedback, only the relevant word was presented on the screen. If the subject did not read the word, then he or she was asked to repeat the task again by the examiner. Only when the child had three failures with the same word, would the examiner press the keyboard and the presentation of a new word was shown. Every eight stimuli the program asked a multiple-choice comprehension question. Each child had to indicate with the mouse which of the pictures showed on the screen, was related to the target word. The children were allowed to use the speech-feedback option. Van Daal and Reitsma (1993) examined whether it is best to give feedback on all words or to allow the disabled readers to choose. It was found that reading disabled children in the intervention who were matched age did not learn less when the computer unsolicitedly delivered the spoken form of all words than when they were allowed to choose. In addition, the results of a series of small quasi-experimental studies indicated positive treatment effects, in which the dyslexics who received computer training with speech feedback, improved their performance in reading and spelling, compared to students who only had access to conventional special education (Lundberg, 1995). Fifteen sessions were the total of the TEDIS program. In each session, the reading materials consisted of 40 nouns and were divided as a function of the different linguistic parameters into (a) word length (short vs. long), (b) word frequency (familiar vs. nonfamiliar) and word linguistic structure (consonant-vowel (CV) vs. consonant-consonant-vowel (CCV)). During the computer-based word reading, we collected information about the number of accurately read words, number of speech feedback, and reading time. The reading time of each stimulus was registered given that the word appeared on the screen until the child pronounced it successfully.

Results

Pretest-posttest measures

A (3x2) Group (dyslexics, GV poor readers, control) x Moment (pretest, posttest) mixed analysis of variance (ANOVA) was performed on the word recognition and phonological awareness tasks. This analysis yielded a main effect of Time [F (1, 67) = 33.47; p<.001, MSE = 185.50, ES = .33]. In addition there was a significant interaction of Group x Moment [F (2, 67) = 4.23; p < .019, MSE = 23.43, ES = .11]. Tests of simple main effect confirmed that there was an improvement on word recognition in dyslexics [F (1, 67) = 23.2; p < .001, MSE = 128.57], and in GV poor readers [F (1, 67) = 10.48; p < .05, MSE = 58.06]. Dyslexics' baseline level was lower than the other groups; however, they reached the same level of performance in post test. Finally, there were no differences between pretest and posttest scores in the control group [F (1, 67) = 2.63; p = .10, MSE = 14.58] (See Figure 1).

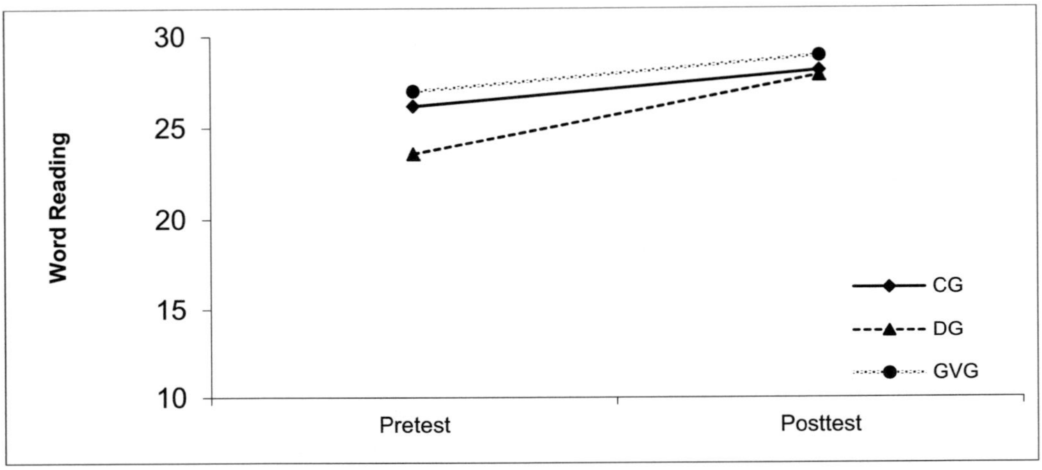

Note: CG = Control Group; DG = Dyslexic Group; GVG= GV Poor Readers Group.

Fig. 1. Interaction between Group and Moment on Word Reading

With regard to phonological awareness measures, both the main effects of Group, [F (6,128) = .82, p <. 04, MSE = 146.56, ES = .09], and of Time, [F (3, 64) = .03, p < .001, MSE = 125.47, ES = .96] were significant. Also, a Group x Time interaction was significant [F (6, 128) = 18.39, p < .04, MSE = 4.0, ES = .09]. Subsequent tests of simple main effects confirmed that there were differences in the posttest between GV poor readers, the control group [F (3, 64) = .85, p < .01, MSE = 150.81], and GV poor readers and dyslexics [F (3, 64) = .87, p < .03, MSE = 125.43]. However, there were no differences between dyslexics and the control group at posttest [F (3, 64) =.91, p = .14, MSE = 109.32]. Again, dyslexic's baseline level was lower than the other groups; however, they reached the same level of performance in post test.

Training sessions measures

A (2x2x15) Group (dyslexics, GV poor readers) x Word Frequency (familiar vs. nonfamiliar) x Word Set (1 vs. 15) mixed analysis of variance (ANOVA) was performed on the number of accurately read words, number of speech feedback, and reading time. A Group x Word Frequency x Word Set interaction was significant [F (13, 767) = 2.11; p < .012, MSE = 36.72,

ES = .35]. Subsequent test of simple main effect revealed that reading time was greater for dyslexics than for GV poor readers in nonfamiliar words during computer-based reading [F (13, 767) = 8.36, p < .001, MSE = 742.62]. A (2x2x15) Group (dyslexics, GV poor readers) x Word Length (short vs. long) x Word Set (1 vs. 15) mixed analysis of variance (ANOVA) was performed on the number of accurately read words, number of speech feedback, and reading time. There was a significant Group x Length x Word Set interaction [F (11, 561) = 3.21; p < .001, MSE = .68, ES = .28] when we analyzed the number of accurately read words. Subsequent test of simple main effect revealed that the dyslexic group was more affected by long words during computer-based reading [F (11, 561) = 5.50, p < .001, MSE = 1.17] (see Figure 2).

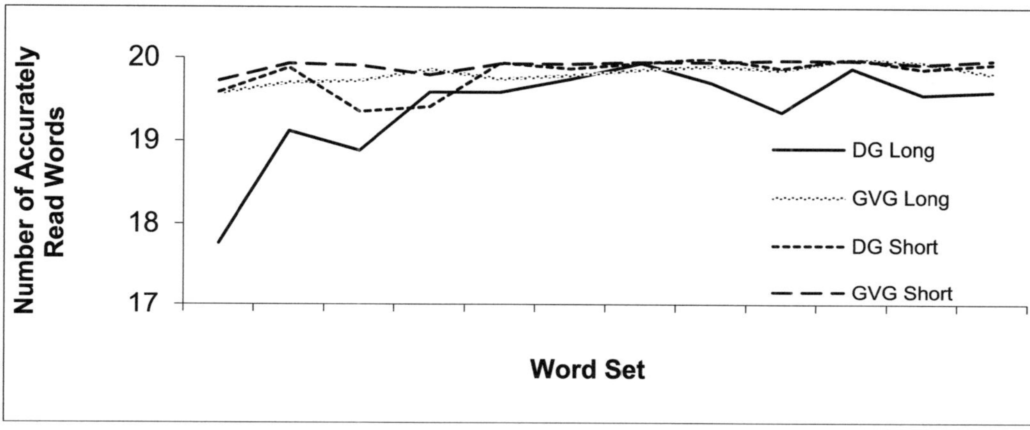

Fig. 2. Interaction between group and word length and word set on the number of accurately read words. DG = long words for dyslexia group; GVC Long = long words for garden-variety poor readers' group; DG Short = short words for dyslexia group; GVG Short = short words for garden-variety poor readers' group.

3.1.1 Discussion

As suggested by Swanson (1999, p. 504) "there have been conceptual shifts regarding what underlies reading problems in children with LD, which in turn raised questions about the best instructional intervention for remediating such problems". Nowadays, there is consensus that many cases of reading disabilities are caused by difficulties in the visual word recognition. The majority of recent research suggests that word identification problems are basically phonological route problems (e.g., Olson, Kliegl, Davidson & Foltz, 1985; Perfetti, 1985; Rack, Snowling & Olson, 1992; Van Den Bos & Spelberg, 1994; Wagner & Torgesen, 1987). As reviewed above, many studies carried out in opaque orthographies using the Reading Level (RL) match design have found empirical evidence in favor of the deficit model in phonological processing, because dyslexics have more difficulty in reading nonwords than normal readers matched in age or in RL (Olson, Wise, Conners, Rack & Fulker, 1989; Stanovich & Siegel, 1994). Moreover, some empirical evidence exists that in languages with a transparent orthography, in which the reading disabled show severe difficulties in the use of the phonological route as they do in the English language (e.g., Jiménez, 1997; Jiménez & Hernández-Valle, 2000; Jiménez & Ramírez, 2002; Jiménez, et al.,

2009), suggesting that a phonemic deficit is curtailing the development of phonological decoding. In addition, the degree of phonological reading deficit is not related to the degree of discrepancy between reading and IQ (for a review see, Stanovich & Siegel, 1994).

The results of this study indicated that computer-assisted practice proved to be as beneficial to the GV poor reader group as for the dyslexic group. We found that reading-disabled children with and without IQ-achievement discrepancy improved their performance on word reading, in comparison to the control group. Nevertheless, dyslexics had more difficulties than GV poor readers during computer-based word reading under conditions that required extensive phonological computation because they were more affected by low frequency words and long words. For another study, Jiménez et al. (2007) assessed the effects of four reading-training procedures for children with reading disabilities (RD) in Spain, with the aim of examining the effects of different spelling-to-sound units in computer speech-based reading. A sample of 82 Spanish children ranging between 7 years 1 month and 10 years 6 months, and whose pseudoword reading performance was below the 25th percentile and IQ >90 were selected. The subjects were randomly assigned to five groups: (1) the Whole-Word training group (WW) (n=16), (2) the Syllable training group (S) (n=16), (3) the Onset-Rime[1] training group (OR) (n=17), (4) the Phoneme training group (P) (n =15), and (5) the untrained control group (n= 18). Children were pre- and post-tested in word recognition, reading comprehension, phonological awareness, and visual and phonological tasks. Results indicated that experimental groups who participated in the phoneme and whole-word condition improved their word recognition compared to the control group. In addition, dyslexics who participated in the phoneme, syllable and onset-rime conditions applied for more number of calls during computer-based word reading under conditions that required extensive phonological computation (low frequency words and long words). However, reading time was greater for long words in the phoneme group during computer-based reading. The authors concluded that reading on the computer with speech feedback can provide a helpful remedial tool for children with RD in a transparent orthography.

Regarding the best instructional intervention for remediating reading disabilities, Swanson (1999) tested in his study whether certain models of instruction (e.g., direct instruction, strategy instruction, etc.) have broad effects across word-recognition and comprehension measures. He found that effect sizes were higher for word recognition when studies included direct instruction. Additionally, an increasing number of researchers have used computers in experiments on the remediation of reading disabilities (e.g., Jones, Torgesen & Sexton, 1987; Olofsson, 1992; Olson & Wise, 1992; Torgesen & Barker, 1995; Van Daal & Reitsma, 1993; Van der Leij, 1994). It has been demonstrated that reading on the computer with speech feedback significantly improved disabled reader's phonological decoding and word recognition. Moreover, studies of computer-aided remediation for reading disabled children demonstrated that word recognition skill improved when different forms of orthographic units were manipulated (Olson & Wise, 1992).

In the teaching of reading, children can be trained on the print-to-sound translation by using linguistic units of different sizes: a word can be taught as a whole unit, in individual letter-sound units, or in sublexical units of intermediate size (syllable, BOSS, onset-rime).

[1] The syllable in Spanish consists of an 'onset' (initial consonant or cluster) plus a 'rime' (vowel and any following consonants).

However, the spelling-to-sound unit used in training may be a critical factor in determining the effectiveness of remedial instruction for RD. Consequently, various remedial studies carried out in English have tried to determine which is the size of the spelling-to-sound unit more optimal for computer speech-based training of RD (e.g., Lovett, Barron, Forbes, Cuksts, & Steinbach, 1994; Olson & Wise, 1992). For Spanish, the Syllable and Onset-Rime condition did not contribute to improve phonological decoding. This finding is not surprising because this type of units does not seem to be as relevant in a language where a direct correspondence between graphemes and phonemes does exist, and where the syllable boundaries are well defined. Therefore, Jiménez et al (2003) suggested that in a transparent orthography such as Spanish, remedial education may be more successful if it concentrates on the phoneme level more than on onset-rime units, in contrast to what has been suggested by Treiman (1992) in the English language. The improvements in the Phoneme group support the idea that the phonemic level plays an important role in dyslexia in a transparent orthography as Spanish. By forcing attention to individual letters within the word and with the speech feedback at the same time during the training, could provide the basis to improve phonemic segmentation skills, and promoting the grapheme-phoneme correspondences, an ability that is not achieved by the severe RD children. In relation to the Whole Word condition, interestingly, this unit also benefited word recognition ability. A possible explanation for this finding has to do with the fact that the dual route model of reading is functional in Spanish despite its orthographic transparency by which, in principle, all the words could be read by the phonological route. Some empirical data support the functionality of both routes in Spanish children (Defior, Justicia & Martos, 1996; Valle-Arroyo, 1989), suggesting no differences between the processes involved in the reading of Spanish and those implicated in opaque orthographies, such as English. In this sense, it is important to note that children who participated in this study were between 7-10 years old, an age in which we would expect the use of the orthographic routine of reading. The reason for the gains after treatment within this experimental condition may be explained by the fact that children could place their attention on the whole word present on the computer screen with the phonological speech feedback. This connection between the word and its individual sounds may have enhanced the connections between their orthographic and phonological forms.

4. Concluding discussion

Wydell and Butterworth (1999) suggested that the effect of a phonological deficit on reading depends on the transparency of the orthography. Probably the most likely source of these difficulties is a deficit in representing phonological information at earlier developing levels of phonology: the syllable, onset, and rime. Goswami (2002) suggested that syllabic representation is basic to many languages, and that children's ability to recognize syllables and rhymes precedes learning a particular spelling system. This developmental view can readily explain cross-language differences in reading acquisition, and it can also explain cross-language differences in the manifestation of developmental dyslexia (see also Wydell & Butterworth, 1999; Wydell & Kondo, 2003 for a similar conclusion). Some of the processes underpinning language acquisition are disrupted in developmental dyslexia leading to deficits in the development of a phonological representation of words before literacy is acquired. According to this theoretical analysis, dyslexic children in all languages appear to have a phonological deficit at the syllable and rhyme levels prior to acquiring literacy. This deficit leads to problems in acquiring letter-sound relationships and in restructuring the phonological lexicon to represent phoneme-level information.

Some linguists have suggested that different phonological units exist in the Spanish language (i.e., syllable, onset and rime). Jiménez and Ortiz (1993) designed a study to verify whether or not such linguistic realities are psychological realities as has been found in the English language. The results obtained suggested that children at the pre-reading stage are more sensitive to syllabic units, than to instrasyllabic and phonemic units. Moreover, they demonstrated that good readers did not differ from disabled readers and non readers at the syllabic awareness level, but they had higher levels of instrasyllabic awareness, and phonemic awareness. In languages like Spanish, onset-rime segmentation is equivalent to phonemic segmentation for many words (e.g., for a word like "loro", the onset-rimes are /l/ /O/ /r/ /O/ and so are the phonemes). In fact, Spanish children with reading disabilities do not use correspondences based on higher level units as onsets and rimes in visual word recognition (Jiménez, Alvarez, Estévez & Hernández-Valle, 2000). Goswami (2002) also suggested that dyslexic children learning to read in languages with a simple syllabic structure would probably have less difficulty in the acquisition of grapheme-phoneme recoding strategies. However, in the first study presented here both Spanish dyslexic subtype samples were impaired as a group relative to the CA group on phonological awareness tasks analyzed. Both dyslexic subtypes performed significantly worse than the RL group on the measures of phonological awareness suggesting that a phonemic deficit is curtailing the development of phonological decoding. We replicated the finding of a dyslexic deficit in an RL match that we found for previous studies conducted in a transparent orthography (i.e., Spanish) (Jiménez, 1997; Jiménez & Hernández-Valle, 2000).

On the other hand, Stanovich et al. (1997b) suggested that surface dyslexia may arise from a milder form of phonological deficit than phonological dyslexia; this type of difficulty could be influenced by the orthographic peculiarities of the language. We suggested that in a transparent orthography the difficulties with the phonological processing emerge more clearly, especially in surface dyslexia. Therefore, we suggest that the existence of dyslexic subtypes could be a consequence of the differences in the orthographic systems.

We would like to conclude this section by pointing out that in studies employing accuracy-based measures of subtypes, the subjects have been selected on the basis of accuracy-based reading scores (Jiménez, 2010). But there is a pool of subjects who might have met rate-based but not accuracy-based criteria for inclusion in a dyslexia study. We do not know what kinds of cognitive and reading profiles rate-disabled children would show, because they are typically not included in subtype studies in English. Until these children are tested, it may be premature to argue that there are differences in the incidence of various subtypes across orthographies. The difference might be due to the accuracy vs. rate criterion of selecting subjects, rather than differences in the orthography, although both could be factors that affect the identification of a reading disability. Consequently, this issue is open to debate and it is exemplified by observations made by Share (2008): 'it remains to be seen to what extent the classic dual-route distinction between phonological and surface dyslexia, a purely accuracy-based dichotomy, relates to accuracy/speed differences, particularly in the case of more conventional (i.e. transparent) orthographies'.

Empirical evidence indicates that computer-assisted practice can improve word recognition for reading disabled children compared to a control group. However, we also found that the performance of dyslexic children during computer-based word reading was also affected by low frequency words and long words.

To conclude, the research findings presented here provide empirical support to the hypothesis based on a phonemic deficit in dyslexia in a transparent orthography. Moreover, the research findings demonstrate that reading by the computer with speech feedback may constitute a helpful remedial tool for children with RD. Consequently, both studies reported here provide empirical evidence about the role of phonological processing in dyslexia in the Spanish language, consistent with other multiple case studies.

The origin of this phonological deficit in developmental dyslexia is also open to debate. Sprenger-Charolles et al. (2006) examined the classical phonological explanation that ascribes dyslexics' reading deficit to a specific cognitive deficiency in phonological processing, primarily in phonemic awareness and in phonological short-term memory. They also examined the current non-phonological explanations that assume that the phonological deficit of dyslexics is secondary to more basic sensori-motor impairment: a deficiency in either rapid auditory processing, or in the visual magnocellular pathway, or in motor skills. The authors show why perceptual explanations of dyslexia should be based on alternative perceptual modes rather than on deficits, and they place the perceptual explanation in the framework of a three-stage model of speech perception. They argue that dyslexics' phonological deficits are secondary to more basic sensori-motor impairments. Overall, they concluded that the non-phonological explanations are rather weak, and they propose a new phonological explanation for dyslexia, based on a specific mode of speech perception. In sum, "allophonic perception offers a new perspective in the study of dyslexia. Therefore, further research is necessary to gain a better understanding of the way dyslexics perceive speech, and especially how they segment the speech stream. While allophonic theory constitutes a first step in this direction, it still has to be articulated with other dimensions of language processing" (p. 172).

5. Acknowledgment

This manuscript has been supported by a grant from Ministerio de Asuntos Exteriores y de Cooperación, AECID, number C/030692/10, Spain. We are grateful to Doris Baker for her careful editing and for the many invaluable corrections she proposed, both in content and on technical and stylistic matters. Correspondence should be addressed to Juan E. Jiménez, Departamento de Psicología Evolutiva y de la Educación, Universidad de La Laguna, Campus de Guajara, 38200 Islas Canarias, España. Electronic mail may be sent to ejimenez@ull.es

6. References

Backman, J., Mamen, M., & Ferguson, H.B. (1984). Reading level design: Conceptual and methodological issues in reading research. *Psychological Bulletin, 96*, 560-568.

Bowey, J.A. y Francis, J. (1991). Phonological analysis as a function of age and exposure to reading instruction. *Applied Psycholinguistics, 12*, 91-121.

Bryant, P.E., & Goswami, U. (1986). Strengths and weakness of the reading level design: A comment on Backman, Mamen, and Ferguson. *Psychological Bulletin, 100,* 101-103.

Castles, A., & Coltheart, M. (1993). Varieties of developmental dyslexia. *Cognition, 47,* 149-180.

Cuetos, F., Rodríguez, B., & Ruano, E, (1996). *Batería de Evaluación de los procesos lectores de los niños de Educación Primaria* (PROLEC) [Assessment test of reading skills for children] Madrid, Spain: T.E.A., Ediciones.

Defior, S., Justicia, F., & Martos, F. (1996). The influence of lexical and sublexical variables in normal and poor Spanish readers. *Reading and Writing: An interdisciplinary Journal, 8,* 487-497.

De Vega, M., Carreiras, M., Gutiérrez, M., & Alonso-Quecuty, M. L. (1990). *Lectura y comprensión. Una perspectiva cognitiva.* Madrid: Alianza Editorial.

Genard, N., Mousty, P., Content, A., Alegria, J., Leybaert, J., & Morais, J. (1998). Methods to establish subtypes of developmental dyslexia. In P. Reitsma & L. Verhoeven (Eds.), *Problems and interventions in literacy development* (pp. 163-176). Netherlands: Kluwer Academic Publishers.

Goswami, U. (2002). Phonology, reading development, and dyslexia: A cross-linguistic perspective. *Annals of Dyslexia,* 52, 141-163.

Goswami, U. (2003). *Phonology, reading development and dyslexia: A cross-language perspective.* Paper presented at the Bangor Dyslexia Conference, Bangor, UK.

Goswami, U., & Bryant, P. E. (1990). *Phonological skills and learning to read.* Hillsdale, N.J. : Erlbaum.

Guzmán, R., & Jiménez, J.E. (2001). Estudio normativo sobre parámetros psicolingüísticos en niños de 6 a 8 años: la familiaridad subjetiva. *Cognitiva, 13,* 153-191.

Ho, F.J. (2001). *Subtypes of dyslexia in Chinese orthography.* Unpublished Doctoral Dissertation. The University of New South Wales, Sidney, Australia.

Jiménez, J.E. (1997). A reading-level match study of phonemic processes underlying reading disabilities in a transparent orthography. *Reading and Writing: An Interdisciplinary Journal, 9,* 23-40.

Jiménez, J.E. (2010). Explaining reading acquisition and developmental dyslexia in alphabetic systems. *The American Journal of Psychology,* 123, 2, 233-236.

Jiménez, J.E., Alvarez, C., Estévez, A., & Hernández-Valle, I. (2000). Onset-rime units in visual word recognition in Spanish normal readers and children with reading disabilities. *Learning Disabilities Research & Practice, 15,* 135-141.

Jiménez, J.E., García, E., Ortiz, M.R., Hernández-Valle, I., Guzmán, R., Rodrigo, M., Estévez, A., Díaz, A., y Hernández, S. (2005). Is the deficit in phonological awareness better explained in terms of task differences or effects of syllable structure? *Applied Psycholinguistics, 26,* 267-283.

Jiménez, J.E., & Hernández-Valle, I. (2000). Word identification and reading disorders in the Spanish language. *Journal of Learning Disabilities, 33,* 44-60.

Jiménez, J.E., Hernández-Valle, I., Ramírez, G., Ortiz, M.R., Rodrigo, M., Tabraue, M., Estévez, A., y O'Shanahan, I. (2007). Computer speech-based remediation for reading disabilities: The size of spelling-to-sound unit in a transparent orthography. *The Spanish Journal of Psychology, 10,* 52-67.

Jiménez, J.E., & Ortiz, M.R. (1993). Phonological awareness in learning literacy. *Cognitiva, 5,* 153-170.

Jiménez, J.E., Ortiz, M.R., Rodrigo, M., Hernández-Valle, I., Ramírez, G., Estévez, A., O'Shanahan, I., Tabraue, M. (2003). Do the effects of computer-assisted practice differ for children with reading disabilities with and without IQ-achievement discrepancy? *Journal of Learning Disabilities, 36*, 34-47.

Jiménez, J. E., & Ramírez, G. (2002). Identifying subtypes of reading disabilities in the Spanish language. *The Spanish Journal of Psychology, 5*, 3-19.

Jiménez, J.E., Rodríguez, C., & Ramírez, G. (2009). Spanish developmental dyslexia: Prevalence, cognitive profile and home literacy experiences. *Journal of Experimental Child Psychology, 103*, 167-185.

Jones, K.M., Torgesen, J.K., & Sexton, M.A. (1987). Using computer guided practice to increase decoding fluency in learning disabled children: A study using the Hint and Hunt Program. *Journal of Learning Disabilities, 20*, 122-128.

Lovett, M.W., Barron, R.W., Forbes, J.E., Cuksts, B., & Steinbach, K.A. (1994). Computer speech-based training of literacy skills in neurologically impaired children: A controlled evaluation. *Brain and Language*, 47, 117-154.

Lundberg, I. (1995). The computer as a tool of remediation in the education of students with reading disabilities: A theory-based approach. *Learning Disability Quarterly, 18*, 89-99.

Manis, F.R., Seidenberg, M.S., Doi, L.M., McBride-Chang,C., & Petersen, A. (1996). On the bases of two subtypes of developmental dyslexia. *Cognition, 58*, 157-195.

Olofsson, A. (1992). Synthetic speech and computer aided reading for reading disabled children. *Reading & Writing: An Interdisciplinary Journal, 4*, 165-178.

Olson, R.K. (1994). Language deficits in specific reading disability. In M.A. Gernsbacher (Ed.), *Handbook of psycholinguistics* (pp. 895-916). New York: Academic Press.

Olson, R.K., Kliegl, R., Davidson, B.J. & Foltz, G. (1985). Individual and developmental differences in reading disability. En G.E. MacKinnon y T.G. Waller (Eds.). *Reading research: Advances in theory and practice* .Vol. 4 (pp. 1-64). New York: Academic Press.

Olson, R., & Wise, B. (1992). Reading on the computer with orthographic and speech feedback: An overview of the Colorado remediation project. *Reading & Writing: An interdisciplinary Journal, 4*, 107-144.

Olson, R.K., Wise, B., Conners, F., Rack, J. & Fulker, D. (1989). Specific deficits in component reading and language skills: Genetic and environmental influences. *Journal of Learning Disabilities*, 22, 339-348.

Perfetti, C.A. (1985). *Reading ability*. Nueva York. Oxford University Press.

Rack, J.P., Snowling, M.J. & Olson, R.K. (1992). The nonword reading deficit in developmental dyslexia: A review. *Reading Research Quarterly, 27*, 29-53.

Rodrigo, M., & Jiménez, J.E. (1999). An análisis of the word naming errors of normal readers and reading disabled children in Spanish. *Journal of Research on Reading*, 22, 180-197.

Share, D. L. (2008). On the Anglocentrism of current reading research and practice: The perils of overreliance on an "outlier orthography". *Psychological Bulletin*, 134, 584-615.

Sprenger-Charolles, L., Colé, P., Lacert, P., & Serniclaes, W. (2000). On subtypes of developmental dyslexia: Evidence from processing time and accuracy scores. *Canadian Journal of Experimental Psychology, 54*, 87-103.

Sprenger-Charolles, L., Colé, P., & Serniclaes, W. (2006). *Reading acquisition and developmental dyslexia*. New York: Psychology Press.

Sprenger-Charolles, L., Siegel, L.S., Jiménez, J.E., & Ziegler, J.C. (2011). Prevalence and reliability of phonological, surface, and mixed profiles in dyslexia: A review of studies conducted in languages varying in orthographic depth. *Scientific Studies of Reading*, 15, 6, 498-521

Stanovich, K.E., & Siegel, L.S. (1994). Phenotypic performance profile of children with reading disabilities: A regression-based test of the phonological-core variable-difference model. *Journal of Educational Psychology, 86*, 24-53.

Stanovich, K.E., Siegel, L.S., & Gottardo, A. (1997a). Progress in the search for dyslexia subtypes. In C.Hulme & M.Snowling (Eds.). *Biology, cognition and intervention* (pp. 108-130). London: Whurr Publishers Ltd.

Stanovich, K.E., Siegel, L.S., & Gottardo, A. (1997b). Converging evidence for phonological and surface subtypes of reading disability. *Journal of Educational Psychology, 89*, 114-127.

Swanson, H.L. (1999). Reading research for students with LD: A meta-analysis of intervention outcomes. *Journal of Learning Disabilities, 32*, 504-532.

Torgesen, J.K., & Barker, T.A. (1995). Computers as aids in the prevention and remediation of reading disabilities. *Learning Disability Quarterly, 18*, 76-87.

Toro, J., & Cervera, M. (1980). *Test de análisis de lectoescritura* [Reading and spelling Test] Madrid: Aprendizaje Visor.

Treiman, R. (1992). The role of intrasyllabic units in learning to read and spell. En P.B. Gough, L. Ehri, & R. Treiman (Eds.), *Reading acquisition* (pp. 65-106). Hillsdale, NJ: LEA.

Valle-Arroyo, F. (1989). Errores de lectura y escritura. Un modelo dual [Errors in reading and spelling. A dual route model] *Cognitiva, 2*, 35-63.

Van Daal, V.H.P., & Reitsma, P. (1993). The use of speech feedback by normal and disabled readers in computer-based reading practice. *Reading and Writing: An Interdisciplinary Journal, 5*, 243-259.

Van den Bos, K.P., & Spelberg, H.C.L. (1994). Word identification routes and reading disorders. In K.P. Van den Bos, L.S. Siegel, D.J. Bakker y D.L. Share (Eds.). *Current directions in dyslexia research* (pp.201-219). Lisse, Netherlands: Swets & Zeitlinger.

Van der Leij, A., (1994). Effects of computer-assisted instruction on word and pseudoword reading of reading-disabled student. In K.P. Van den Bos, L.S. Siegel, D.J. Bakker y D.L. Share (Eds.). *Current directions in dyslexia research* (pp.251-267). Lisse, Netherlands: Swets & Zeitlinger.

Wagner, R.K., & Torgesen, J.K., (1987). The nature of phonological processing and its causal role in the acquisition of reading skills. *Psychological Bulletin, 101*, 192-212.

Wydell, T.N. & Butterworth, B.L. (1999). A case study of an English-Japanese bilingual with monolingual dyslexia. *Cognition*, 70, 273–305.

Wydell, T. N., & Kondo, T. (2003). Phonological deficit and the reliance on orthographic approximation for reading: A follow-up study on an English-Japanese bilingual with monolingual dyslexia. *Journal of Research in Reading, 26*, 33–48.

4

Phonological Restriction Knowledge in Dyslexia: Universal or Language-Specific?

Norbert Maïonchi-Pino
Tohoku University, Institute of Development, Aging and Cancer, Department of Developmental Cognitive Neuroscience & Department of Functional Brain Imaging, Sendai, Japan

1. Introduction

Developmental dyslexia is the most studied and well-documented of the specific learning disabilities in school-age children across languages, which reaches from 5-to-17.5% individuals (e.g., Shaywitz & Shaywitz, 2005; Snowling, 2001). There is now a consensus that developmental dyslexia stems from a genetic neurodevelopmental disorder that does not depend on inadequate intellectual or educational backgrounds (e.g., Lyon, Shaywitz, & Shaywitz, 2003; Sprenger-Charolles, Colé, Lacert, & Serniclaes, 2000; Vellutino, Fletcher, Snowling, & Scanlon, 2004). There is considerable evidence for a phonological deficit as the major correlate of language disabilities in dyslexia, which underpins the cognitive disorder (e.g., Ramus, Rosen, Dakin, Day, Castellote, White, & Frith, 2003; Ziegler & Goswami, 2005). However, an outstanding, long-lasting question that remains unclear, even unanswered, is what underlies the phonological deficit in dyslexia (e.g., Ramus, 2001). Three main directions have been proposed to account for the phonological deficit: 1) limited phonological short-term memory; 2) degraded, under-specified or, conversely, over-specified phonological representations; 3) speech perception disorders. However, the degraded, under-specified phonological representation hypothesis that is basically referred to accounts for the dyslexics' phonological deficit has been recently challenged: it has been suggested that the dyslexics' phonological deficit relies on difficulties to store, access, and retrieve the phonological representations (e.g., Ahissar, 2007; Ramus & Szenkovits, 2008; Szenkovits & Ramus, 2005). To date, to reconcile both views, it has been proposed that the phonological deficit results in multi-dimensional difficulties that include difficulties to learn and manipulate the speech units as well as difficulties to store, access, and retrieve the phonological representations (e.g., Snowling, 2001; Ziegler, Castel, Pech-Geogel, George, Alario, & Perry, 2008). Despite this tentative proposal, there is no consensus. Here, I propose to draw an up-to-date portrait of an alternative option that has not been studied so far to disentangle whether another possible source of the phonological deficit in dyslexia may be envisaged: Are dyslexics sensitive to *universal* phonological knowledge?

2. On the possible origins of the phonological deficit

Overall, what the past studies have revealed is that the phonological deficit has no clear-cut well-specified origins. Within the phonological deficit hypothesis, typically, it has been suggested that the core deficit children face is rooted in degraded, under-specified phonological representation (e.g., Boada & Pennington, 2006; Elbro & Jensen, 2005; Snowling, 2001).

In a non-negligible proportion, dyslexics' phonological deficit originates in impairments to process auditory information (i.e., ≈ 50%; Ramus et al., 2003). Typically, to account for the degraded nature of the phonological representations, it has been hypothesized that the dyslexics' perceptual system could not turn to be attuned to the native phonemic categories as shown with impairments in categorical perception (e.g., Adlard & Hazan, 1998; Mody, Studdert-Kennedy, & Brady, 1997; Veuillet, Magnan, Écalle, Thai-Van, & Collet, 2007). The categorical perception refers to the tendency to perceive a sound as a member of a category (e.g., /b/ or /p/). Thus, the variants of the same phoneme within a category are more likely perceived as being similar to each other compared to phonemes from other categories (i.e., /bʰ/ is more likely judged as similar to /b/ than /p/ while /pʰ/ is more likely judged as similar to /p/ than /b/. Scientifically-speaking, the categorical perception can be described as "the degree to which acoustic differences between variants of the same phoneme are less perceptible than differences of the same acoustic magnitude between two different phonemes" (Serniclaes et al., 2004, p. 337). Indeed, dyslexics have been shown to be impaired the processing of relevant acoustic-phonetic characteristics in their native language such as the voicing (e.g., /ba/ - /pa/; Bogliotti, Serniclaes, Messaoud-Galusi, & Sprenger-Charolles, 2008; Hoonhorst, Colin, Markessis, Radeau, Deltenre, & Serniclaes, 2009; Serniclaes, Sprenger-Charolles, Carré, & Démonet, 2001; Serniclaes, van Heghe, Mousty, Carré, & Sprenger-Charolles, 2004). Lower performances in between-categories perception but higher performances in within-categories perception compared to both chronological age-matched and reading level-matched controls have been interpreted as an allophonic mode of speech perception[1]. In other words, dyslexics have difficulties to discriminate two phonemes that belong to two different categories as determined by the voicing (i.e., /ba/ vs. /pa/; low between-boundaries performance) whereas they can discriminate two variants of a same phoneme even if one of the variant does not exist in the native language (e.g., /p/ and /pʰ/; high within-boundaries performance). Hence, dyslexics' phonological representations would be over-specified since dyslexics would maintain acoustic-phonetic contrasts that are irrelevant in their native language and should be deactivated early in life (e.g., Saffran, Werker, & Werner, 2006; Werker & Tees, 1984). To be unable to discriminate relevant acoustic-phonetic duration-based contrasts in their native language (i.e., voicing; e.g., /b/ vs. /p/) would induce degraded, under-specified phonological representations and subsequent difficulties to use grapheme-to-phoneme correspondences (e.g., Bogliotti et al., 2008; Serniclaes et al., 2004). Alternatively, the phonological deficit could stem from difficulties in the time-course aspects of pre-lexical phonetic-phonological processing rather than from impaired phonological-lexical representations (e.g., Blomert, Mitterer, & Paffen, 2004; Nittrouer, 1999).

To determine whether the dyslexic's perceptual system is tuned to process finely-sharpened universal phonological representations (i.e., sound sequences that respect or not the

[1] An allophone is a contextual variant of a same phoneme which may be not distinguished within a same phonemic category (e.g., /r/ and /ʁ/ in French). For instance, in French, replacing /r/ with /ʁ/ in /pri/ 'price' will not change its meaning while replacing /r/ or /ʁ/ with /l/ will, i.e., /pli/ , wrinkle'. Allophones are language-dependent.

universal phonological well-formedness), I here envisage the universal phonological sonority-related *markedness* to provide further arguments on the origin of the dyslexics' phonological deficit: universal or language-dependent and degraded/under-specified phonological representations or difficulties to access them?

3. Why the phonological grammar is of interest?

3.1 A phonological grammar?

Native phonological knowledge includes a phonological grammar that embeds language-specific phonemes and phonotactic restrictions that constrain the co-occurrence of sound sequences to perceive and produce sentences (e.g., de Lacy, 2007). In normally-developing newborns and adults, this is a well-known phenomenon that listeners tend to misperceive and repair phonotactically-illegal sound sequences in their native language. Given that the perceptual system becomes, early-on, attuned to sounds and phonotactic restrictions relevant to the native language (e.g., Jusczyk, Friederici, Wessels, Svenkerud, Jusczyk, 1993; Kuhl, Andrusko, Chistovich, Chistovich, Kozhevnikova, Ryskina, Stolyarova, Sundberg, Lacerda, 1997), it has been argued that the perceptual repair could result from: 1) a perceptual assimilation of acoustic-phonetic properties of nonnative sound sequences into native ones or to the phonetically-close ones (e.g., /dla/ in /gla/; in English: Best, 1995; in French: Hallé, Seguí, Frauenfelder, & Meunier, 1998); 2) a compensation for coarticulation since sound sequences such as /dla/ are more difficult to perceive and articulate than /gla/ (e.g., Wright, 2004); 3) a perceptual fit to the phonotactic probablities (e.g., Bonte, Mitterer, Zellagui, Poelmans, & Blomert, 2005); 4) an *illusory epenthetic vowel*; an epenthesis may be a consonant or a vowel present in the phoneme inventory of a target-language, which is inserted to restore a native phonotactically-legal sound sequence (e.g., /dəl/ in English: Berent, Steriade, Lennertz, & Vaknin, 2007; /buz/ in Japanese: Dupoux, Kakehi, Hirose, Pallier, & Mehler, 1999; /dil/ in Portuguese: Dupoux, Parlato, Frota, Hirose, & Peperkamp, 2011). However, in dyslexic adults or children, data remain rare, and focus on phonotactic probabilities (e.g., Bonte, Poelmans, & Blomert, 2007) or, recently, on compensation for place assimilation (e.g., Marshall, Ramus, & van der Lely, in press) and voicing assimilation (e.g., Szenkovits, Darma, Darcy, & Ramus, submitted). Ramus and collaborators thus showed that French dyslexics assimilated phonotactically-illegal sound sequences into phonotactically-legal ones to the same extent as controls. This suggests that dyslexics are able to normally acquire native phonological grammar, and questions the degraded phonological grammar and representations (for counter-arguments, see Bonte et al., 2007).

3.2 An unexplored alternative

As hypothesized within the Optimality Theory framework (Prince & Smolensky, 1993; 1997; 2004), sound sequences that are phonotactically-illegal clusters such as /ʁb/ are more likely rejected compared to phonotactically-legal clusters such as /bʁ/ since all speakers are supposed to have universal phonological knowledge on grammatical restrictions irrespective to their (acoustic-)phonetic properties and phonotactic probabilities. However, whether dyslexics have universal phonological knowledge on grammatical restrictions remain unexplored.

3.2.1 Phonological *markedness* and sonority profile

Phonotactic restrictions straightforwardly rule how sound sequences co-occur. It has been shown that sound sequences depend on the sonority of phonemes (e.g., Clements, 1990). Sonority is a scalar acoustic-phonetic property that refers to the sound's "[...] loudness relative to that of other sounds with the same length, stress, and pitch" (Ladefoged, 1975, p. 221). Under this definition, Fig. 1 presents that sonority hierarchically ranks consonants from the high-sonority phonemes (i.e., from liquid to nasal) to low-sonority ones (i.e., from fricative, /f/, /z/, /ʃ/... to occlusive, /b/, /t/, /g/...). Also, the linguistic structures are supposed to conform to a sonority-based organization as proposed by the *sonority sequencing principle* (e.g., Clements, 1990; Selkirk, 1984): syllables favor a structure with an onset maximally growing in sonority towards the vowel and falling minimally to the coda. Hence, universally-optimal CV syllables that bear high-sonority onsets (e.g., /la/) tend to be avoided in the phonotactics of languages to favor low-sonority ones (e.g., /ta/) whereas, in syllables that do contain a coda, high-sonority codas (e.g., /al/) tend to be preferred to low-sonority ones (e.g., /at/; see Selkirk, 1984). Using a sonority-based distribution of syllables which combines the sonority and the sonority sequencing principle, it is possible to assess the universal phonological knowledge on grammatical restrictions.

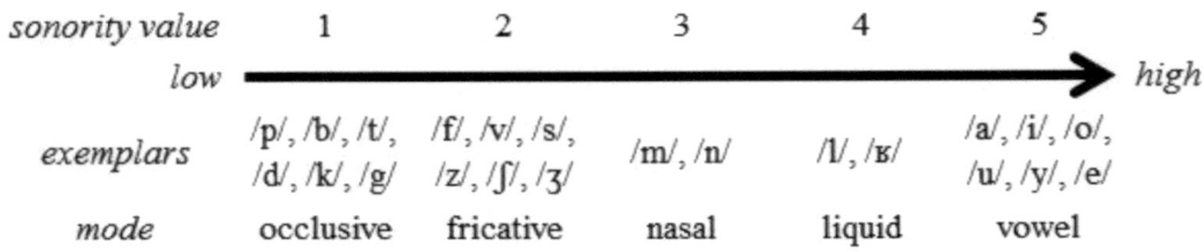

Fig. 1. Sonority scale adapted from Clements (1990) and Selkirk (1984).

3.2.2 Sonority-related *markedness* as a universal phonological knowledge

As proposed within the Optimality Theory framework (Prince & Smolensky, 1993; 1997; 2004), all listeners undergo universal *markedness* and *faithfulness constraints*. Markedness constraints are phonological grammatical restrictions that disfavor some grammatically ill-formed structures (e.g., /ʁb/) whereas faithfulness constraints are constraints that require mapping the input to the output (e.g., mapping the input /ʁb/ to the output /ʁb/). If the input is grammatically well-formed (e.g., /bʁ/), its acoustic-phonetic properties are faithfully encoded and mapped to the output /bʁ/. But, if the input is grammatically ill-formed (e.g., /ʁb/), the input fails to be faithfully encoded and mapped to the output /ʁb/. Accordingly, a grammatically ill-formed input is recoded as a grammatically well-formed output that could trigger a perceptual confusion (e.g., the insertion of an illusory vowel; i.e., an epenthetic vowel such as /ə/). In the view of the Optimality Theory (Prince & Smolensky, 1993; 1997; 2004), universal low-frequency structures -the grammatically ill-formed ones- (e.g., /ʁb/) that transgress markedness constraints are labeled as *marked* whereas universal high-frequency structures -the grammatically well-formed ones- (e.g., /bʁ/) are labeled as *unmarked*. Thus, onset clusters with a sonority high-rise (e.g., /bʁ/, s = +3) are less marked than onset clusters with a sonority low-rise (e.g., /sm/, s = +1), which are less marked than onset clusters with a sonority plateau (e.g., /kb/, s = 0). Then, onset clusters with a sonority plateau are less marked than onset clusters with a sonority low-fall (e.g., /ft/, *s* = -1), which are less marked than onset clusters with a sonority high-fall (e.g., /ʁb/, *s* = -3). Hence, monotically, markedness increases and well-formedness decreases from sonority high-rise (unmarked structures) to sonority high-fall (marked structures).

4. The present study

As I mentioned above, there is plenty of work to refine our understanding of where the phonological deficit comes from. Does the phonological deficit arise from degraded, under-specified phonological representations? If the phonological representations are intact, do dyslexic children have intact universal phonological representations? To provide innovative arguments in speech perception in dyslexia, I designed a preliminary syllable count task to pit the universal phonological knowledge on grammatical restrictions in French dyslexic children. I tested the (mis)perception of marked, grammatically ill-formed unattested onset clusters in French dyslexic compared to chronological age-matched controls and reading level-matched controls. Children were aurally-administered monosyllabic $C_1C_2VC_3$ pseudowords (e.g., /pkal/) and their disyllabic $C_1uC_2VC_3$ counterparts (e.g., /pukal/). All C_1C_2 clusters within monosyllabic pseudowords were constructed by splicing out the /u/. Onset clusters (C_1C_2) were classified as high-fall, low-fall, plateau, low-rise or high-rise.

Given the markedness constraints (i.e., avoid marked, grammatically ill-formed outputs such as /ʁb/) and the faithfulness constraints (i.e., map the input /ʁb/ to the output /ʁb/), the misperception of C_1C_2 clusters should increase as markedness increases. Hence, if perceptual confusion depends on universal markedness-related knowledge as determined by sonority profiles, /gmal/ (high-rise SP, the most marked) should be more misperceived as disyllabic than /pkal/ (plateau SP), which in turn, should be more misperceived than /ʁbal/ (high-fall SP, the least marked) in both chronological age-matched and reading level-matched controls. However, since dyslexics are supposed to have degraded, under-specified phonological representations, phonological sonority-related markedness effects and phonological repair with an illusory epenthetic vowel should not be observed.

5. Experiment 1

5.1 Method

5.1.1 Participants

Five French dyslexic children with no comorbid attention deficit hyperactivity disorder (ADHD) were tested in this experiment. Dyslexic children were compared to five chronological age-matched controls and five reading level-matched controls. Control children were recruited from an urban public elementary school. All children were tested after parents returned a consent form. Dyslexic children were diagnosed as dyslexics around two years prior this experiment (*M* = 29 months; *SD* = 4 months) by a speech and language therapist. All children were French native speakers with no second language learning, middle class, and right-handed[2]. They reported no hearing disorders. Reading level and IQs

[2] Children's right-handedness was assessed with the Edinburgh Handedness Inventory (Oldfield, 1971) and all scored between +0.80 and +1.

were assessed prior to the experiment. Student t tests confirmed that verbal and performance IQs significantly differed between dyslexics and chronological age-matched controls, $t(8) = -3.96$, $p < .005$, $t(8) = 3.10$, $p < .02$ respectively; they also differed on reading level, $t(8) = 9.09$, $p < .0001$, but did not differ on chronological age, $p > .1$. Chronological age significantly differed between dyslexic children and reading level-matched controls, $t(8) = 8.71$, $p < .0001$; neither reading level nor verbal and performance IQs significantly differed, $p > .1$.Chronological age as well as reading level and verbal IQ significantly differed between chronological age-matched and reading level-matched controls, $t(8) = 8.92$, $p < .0001$, $t(8) = 10.56$, $p < .0001$, $t(8) = 2.33$, $p < .05$, respectively. Difference was marginally significant for the performance IQ, $t(8) = 2.01$, $p < .08$. Our research was approved by the Regional School Management Office. Profiles are presented in Table 1[3].

Group	N (boys/girls)	Chronological age	Range	Reading level	PIQ	VIQ
Dyslexic children	5 (4/1)	138.0 (5.1)	11;5-12;0	101.4 (6.1)	97.8 (2.9)	95.2 (4.8)
Chronological age-matched controls	5 (3/2)	137.2 (4.3)	10;11-11;10	133.4 (5.0)***	105.8 (5.0)*	107.4 (4.9)**
Reading level-matched controls	5 (5/0)	101.2 (7.9)***	7;7-9;2	102.4 (4.2)	100.0 (4.1)	101.2 (3.3)

Table 1. Chronological and reading level ages, range, verbal and performance IQs for dyslexic children, chronological age-matched, and reading level-matched controls.

5.1.2 Stimuli

Forty stimuli were selected. They were twenty monosyllabic $C_1C_2VC_3$ pseudowords and their disyllabic $C_1uC_2VC_3$ counterparts, which shared their VC_3 rhyme (i.e., /al/) but differed on the structure of their C_1C_2 clusters (Table 2). Onset clusters were unattested in French. I subdivided them into five sonority profiles (SPs) as follows: high-fall (e.g., /ʁbal/), low-fall (e.g., /fkal/), plateau (e.g., /pkal/), low-rise (e.g., /kfal/), and high-rise (e.g., /zʁal/). Onset cluster markedness progresses from high-fall SPs (the most marked, the grammatically worst ill-formed) to high-rise SPs (the least marked, the grammatically most well-formed). Each SP contained four different C_1C_2 clusters, repeated eight times within each SP; overall, there were 4 C_1C_2 x 5 SPs x 8 repetitions x 2 conditions (mono- and disyllabic pseudowords) = 320 stimuli. To exclude some possible phonological biases such as compensation for assimilation or coarticulation, I did not include homorganic consonants (i.e., consonants that share the same place of articulation) and consonants that differ in voicing within C_1C_2 onset clusters. However, C_1 and C_2 could differ in mode of articulation. Disyllabic $C_1uC_2VC_3$ counterparts were recorded by a female native speaker of French. All sounds were digitally recorded with a Sennheiser e865s microphone through a Tascam US-144MK II external audio interface, sampled at a 44 kHz rate, converted with a 16-bit resolution, and bandpass filtered (0 Hz to 5,000 Hz). C_1u first syllable in disyllabic pseudowords systematically carried stress. Monosyllabic $C_1C_2VC_3$ pseudowords were

[3] Note: N: number of participants; chronological and reading level ages are in months; ranges are years, months; standard deviations within parentheses; significant difference with dyslexic children: *** $p < .0001$, ** $p < .005$, * $p < .02$; Reading level as determined by the Alouette test (Lefavrais, 1967); PIQ as measured by Raven's Progressive Matrices for French children (PM 38; Raven, 1998); VIQ as measured by WISC-III for French children (Wechsler, 1996).

obtained by splicing out step-by-step the vowel /u/ with Praat software (Boersma & Weenink, 2011). Visual and auditory inspection of the waveforms minimized the /u/ coarticulation-based traces in the C_1 and C_2. Mean duration was 197.3 ms (*SD* = 16.1) for the C_1C_2 clusters and 79.8 ms (*SD* = 11.2) for the vowel /u/.

Sonority profiles				
high-fall	low-fall	plateau	low-rise	high-rise
/ʁbal/,	/fkal/,	/pkal/,	/bzal/,	/zʁal/,
/ʁzal/,	/ʒgal/,	/tpal/,	/tfal/,	/ʒʁal/,
/lval/,	/mʒal/,	/bdal/,	/dval/,	/gmal/,
/lgal/	/ʃpal/	/vzal/	/kfal/	/dmal/

Table 2. Monosyllabic pseudowords used as a function of sonority profiles.

5.1.3 Procedure

This experiment was designed, compiled and run using E-Prime 2.0 Professional software (Schneider, Eschman, & Zuccolotto, 2002) on Sony X-series laptop computers under Windows 7 OS. Children wore Sennheiser HD 25-1 II headphones (16 Hz-22 kHz range, 70 Ω impedance) and were presented pseudowords binaurally at 70 dB SPL. Trials consisted in the presentation of a vertically-centered exclamation mark (i.e., '+') for 500 ms, followed after a 200-ms blank screen by a pseudoword. A 1,000-ms delay separated two consecutive trials. Children were requested to decide as quickly and as accurately as possible whether the pseudoword had one or two syllables (numpad 1 = one syllable, numpad 2 = two syllables). Children were first trained with a practice list of 16 trials with corrective feedback. No feedback was given for the experimental trials. Trials were randomized. The software automatically recorded response times and response accuracy.

5.2 Results

I report first the results from two 5 x 2 x 3 mixed-design repeated measures ANOVAs with Statistica software by subject (*F*1) and by item (*F*2) on response times and response accuracy (~ 84.1% of the data). ANOVAs were run with Group (dyslexics vs. chronological age-matched controls vs. reading level-matched controls) as between-subject factor and Sonority profile (high-fall vs. low-fall vs. plateau vs. low-rise vs. high-rise) and Syllable structure (monosyllabic vs. disyllabic) as within-subject factors.

The *d'* (Tanner & Swets, 1954) was calculated to assess the discrimination sensitivity threshold. Student *t* tests on the *d'* computed for each group show that the discrimination sensitivity threshold does not differ between dyslexic children (M = 1.94, SD = 0.12), chronological age-matched controls (M = 2.18, SD = 0.18) and reading level-matched controls (M = 1.92, SD = 0.27), $p_s > .1$. No children had a $d' = 0 \pm 5\%$ (i.e., random responses). The β, which estimates the criterion decision, did not differ between children, $ps > .1$. Response times and response accuracy were correlated in dyslexic children, $r = -.68$, $t(4) = -3.30$, $p < .006$, in chronological age-matched controls, $r = -.73$, $t(4) = -4.02$, $p < .001$, and in reading level-matched controls, $r = -.72$, $t(4) = -3.88$, $p < .008$.

The analysis revealed a significant main effect of Group in response times only, $F1(4, 48) = 40.09$, $p < .0001$, $\eta^2_p = 0.62$, $F2\ (4, 310) = 31.21$, $p < .0001$, $\eta^2_p = 0.36$; indicating that dyslexic children (1,759 ms) were systematically slower to respond compared to chronological age-matched controls (1,213 ms) and reading level-matched controls (1,509 ms), $t(8) = 29.11$, $p < .0001$, $t(8) = 13.46$, $p < .001$, respectively.

The Sonority profile x Syllable structure interaction was significant in response times (Fig. 2), $F1(4, 48) = 40.09$, $p < .0001$, $\eta^2_p = 0.62$, $F2\ (4, 310) = 31.21$, $p < .0001$, $\eta^2_p = 0.36$ and response accuracy (Fig. 3), $F1\ (4, 48) = 32.69$, $p < .0001$, $\eta^2_p = 0.73$, $F2(4, 310) = 28.55$, $p < .0001$, $\eta^2_p = 0.29$. Fisher's LSD post-hoc tests (Bonferroni's adjusted α-level for significance, $p < .001$) revealed that responses to more marked onset clusters with high-fall SPs (e.g., /ʁbal/) were slower and less accurate relative to the less marked onset clusters with plateau SPs (e.g., /pkal/), which in turn, were slower and less accurate than high-rise SPs (e.g., /gmal/). Responses to low-fall SPs (e.g., /fkal/) were slower and less accurate than low-rise SPs (e.g., /kfal/). Responses to disyllabic counterparts of grammatically worst ill-formed onset clusters with high-fall SPs (e.g., /ʁubal/) were faster and more accurate relative to disyllabic counterparts of less marked onset clusters with plateau SPs (e.g., /pukal/), which in turn, were faster and more accurate than high-rise SPs (e.g., /gumal/). Responses to low-fall SPs (e.g., /fukal/) were faster and more accurate than low-rise SPs (e.g., /kufal/).

Neither the Group nor the Syllable structure main effects were significant in response accuracy. The three-way Sonority profile x Syllable structure x Group interaction did not significantly interact in response times, $Fs < 1$, $p > .1$ and response accuracy, $Fs < 1$, $p > .1$.

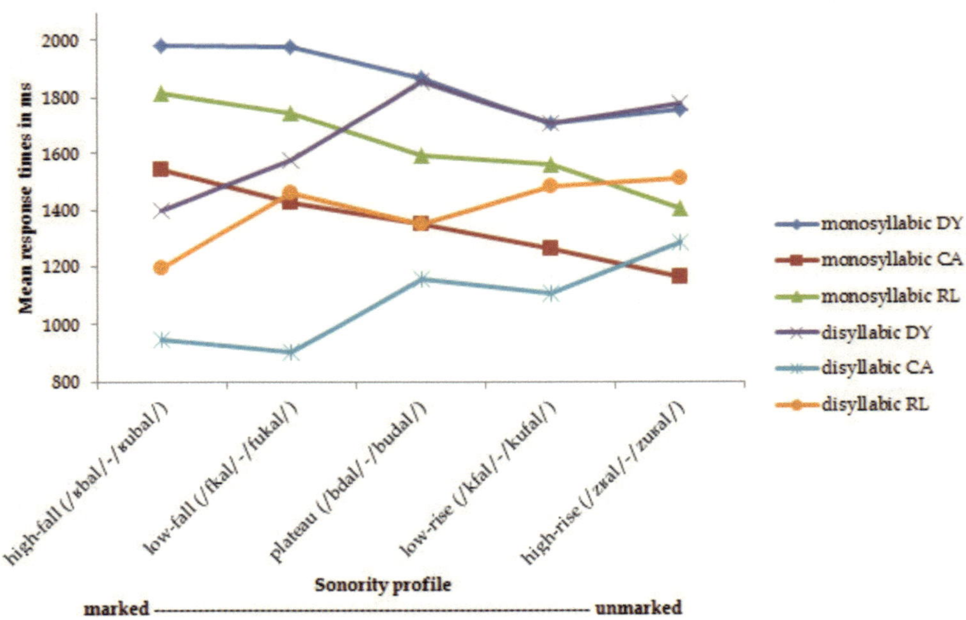

Fig. 2. Mean response times (in ms) to the Sonority profile x Syllable structure interaction for the dyslexic children (DY), chronological age-matched controls (CA) and reading level-matched controls (RL).

To ensure that the perceptual confusion response patterns are not due to coarticulation-based artifacts relative to traces of spliced /u/ from the C_1uC_2 clusters, I examined the nature of the misperception *a posteriori*. Dyslexic children as well as controls were post-tested. Children were asked to report whether or not they heard a vowel, and if so, which one, within monosyllabic pseudowords (n = 160). The task was quite similar, except that for each error, a visual feedback was displayed and children were therefore asked to press on the vowel they thought they heard (i.e., /a/, /i/, /u/, /o/, /e/, /ɛ/, /y/, /ə/, or not a vowel). Response patterns showed that when French dyslexic children misperceived the C_1C_2 clusters, they reported an epenthetic /ə/ ($M = 80.0 \pm 4.4$) more frequently than other vowels ($M = 3.5 \pm 4.7$), $t(4) = 24.69$, p <.0001). Response patterns were similar in chronological age-matched controls ($M = 83.9 \pm 5.5$ vs. $M = 5.8 \pm 2.9$, $t(4) = 18.37$, $p < .0001$) and in reading level-matched controls ($M = 81.7 \pm 6.2$ vs. $M = 2.6 \pm 3.8$, $t(4) = 27.00$, $p < .0001$).

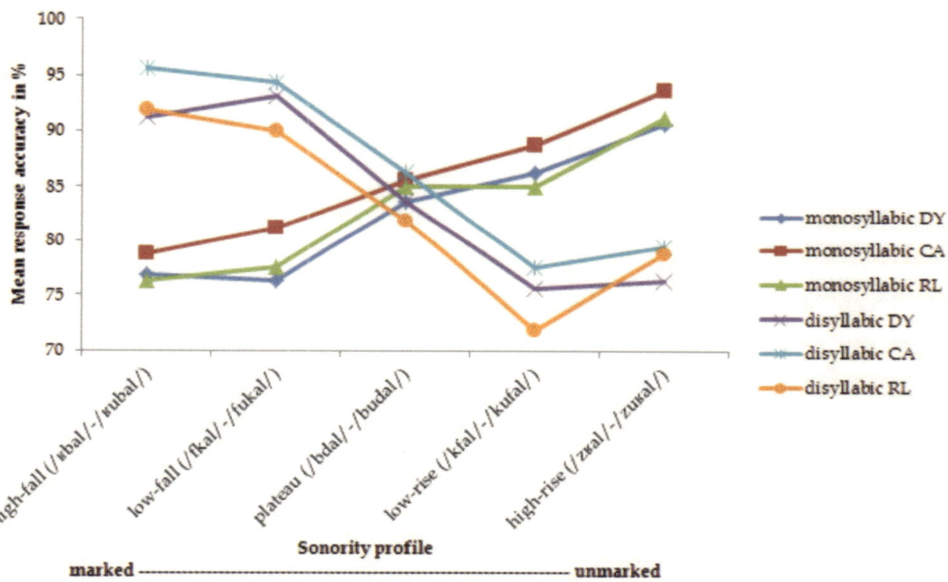

Fig. 3. Mean response accuracy (in %) to the Sonority profile x Syllable structure interaction for the dyslexic children (DY), chronological age-matched controls (CA) and reading level-matched controls (RL).

As in the Berent et al.'s studies (2007; 2008), I submitted children' response accuracy to the C_1C_2 clusters to a linear hierarchically-forced stepwise regression analysis[4]. I first forced in the C_1C_2 cluster length (in ms); then, I forced in the statistical properties of biphones and triphones respectively (I considered C_1VC_2 triphones with a vowel /ə/ that was the most reported epenthetic vowel in children), the bigram frequency (Peereman, Lété, & Sprenger-Charolles, 2007), and the phonotactic transitional probabilities (Crouzet, 2000). The analysis revealed that markedness, which was entered last, accounts for significant unique variance in dyslexic children (Adjusted $R^2 = .276$, $p < .0001$, $\beta = .62$),, chronological age-matched

[4] I used the statistical properties extracted from an oral frequency-based database in French (Gendrot, 2011).

controls (Adjusted $R^2 = .258$, $p < .005$, $\beta = .55$) and reading level-matched controls (Adjusted $R^2 = .394$, $p < .0001$, $\beta = .76$).

6. Discussion

As can be seen throughout this chapter, the dyslexics' phonological deficit has unresolved issues. However, the degraded, under-specified phonological representation hypothesis as a failure in the perception of finely-sharped acoustic-phonetic cues appears to be somehow misleading (e.g., Ramus & Szenkovits, 2008). To solve the intricate problem of the nature of the dyslexics' phonological deficit, I tried to assess whether -and how- the phonological representations are difficult to be accessed, either language-specific or universal, in French dyslexic children compared to chronological age-matched and reading level-matched controls.

The results provide major, innovative responses to a twofold debate: about the nature of the phonological deficit in dyslexics and about the universal phonological knowledge on grammatical restrictions. Crucially, I first observed that the (mis)perception of unattested onset clusters relies on universal sonority-related phonological knowledge on grammatical restrictions. Indeed, response patterns indicate a markedness-modulated misperception of monosyllabic pseudowords as disyllabic ones: as markedness increased from high-rise SP to high-fall SP, perceptual confusion was prone to increase. Also, response patterns were reversed to their disyllabic counterparts: as markedness increased, perceptual confusion decreased. Furthermore, there was no speed-accuracy trade-off: as response accuracy increased, response times decreased.

A posteriori measures confirmed that monosyllabic pseudowords were not perceptually-confused due to coarticulation-based artefacts relative to traces of the spliced vowel /u/: monosyllabic pseudowords are more likely phonologically-repaired with an illusory epenthetic vowel /ə/. Since the vowel /ə/ represents a high-frequency vowel in French, a linear hierarchically-forced stepwise regression analysis discarded a straightforward influence of statistical properties and acoustic-phonetic cues on the misperception and the phonological repair by an illusory epenthetic vowel. Neither the C_1C_2 cluster length, nor the frequency of biphones and triphones explain our results: sonority-related markedness accounts for significant unique variance.

Surprisingly, Group effects were absent; French dyslexic children were as sensitive as both chronological age-matched and reading level-matched controls to the phonological sonority-related markedness of C_1C_2 onset clusters and, as well as controls, they phonologically repaired unattested marked C_1C_2 clusters into attested unmarked ones with an epenthetic /ə/ vowel: this is in accordance with recent results of Maïonchi-Pino, Yokoyama, Takahashi, Écalle, Magnan, & Kawashima (2011) in French adult native speakers (in English, also see Berent et al., 2007; 2008). Of interest, dyslexic children did not differ from both control groups on their response accuracy and discrimination sensitivity threshold (d'); however, response times were slower. This suggests that dyslexic children have normal, intact universal phonological constraints and robust phonological representations of their native language; they are able to efficiently recode grammatical ill-formed sequences (i.e., to do that, children insert an epenthetic vowel /ə/ that tends to restore an attested, grammatical well-formed, phonological sequence) and universal phonological representations to avoid a transgression of grammatical well-formedness of phonological sequence. Thus, the children' misperception of marked onset clusters could be attributed to universal phonologically-constrained preferences that follow sonority-related markedness constraints. Since sonority-related markedness relies on acoustic-phonetic cues that might require efficient abilities to perceive, store and process brief acoustic-phonetic information (e.g., Hayes & Steriade, 2004; for counter-argument on the phonetic basis of sonority, see Clements, 2006), and since dyslexic children are as sensitive as controls to this phonological marker, our results compete to reconsider the degraded, under-specified phonological representation hypothesis to further explore the phonological access deficit hypothesis (e.g., Ramus & Szenkovits, 2008).

7. Conclusion

Dyslexic children therefore have intact universal phonological sonority-related sensitivity and efficient language-dependent abilities to underlie both the (mis)perception of phonotactically-illegal clusters and the phonological repair processes, respectively. Further, acoustic-phonetic cues as well as statistical properties do not exhibit straightforward influence, but I do not discard that both contribute to the markedness-related misperception. Further, in our experiment, it remains unresolved whether Peperkamp's position (2007, p. 634-635) is true: "the role of the grammar in phonological perception is not to repair phonologically illegal structure but rather to undo the effect of native phonological processes, and that perceptual repairs take place at a lower, phonetic, processing level". Although I acknowledge that extensive research is important to refine our results, I point out that, as suggested by Ramus & Szenkovits (2008) or Szenkovits et al. (submitted) dyslexics' phonological deficit accommodates with a deficit in storing and accessing the phonological representations.

8. Acknowledgments

I thank gratefully the head teachers, teachers, speech and language therapists, parents and children who participated in these experiments. I also thank gratefully Pr. Yasuyuki Taki and Dr. Hiroshi Hashizume from the Dept. of Developmental Cognitive Neuroscience (Tohoku University), Drs. Satoru Yokoyama and Kei Takahashi as well as Pr. Ryuta Kawashima from the Dept. of Functional Brain Imaging (Tohoku University), and Prs. Annie Magnan and Jean Écalle from the Laboratoire d'Étude des Mécanismes Cognitifs (Université Lyon 2) for supporting this study. This work was supported by the Japan Society for the Promotion of Science via a 2-year Postdoctoral Fellowship for Foreign Researcher awarded to Norbert Maïonchi-Pino.

9. References

Adlard, A. & Hazan,V. (1998). Speech perception abilities in children with developmental dyslexia. *The Quarterly Journal of Experimental Psychology, 51A,* pp. 153-177.

Ahissar, M. (2007). Dyslexia and the anchoring-deficit hypothesis. *Trends in Cognitive Sciences, 11,* pp. 458-465.

Berent, I.; Lennertz, T.; Jun, J.; Moreno, M., & Smolensky, P. (2008). Language universals in human brains. *Proceedings of the National Academy of Sciences, 105,* pp. 5321-5325.

Berent, I.; Steriade, D.; Lennertz, T., & Vaknin, V. (2007). What we know about what we have never heard: Evidence from perceptual illusions. *Cognition,* 104, pp. 591-630.

Best, C. (1995). A direct realist perspective on cross-language speech perception. In W. Strange & J. J. Jenkins (Eds.), *Speech perception and linguistic experience: Issues in cross-language research* (pp. 171-204). Timonium: York Press.

Blomert, L.; Mitterer, H., & Paffen, C. (2004). In search of the auditory, phonetic, and/or phonoloigcal problems in dyslexia: Context effects in Speech Perception. *Journal of Speech, Language, and Hearing Research, 47,* pp. 1030-1047.

Boada, R. & Pennington, B. (2006). Deficient implicit phonological representations in children with dyslexia. *Journal of Experimental Child Psychology, 95,* pp. 153-193.

Bogliotti, C.; Serniclaes, W. ; Messaoud-Galusi, S., & Sprenger-Charolles, L., (2008). Discrimination of speech sounds by dyslexic children: comparisons with chronological age and reading level controls. *Journal of Experimental Child Psychology, 101,* pp. 137-155

Boersma, P. & Weenink, D. (2011). Praat: Doing phonetics by computer. Version 5.2.15, http://www.praat.org/.

Bonte, M.; Mitterer, H.; Zellagui, N.; Poelmans, H., & Blomert, L. (2005). Auditory cortical tuning to statistical regularities in phonology. *Clinical Neurophysiology, 116,* pp. 2765-2774.

Bonte, M.; Poelmans, H., & Blomert, L. (2007). Deviant neurophysiological responses to phonological regularities in speech in dyslexic children. *Neuropsychologia, 45,* pp. 1427-1437.

Clements, G. (1990). The role of the sonority cycle in core syllabification. In J. Kingston & M. Beckman (Eds.), *Papers in laboratory phonology I: Between the grammar and physics of speech* (pp. 282-333). Cambridge: Cambridge University Press.

Clements, G. (2006). Does sonority have a phonetic basis? In E. Raimy & C. Cairns (Eds.), *Contemporary Views on Architecture and Representations in Phonological Theory*. Cambridge: MIT Press.

Crouzet, O. (2000). Segmentation de la parole en mots et régularités phonotactiques: effets phonologiques, probabilistiques ou lexicaux ? *Unpublished doctoral dissertation,* http://olivier.crouzet.free.fr/reprints/phd/phd.pdf

de Lacy, P. (2007). *The Cambridge Handbook of Phonology*. Cambridge: Cambridge University Press.

Dupoux, E., Kakehi, K., Hirose, Y., Pallier, C., & Mehler, J. (1999). Epenthetic vowels in Japanese: A perceptual illusion? *Journal of Experimental Psychology: Human Perception and Performance, 25,* pp. 1568-1578.

Dupoux, E., Parlato, E., Frota, S., Hirose, Y., & Peperkamp, S. (2011). Where do illusory vowels come from? *Journal of Memory and Language, 64,* pp. 199-210.

Elbro, C. & Jensen, M. (2005). Quality of phonological representations, word learning, and phoneme awareness in dyslexic and normal readers. *Scandinavian Journal of Psychology, 46,* pp. 375-384.

Gendrot, C. (2011). Fréquence phonemes, diphones, triphones. Version 1.00, http://www.lexique.org/public/freq_phonemes_diphones_triphones.php.

Hallé, P.; Seguí, J.; Frauenfelder, U., & Meunier, C. (1998). Processing of illegal consonant clusters: A case of perceptual assimilation? *Journal of Experimental Psychology: Human Perception and Performance, 24,* pp. 592-608.

Hayes, B. & Steriade, D. (2004). A review of perceptual cues and cue robustness. In D. Steriade (Ed.), *Phonetically based phonology* (pp. 1-33). Cambridge: Cambridge University Press.

Hoonhorst, I.; Colin, C.; Markessis, E.; Radeau, M.; Deltenre, P., & Serniclaes, W. (2009). French native speakers in the making: From language-general to language-specific voicing boundaries. *Journal of Experimental Child Psychology, 104,* pp. 353–366.

Jusczyk, P.; Friederici, A.; Wessels, J.; Svenkerud, V., & Jusczyk, A. (1993). Infants' sensitivity to the sound pattern of native language words. *Journal of Memory and Language, 32,* pp. 402-420.

Kuhl, P.; Andrusko, J.; Chistovich, I.; Chistovich, L.; Kozhevnikova, E.; Ryskina, N.; Stolyarova, E.; Sundberg, U., & Lacerda, F. (1997). Crosslanguage analysis of phonetic units in language addressed to infants. *Science, 277,* pp.684-686.

Ladefoged, P. (1975). *A course in phonetics.* New York: Harcourt, Brace, Jovanovich.

Lefavrais, P. (1967). *Test de l'Alouette. [Alouette test].* Paris: ECPA.

Lyon, G.; Shaywitz, S. & Shaywitz, B. (2003). Defining dyslexia, comorbidity, teacher's knowledge of language and reading. *Annals of Dyslexia,* 53, pp. 1-14.

Maïonchi-Pino, N.; Takahashi, K.; Yokoyama, S.; Écalle, J.; Magnan, A; & Kawashima, R. (2011). Is phonological knowledge on linguistic restrictions universal? A French-Japanese cross-linguistic approach. Poster presented at the XVIIth ESCOP conference, San Sebastian, Spain, September 29th - October 2nd.

Marshall, C.; Ramus, F., & van der Lely, H. (in press). Do children with SLI and/or dyslexia compensate for place assimilation? Insight into phonological grammar and representations. *Cognitive Neuropsychology.*

Mody, M.; Studdert-Kennedy, M., & Brady, S. (1997). Speech perception deficits in poor readers: auditory processing or phonological coding? *Journal of Experimental Child Psychology, 64,* pp. 199-231.

Nittrouer, S. (1999). Do temporal processing deficits cause phonological problems? *Journal of Speech, Language, and Hearing Sciences, 42,* pp. 925–942.

Oldfield, R. (1971). The assessment and analysis of handedness: The Edinburgh inventory. *Neuropsychologia, 9,* 97-113.

Peereman, R., Lété, B., & Sprenger-Charolles, L. (2007). Manulex-Infra: Distributional characteristics of grapheme-phoneme mappings, infra-lexical and lexical units in child-directed written material. *Behavior Research Methods, Instruments, & Computers, 39,* 579–589.

Peperkamp, S. (2007). Do we have innate knowledge about phonological markedness? Comments on Berent, Steriade, Lennertz, and Vaknin. *Cognition, 104,* pp. 631-637.

Prince, A. & Smolensky, P. (1993). *Optimality Theory: Constraint Interaction in Generative Grammar.* Rutgers University Center for Cognitive Science, Technical Report 2.

Prince, A. & Smolensky, P. (1997). Optimality: From neural networks to universal grammar. *Science, 275,* pp. 1604-1610.

Prince, A. & Smolensky, P. (2004). *Optimality Theory: Constraint interaction in generative grammar.* Malden: Blackwell Publishers.

Ramus, F. (2001). Outstanding questions about phonological processing in dyslexia. *Dyslexia, 7,* pp. 197-216.

Ramus, F.; Rosen, S.; Dakin, S.; Day, B.; Castellote, J.; White, S., & Frith, U. (2003). Theories of developmental dyslexia: insights from a multiple case study of dyslexic adults. *Brain, 126,* pp. 841-865.

Ramus, F. & Szenkovits, G. (2008). What phonological deficit? *Quarterly Journal of Experimental Psychology, 61,* pp. 129-141.

Raven, J. (1998). *Progressive Matrices Couleurs (PM 38), Progressive Matrices Standard (PM 47), étalonnage français. [Raven's Colored Progressive Matrices (PM 38), Standard Progressive Matrices (PM 47), French standardization].* Paris: ECPA.

Saffran J.; Werker, J., & Werner, L. (2006). The infant's auditory world: Hearing, speech, and the beginning of language. In R. Siegler & D. Kuhn (Eds.), *Handbook of child development* (pp. 58-108). New York: Wiley.

Schneider, W.; Eschman, A., & Zuccolotto, A. (2002). *E-Prime user's guide.* Pittsburgh: Psychology Software Tools, Inc.

Selkirk, E. (1984). On the major class features and syllable theory. In M. Arnolf & R. Octyle (Eds.), *Language and sound structure* (pp. 107-136). Cambridge: MIT Press.

Serniclaes, W.; Sprenger-Charolles, L.; Carré, R., & Démonet, J.-F. (2001). Perceptual categorization of speech sounds in dyslexics. *Journal of Speech, Language, and Hearing Research, 44,* pp. 384-399.

Serniclaes, W.; Van Heghe, S.; Mousty, P.; Carré, R., & Sprenger-Charolles, L. (2004). Allophonic mode of speech perception in dyslexia. *Journal of Experimental Child Psychology, 87,* pp. 336-361.

Shaywitz, S. & Shaywitz, B. (2005). Dyslexia (Specific Reading Disability). *Biological Psychiatry, 57,* pp. 1301-1309.

Snowling, M. (2001). From language to reading and dyslexia. *Dyslexia, 7,* pp. 37-46.

Sprenger-Charolles, L.; Colé, P.; Lacert, P., & Serniclaes, W. (2000). On subtypes of developmental dyslexia: evidence from processing time and accuracy scores. *Canadian Journal of Experimental Psychology, 54,* pp. 88-104.

Szenkovits, G.; Darma, Q.; Darcy, I., & Ramus, F. (submitted). Exploring dyslexics' phonological deficit II: Phonological grammar.

Szenkovits, G. & Ramus, F. (2005). Exploring dyslexics' phonological deficit I: Lexical vs. sub-lexical and input vs. output processes. *Dyslexia, 11,* 253-268.

Tanner, W. & Swets, J. (1954). A decision-making theory of visual detection. *Psychological Review, 61,* pp. 401-409.

Vellutino, F.; Fletcher, J.; Snowling, M., & Scanlon, D. (2004). Specific reading disability (dyslexia): What have we learned in the past four decades? *Journal of Child Psychology and Psychiatry, 45,* pp. 2-40.

Veuillet, E.; Magnan, A.; Écalle, J. ; Thai-Van, H., & Collet, L. (2007). Auditory processing disorder in children with reading disabilities: effect of audiovisual training. *Brain, 130,* pp. 2915-2928.

Wechsler, D. (1996). *Manuel du WISC-III. [Manual of the WISC-III].* Paris: ECPA.

Werker, J. & Tees, R. (1984). Cross-language speech perception: evidence for perceptual reorganization during the first year of life. *Infant Behavior and Development, 7,* pp. 49–63.

Wright, R. (2004). A review of perceptual cues and robustness. In D. Steriade, R. Kirchner, & B. Hayes (Eds.), *Phonetically based phonology* (pp. 34-57). Cambridge: Cambridge University Press.

Ziegler, J. & Goswami, U. (2005). Reading acquisition, developmental dyslexia, and skilled reading across languages: A psycholinguistic grain size theory. *Psychological Bulletin, 131,* pp. 3-29.

Ziegler, J.; Castel, C.; Pech-Georgel, C.; George, F.; Alario, F.-X., & Perry, C. (2008). Developmental dyslexia and the dual route model of reading: Simulating individual differences and subtypes. *Cognition, 107,* pp. 151–178.

5

Antisaccades in Dyslexic Children: Evidence for Immaturity of Oculomotor Cortical Structures

Maria Pia Bucci[1], Naziha Nassibi[1], Christophe-Loic Gerard[2], Emmanuel Bui-Quoc[3] and Magali Seassau[4]
[1]*Laboratoire de Psychologie et Neuropsychologie Cognitives, FRE 3292 CNRS - Université Paris Descartes, Paris,*
[2]*Service de Psychopathologie de l'enfant et de l'adolescent. Hôpital Robert Debré, Paris,*
[3]*Service OPH, Hôpital Robert Debré, Paris,*
[4]*e(ye)BRAIN, Ivry-sur-Seine,*
France

1. Introduction

The antisaccade task has been introduced for the first time by Hallet (1978) in order to explore the ability of the brain to control behaviour flexibly. Antisaccades are voluntary saccades during which subjects have to inhibit the movement towards a peripheral visual target. Usually subjects fixate a central fixation point, which is then extinguished and the peripheral target is presented. Subjects are instructed to generate a saccade of the same amplitude to the opposite direction, as quickly and accurately as possible. It is generally assumed that the sudden appearance of the target in an antisaccade task automatically triggers a motor program for a prosaccade in this direction, and that errors occur when certain endogenous processes fail to inhibit or cancel this program (Everling & Fischer, 1998). It is argued that correct antisaccade latencies are increased compared to prosaccade latencies because the application of the inhibitory processes is time consuming (Olk & Kingstone, 2003). Everling and Fischer (1998) argued that antisaccade performance requires two intact subprocesses: 1) the ability to suppress a reflexive saccade towards the target; 2) the ability to generate a voluntary saccade in the opposite direction. In clinical research, increased antisaccade error rates are often interpreted as reflecting failures in inhibitory processing (Crawford, Bennett, Lekwuwa, Shaunak, & Deakin, 2002; Hutton et al., 2008).

Neuropsychological studies have shown an important role of the frontal cortices during performing antisaccades. For instance, Everling and Munoz (2000), and Funahashi et al. (1993) revealed that several frontal structures (frontal eye field, dorsolateral cortex and supplementary eye field) are more activated during antisaccade tasks than during prosaccades (a saccade made towards the peripheral target). Furthermore, Matsuda et al. (2004) reported increased activity in the inferior parietal cortex during antisaccade tasks compared to prosaccades. Interestingly, Ettinger et al. (2008) showed activity in such area during a period preceeding the antisaccade generation, suggesting an inhibitory role of this region. Other studies found out that the parietal cortex (some regions in the intraparietal sulcus) is responsible for the vector inversion required to generate an antisaccade to the correct location (Clementz et al., 2007; Zhang & Barash, 2000).

Several researchers have focused on the development of the ability to perform antisaccades. For example, as suggested in Luna's exhaustive review (Luna et al., 2008) exhaustive review, the maturity of the cortical structures devoted to eye movement performances is reached at 14-15 years. Consequently, the improvements in antisaccade performance continue during adolescence even though the ability to successfully inhibit a saccade toward a new target is already present at 8 years old (Johnson, 1995).

Moreover, the antisaccade task has also been used as important clinical tool for investigating dysfunction in various neurological and psychiatric disorders (Leigh and Kennard, 2004). Patients with discrete lesions of the dorsolateral cortex and in the frontal eye field have difficulty in performing correctly the antisaccade task (Guitton et al., 1985; Walker et al., 1998; Gaymard et al., 1999; Davidson et al., 1999).

The antisaccade task has been extensively studied in dyslexic children by the Fischer's group. Indeed, Biscaldi et al. (2000) and Fischer & Hartnegg (2000a) compared the performance in an antisaccade task between dyslexic children and non-dyslexic children of similar age. These authors reported an increased number of directional errors and several saccades being missed in dyslexic children. Furthermore, Fischer and Hartnegg (2000b) showed that this poorer performance in dyslexic children could be improved by training, leading to obtain a performance similar to that reported in non-dyslexic children. Therefore, although some evidence exists suggesting impaired inhibitory processing in dyslexic children, such a deficit can be overcome by training.

Based on all these findings we aimed to explore whether the poor antisaccade performance reported in dyslexic children could be a consequence of immaturity of cortical structures responsible of triggering and execution of saccadic eye movements rather than a congenital deficit of these areas. Indeed, the fact that dyslexic children are able to improve antisaccade performance with training as shown by Fischer and Hartnegg (2000b) is in line with the hypothesis of a delayed maturation of the oculomotor system in such type of subjects (Bucci et al., 2008).

In the present study we compared antisaccade performance in three different groups of children: (i) dyslexic children; (ii) age-matched non-dyslexic children; (iii) reading age-matched non-dyslexic children.

2. Materials and methods

2.1 Participants

Twenty-one dyslexic children were recruited from the pediatric hospital where they were referred for a complete evaluation of their dyslexia state with an extensive examination including neurological/psychological and phonological capabilities. For each child the time required to read a text, its comprehension, and the capacity of reading word/pseudowords was evaluated by using the L2MA battery (Chevrie-Muller et al., 1997). This is a standard test developed by the Applied Psychology Centre of Paris (Centre de Psychologie Appliquée de Paris), and is used everywhere in France. Inclusion criteria for dyslexic were: scores on this test below 2 standard deviations of normalized values; and a normal mean intelligence quotient, between 85 and 115 (IQ, evaluated with WISC IV). The mean age of the dyslexic children was 11.19 ± 0.2 years, the mean IQ was 100 ± 6 and the mean reading age was 8 ± 1 years. A carefully selected age-matched (29 children, mean age 11.6 ± 0.17) and reading age-matched (24 children, mean age 7.8 ± 0.19) groups of non-dyslexic children were selected. These children had to satisfy the following criteria: no known neurological or psychiatric abnormalities, no history of reading difficulty, no visual impairment or difficulty with near vision. For the two groups of non-dyslexic children reading capabilities were in normal range. Both the similitude test of the WISC IV assessing the verbal capability, and the matrix test of the WISC IV assessing the logic capability were performed. Normal range for both tests is 10 ± 3 (Wechsler intelligence scale for children—fourth edition, 2004). The selected reading age-matched group was normal for verbal (11.78 ± 0.8) and for logic (9.97 ± 0.6) capabilities. The selected age-matched group was also normal (10.36 ± 0.4 for verbal and 11.89 ± 0.5 for logic).

Both non-dyslexic and dyslexic children underwent an ophthalmologic and orthoptic examination in order to evaluate their visual function (median values shown in Table 1). All children had normal binocular vision (60 sec of arc or better), which was evaluated with the TNO random dot test. Visual acuity was normal (≥20/20) for all children, dyslexic as well as non dyslexic. The near point of convergence was normal for all three groups of children tested (≤ 5 cm). Moreover, an orthoptic evaluation of vergence fusion capability using prisms and Maddox rod was carried out at far and at near distance. At far distance, the divergence and convergence amplitudes were similar in the three groups of children examined. In contrast, at near distance, the divergence and convergence amplitudes were significantly different in the dyslexic group with respect to the other two groups of non dyslexic children. ANOVA showed significant main effects of group, $F_{(2,71)} = 6.36$, $p < 0.003$ and of the divergence and convergence amplitudes, $F_{(2,71)} = 3.18$, $p < 0.04$., respectively). The LSD test showed that the dyslexic group had significantly smaller value of divergence and convergence amplitudes with respect to the two groups of non-dyslexic children (younger and older).

Finally, phoria (i.e. latent deviation of one eye when the other eye is covered, using the cover-uncover test) was normal for all three groups of children tested.

	TNO	NPC	Phoria Far	Phoria Near	Div Far	Div Near	Conv Far	Conv Near
D 10-13	63	3	0	Exo 1	4	10	15	32
ND 7-9	45	2	0	Exo 2	4	14*	16	40*
ND 10-13	40	2	0	Exo 2	6	13*	17	40*

Note: dyslexic children, D 10-13; non-dyslexic children chronological age matched, ND 10-13; and non-dyslexic children reading age matched, ND 7-9. Median values of: binocular vision (Stereoacuity test, TNO measured in seconds of arc); near point of convergence, NPC measured in cm; Heterophoria at far and near distance, measured in prism diopters; Exo = exophoria; Vergence fusional amplitudes (divergence and convergence) at far and at near distance, measured in prism diopters. Asterisks indicate that value is significantly different with respect to the group of dyslexic children ($p<0.01$).

Table 1. Clinical characteristic of the three groups of children examined

The investigation adhered to the principles of the Declaration of Helsinki and was approved by our Institutional Human Experimentation Committee. Informed consent was obtained from the children's parents after explaining the procedure for the experiment to them.

2.2 Oculomotor paradigm

Stimuli were presented on a PC screen of 22", its resolution was 1920×1080 and the refresh rate was 60 Hz. The stimulus consisted in a red filled circle subtending a visual angle of 0.5 deg. The trial consisted of a target positioned at the center of the screen for a variable delay between 2000 and 3500 ms. The central target disappeared and after a period of 200 ms (= gap period), a lateral target (green filled circle) appeared at 22.8 degrees, randomly to the left or to the right of the center, and stayed on for 1000 ms. After this duration, the central fixation target appeared again, signalling the beginning of the next trial as shown in Figure 1. The lateral target appeared randomly to the left or right and each direction was presented an equal number of times (i.e., 15 each). Children were instructed to look at the central fixation point, then to trigger a saccade as soon as possible in the opposite direction and symmetrically to the lateral target. Thus, when the target moved to the right, the child had to look at the same distance to the left side. When the target returned to the center, the child was instructed to follow it back to the center. An initial training block of trials was given to ensure that the instructions were understood.

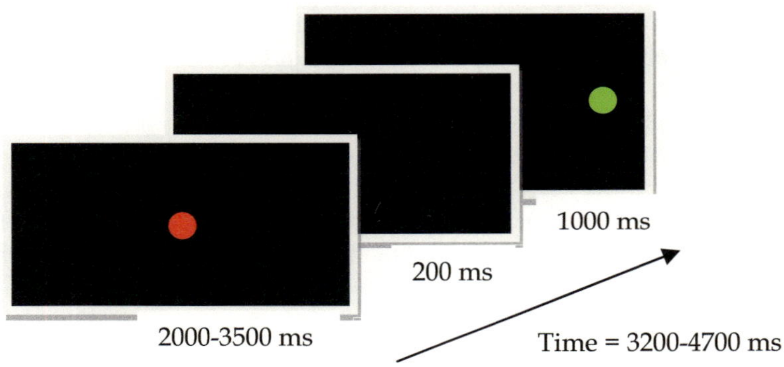

Note: When the green target appears, the child has to make a saccade to it mirror position as quickly as possible. The duration of each trial was between 3200 and 4700 ms.

Fig. 1. Schematic trial of the antisaccade task.

2.3 Eye movements recording

Eye movements were recorded with the Mobile Eyebrain Tracker (Mobile EBT®, e(ye)BRAIN, www.eye-brain.com), an eye-tracking device CE marked for medical purpose (see Figure 2). The Mobile EBT® benefits from cameras that capture the movements of each eye independently. Recording frequency was set up to 300 Hz.

2.4 Procedure

Children were seated in a chair in a dark room with the head leaning on a forehead and chin support; viewing was binocular; the viewing distance was 58 cm. Calibration was carried out at the beginning of eye movements recordings. During the calibration procedure, children were asked to fixate a grid of 13 points (diameter 0.5 deg) mapping the screen. Each calibration point required a fixation of 250 ms to be validated. A polynomial function with five parameters was used to fit the calibration data and to determine the visual angles. After the calibration procedure, the antisaccade task was presented to the child. Duration of the task was kept short (lasting a couple of minutes) allowing an accurate evaluation of eye movement recordings.

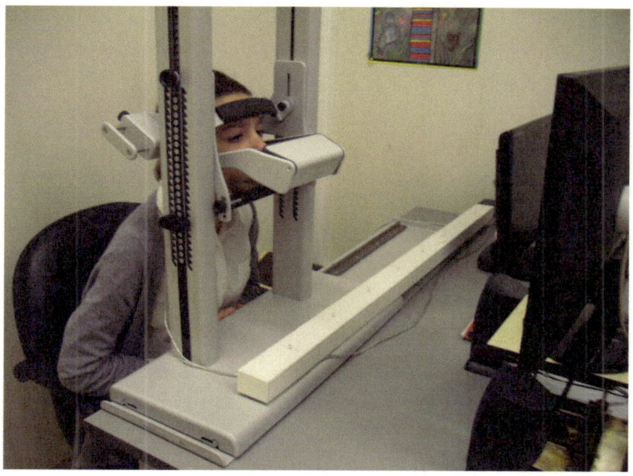

Fig. 2. Mobile Eyebrain Tracker (Mobile EBT®) used to record eye movements from both eyes in children.

2.5 Data analysis

The software MeyeAnalysis (provided with the eye tracker) was used to extract saccadic eye movements from the data. It determines automatically the onset and the end of each saccade. All detected saccades were verified afterwards by the investigator and corrected/discarded if necessary.

The latency and the gain (saccade amplitude/mirror target amplitude) of correct responses and of wrong responses, as well as the percentage of correct antisaccade responses were analyzed in the three different groups of children. Saccades with latencies inferior to 100 ms were counted but not included in the analysis.

Statistical analysis was performed by a three-way ANOVAs using the three groups of children (dyslexics and non-dyslexics, chronological and reading-age matched) as inter-subject factor.

3. Results

The ANOVA showed a main effect of age ($F_{(2,71)}=130.9$, $p<0.001$). Post hoc comparisons showed that reading age matched non-dyslexic children (ND 7-9) were significantly younger than the two other groups ($p<0.001$). There was no age difference between the group of dyslexic children (D 10-13) and the group of chronological age-matched non dyslexic children (ND 10-13) ($p=0.22$).

Figure 3 shows the mean latency of antisaccades for each group of children examined (dyslexic children 10-13 years (D 10-13), non dyslexic children, 7-9 (ND 7-9), and 10-13 years old (ND 10-13) respectively).

The mean latency value for correct antisaccades was 337 ± 14.7 ms for the group of dyslexic children and 353 ± 14.0 ms and 282 ± 12.5 ms for the group of younger and older non dyslexic children respectively.

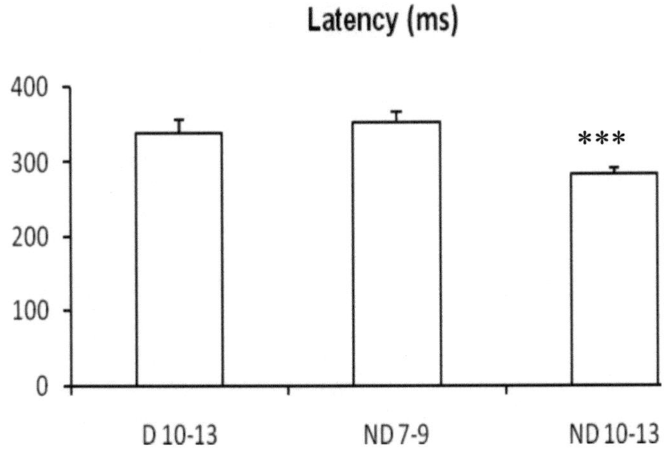

Note: Vertical lines indicate standard error. *** = p<0.01.

Fig. 3. Mean latency of antisaccades for dyslexic children 10-13 years old (D 10-13) and non dyslexic children 7-9 years old (ND 7-9) and 10-13 years old (ND 10-13), respectively.

The ANOVA showed a significant main effect of group, $F_{(2,71)} = 8.18$, $p<0.0006$ on the latency of antisaccades. Post hoc comparison showed that the latency of antisaccades of the older group of non-dyslexic children was significant shorter with respect to the group of dyslexic children ($p<0.01$) and to the younger group of non dyslexics ($p<0.0001$). The latency of dyslexics was similar to that of non-dyslexic reading age matched children (ND 7-9) ($p=0.73$).

The mean latency value measured for saccades in the wrong direction (prosaccades towards the target) is showed in Figure 4. The mean value was 196 ± 10.2 ms for the group of dyslexic children and 182 ± 9.5 ms and 175 ± 8.8 ms for the group of younger and older non dyslexic children. The ANOVA showed no significant main effect of group ($F_{(2,71)} = 1.18$, $p=0.31$).

For each group of children tested we counted also the frequency of anticipatory saccades (latency < 100 ms). The ANOVA did not show group effect ($F_{(2,71)}=1.60$, $p=0.20$). Dyslexic children (D 10-13) made 5.7 ± 1.4 % of anticipatory saccades; while reading age matched (ND 7-9) and chronological age matched non-dyslexic children (ND 10-13) made 3.8 ± 1.3 and 2.4 ± 1.2 % of anticipatory saccades, respectively.

In Figure 5 the gain of correct and wrong antisaccade trials are shown for the different groups of children. The ANOVA revealed that a main effect of group was approaching significant for the gain of the antisaccades ($F_{(2,71)} = 2.97$, $p<0.057$) but this was not significant for the wrong prosaccades ($F_{(2,86)} = 0.72$, $p=0.48$).

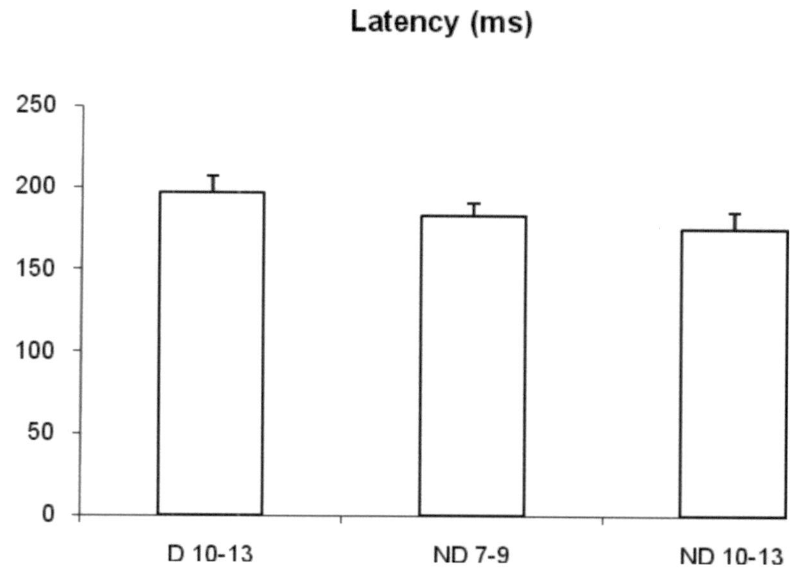

Note: Vertical lines indicate standard error.

Fig. 4. Mean latency of wrong prosaccades (towards the target) for dyslexic children 10-13 years old (D 10-13) and non dyslexic children 7-9 years (ND 7-9) and 10-13 years old (ND 10-13).

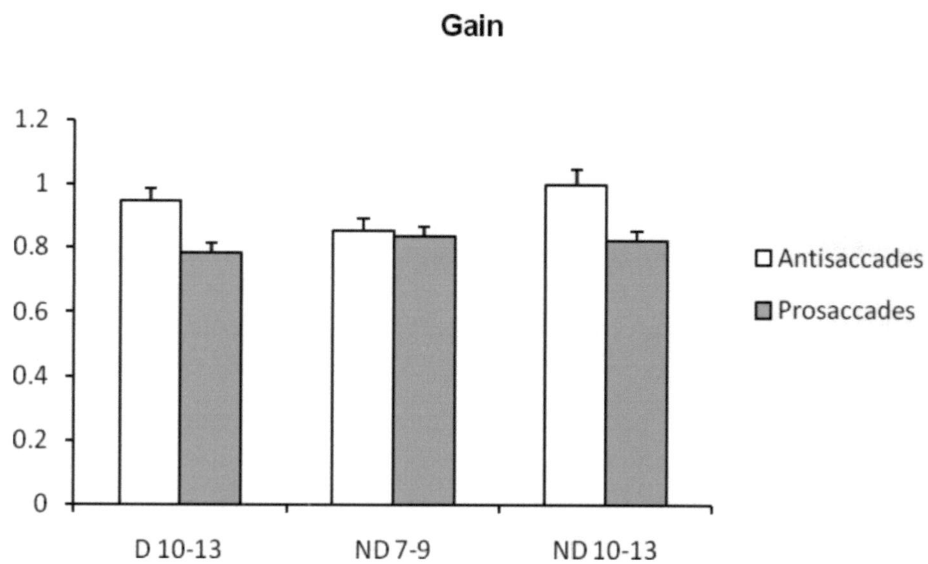

Note: Vertical lines indicate standard error.

Fig. 5. Gain (amplitude of eye movements/amplitude of the attended position target) for antisaccades and wrong prosaccades for dyslexic children 10-13 years old (D 10-13) and non dyslexic children (younger and older, 7-9 (ND 7-9) and 10-13 years old (ND 10-13), respectively).

The mean error rate was also examined (see Figure 6). The mean error rate was 50.8 ± 4.4 % for the group of dyslexic children and 63.3 ± 4.2 % and 30.3 ± 3.8% respectively for the group of younger and older non dyslexic children.

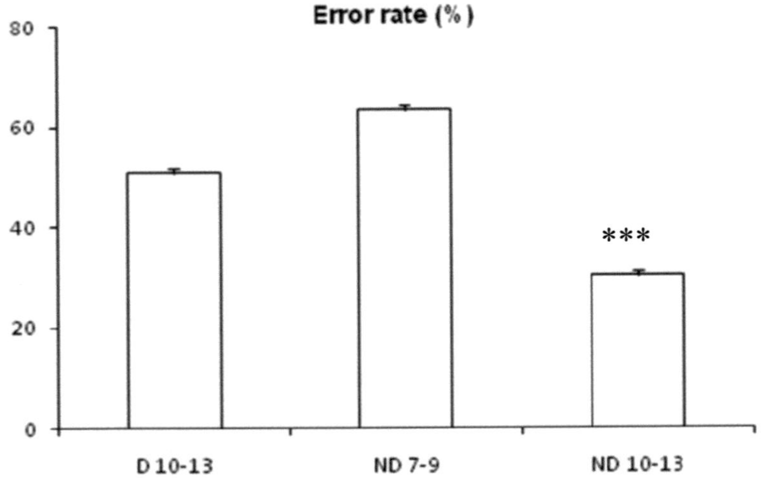

Note: Vertical lines indicate standard error. *** = p<.0003.

Fig. 6. Mean error rate in antisaccades for dyslexic children 10-13 years old (D 10-13) and non dyslexic children (younger and older, 7-9 (ND 7-9) and 10-13 years old (ND 10-13), respectively).

The ANOVA on error rate showed a significant main effect of group, $F_{(2,86)} = 17.88$, $p<0.0001$. Post hoc comparison showed that the error rate for the older group of non-dyslexic children was significantly lower with respect to the other groups of children: $p<0.003$ for the dyslexics and $p<0.0001$ for the younger non dyslexic children. There was no difference between the non-dyslexic younger group and the dyslexic group ($p=0.10$).

4. Discussion

The present study showed first that dyslexic children performed the antisaccade task differently to chronological age matched non-dyslexic children: the latency values of correct antisaccades were longer; furthermore the error rate for dyslexic children was significantly higher compared to that of non dyslexic children of similar age. Secondly, this study showed that in non-dyslexic children the performance in the antisaccade task improved with age.

Both results lend support to the previous studies conducted by Fischer's group with dyslexic children (Biscaldi et al., 2000; Fischer & Hartnegg, 2000a) and also other studies with normal children conducted by Fukushima et al. (2000) and by Irving et al. (2009). Note also that in this study the mean latency values of wrong prosaccades were similar in all three groups of children tested. This finding is only apparently in contrast with developmental evidences showing that latency of saccades is age dependent (see Leigh & Zee, 2006 for review). Indeed, in all developmental studies exploring latency of saccades, children had to saccades as quickly as possible to the target (by making a prosaccade) and it is well known, particularly in the case of children, that latency value depends on the subject's attention and motivation (Clark, 1999). In the present study child had to perform an antisaccade task and the latency here reported for prosaccades is due to a wrong response. Note that a similar finding has been also reported from the study of Munoz et al. (1998).

The new important finding of the present study comes from the comparison between dyslexic children with reading age matched non-dyslexic children. Indeed, the oculomotor behavior of the group of dyslexic children 10-13 years old was similar to that observed in the group of reading age matched non-dyslexic children (7-9 years old). Both the latency values of correct antisaccades and the error rate in the antisaccade task of dyslexic children 10-13 years old were similar to those found in reading age matched non dyslexic children (7-9 years old).

During saccade latency, it is assumed that several processes occur such as the shift of the visual attention to the new stimulus, the disengagement of oculomotor fixation, and the computation of the new parameters (Fischer & Ramsperger, 1984; Findlay & Walker, 1999). These processes involve different cortical and sub-cortical areas (see Leigh & Zee, 2006 for a full review). The longer saccade latency has frequently been attributed to an underdeveloped related cortex, and some investigations have also suggested that increased latency of saccades is related to difficulty in controlling visual fixation (Munoz et al., 1998).

To perform an antisaccade it is necessary to first inhibit the reflexive response towards the stimulus, and then to prepare a voluntary saccade in the opposite direction (antisaccade). Klein (2001), and Klein and Foerster (2001) reported that the capability to inhibit this type of saccade as well as the circuitry controlling cognitive processes is present as early as at 6 years old. They suggested that what is immature in young children is the capability to use such cognitive facilities, leading to a partially correct antisaccade response but to an overall impaired general performance for this task.

Malone and Iacono (2002) hypothesized that although young children have adequate working memory capability to perform correctly on the antisaccade task, they might not be capable of maintaining these instructions continuously throughout the course of the experiment. This may explain why young children in the current study showed long latencies and a high error rate in the antisaccade task.

On the other hand, it is also well known that the parietal cortex, the frontal eye field, the supplementary eye fields and the prefrontal cortex play important roles in antisaccade performance (Luna et al., 2008; McDowell et al., 2008). Further, the inferior parietal cortex has been suggested to be important for the inhibitory period preceding an antisaccade movement (Ettinger et al., 2008) and regions in the intraparietal sulcus (within parietal cortex) could be responsible for generating a correct antisaccade response (Clementz et al., 2007; Nyffeler et al., 2007).

Based on all the available evidences, we postulate the hypothesis that in dyslexic children the delayed maturation of all these structures could lead to longer latencies and increased error rate in the antisaccade task, similar to those reported in reading age matched non-dyslexic children.

Furthermore, it should be noted that the limited fusional amplitude in divergence and convergence capabilities reported in dyslexic children with respect to the two groups of non dyslexic children found with the orthoptic tests is also in favour of a general immaturity of the cortical structures controlling the oculomotor system. Indeed, fusional vergence capabilities are age dependent (Scheiman et al., 1989; von Norrden and Campos, 2006) and at the cortical level some studies showed evidence of vergence control. For instance, the study of Gamlin & Yoon (2000) identified an area close to frontal eye field containing cells that discharge before and during vergence movements. More recently, Quinlan and Culham (2007) with an fMRI study showed an activation of parietal and occipital cortex while humans performed convergence. Thus, in the light of the existing physiological evidence for cortical control of vergence both in monkeys and in humans, the results of the clinical tests presented here in dyslexics suggest immaturity of the neuro-physiological circuitry responsible for generating vergence movements that are closer to the structures for generating saccades.

Finally, it should be noted that orthoptic training is widely used by clinicians for improving vergence capabilities (e.g., von Noorden & Campos, 2006). van Leeuven et al. (1999) and Bucci et al. (2004) reported objective studies on eye movements recordings in children, showing an improvement of vergence eye movements performance after orthoptic training. Consequently, orthoptic training could be applied also for dyslexic population.

5. Conclusion and future directions

The deficits in oculomotor behavior reported in dyslexic children seem to be due to the immaturity of their adaptive mechanism. We believe that visual attentional training along with oculomotor training could help dyslexic children to override such deficiencies allowing an appropriate control of the triggering and execution of saccadic eye movements. We hope to develop new training techniques resulting from this principle to help dyslexic children.

6. Acknowledgments

We thank the medical doctor and nurses of "Service de Psychopathologie de l'enfant et de l'adolescent", Robert Debré Hospital (Paris, France), Eliane Delouvrier, Camille de Solages, teachers, parents and children for their participation.

7. References

Biscaldi M, Fischer B & Hartnegg K. (2000). Voluntary saccadic control in dyslexia. Perception, 29, 509–521.

Bucci MP, Kapoula Z, Yang Q, Bremond-Gignac D & Wiener-Vacher S. (2004). Speed-accuracy of saccades, vergence and combined movements in children with vertigo. Exp. Brain Res. 157 (3), 286-295.

Bucci MP, Kapoula Z & Brémond-Gignac D. Poor binocular coordination of saccades in dyslexic children. *Graefe's Archive for Clinical and Experimental Ophthalmology* 246(3): 417-428, 2008.

Chevrie-Muller C, Simon AM & Fournier S. (1997). Batterie Langage oral écrit. Mémoire. Attention (L2MA) Paris, Editions du Centre de Psychologie appliquée.

Clark JJ. (1999). Spatial attention and latencies of saccadic eye movements. Vision Res. 39, 585–602.

Clementz BA, Brahmbhatt S B, McDowell J E, Brown R & Sweeney J A. (2007). When does the brain inform the eyes whether and where to move? An EEG study in humans. Cerebral Cortex, 17(11), 2634–2643.

Crawford TJ, Bennett D, Lekwuwa G, Shaunak S & Deakin J F W. (2002). Cognition and the inhibitory control of saccades in schizophrenia and Parkinson's disease. Progress in Brain Research 140, 449-466.

Davidson, M. C., Everling, S. L. A. & Munoz, D. P. (1999). Comparison of pro- and anti-saccades in primates. III. Reversible activation/inactivation of frontal eye field and superior colliculus. Soc. Neurosci. Abstr. 25, 147.9.

Everling S & Fischer B. (1998). The antisaccade: a review of basic research and clinical studies. Neuropsychologia, *36*(9), 885-899.

Everling S & Munoz DP. (2000). Neuronal correlates for preparatory set associated with pro-saccades and anti-saccades in the primate frontal eye field. Journal of Neuroscience, 20(1), 387–400.

Ettinger U, Ffytche D H, Kumari V, Kathmann N, Reuter B, Zelaya F, et al. (2008). Decomposing the neural correlates of anti-saccade eye movements using event-related FMRI. Cerebral Cortex, 18(5), 1148–1159.

Findlay JM, Walker R. (1999). A model of saccade generation based on parallel processing and competitive inhibition. Behav Brain Sci 22, 661-674.

Fischer B & Hartnegg K. (2000a). Stability of gaze control in dyslexia. Strabismus, 8, 119–122.

Fischer B & Hartnegg K. (2000b). Effects of visual training on saccade control in dyslexia. Perception, 29, 531–542.

Fischer B & Ramsperger E. (1984) Human express saccades: extremely short reaction times of goal directed eye movements. Exp Brain Res 57(1), 191-195.

Funahashi S, Chafee M V & Goldman-Rakic PS. (1993). Prefrontal neuronal activity in rhesus monkeys performing a delayed anti-saccade task. Nature, 365(6448), 753–756.

Gaymard, B., Ploner, C. J., Rivaud-Pechoux, S. & Pierrot- Deseilligny, C. (1999). The frontal eye field is involved in spatial short term memory but not in reflexive saccade inhibition. Exp. Brain Res. 129, 288–301.

Gamlin PD & Yoon K. (2000). An area for vergence eye movement in primate frontal cortex. Nature 407 (6807), 1003-1007.

Guitton, D., Buchtel, H. A. & Douglas, R. M. (1985). Frontal lobe lesions in man cause difficulties in suppressing reflexive glances and in generating goal-directed saccades. Exp. Brain Res. 58, 455–472.

Hallet P. (1978). Primary and secondary saccades to goals defined by instructions. Vision Research. 18, 1279-1296.

Klein C. (2001). Developmental functions for saccadic eye movement parameters derived from pro- and antisaccade tasks. Experimental Brain Research, 139, 1–17.

Klein C & Foerster F. (2001). Development of prosaccade and antisaccade task performance in participants aged 6 to 26 years. Psychophysiology 38, 179–189.

Johnson MH. (1995). The inhibition of automatic saccades in early infancy. Dev Psychobiol, 28(5):281-91.

Leigh RJ, Kennard C. Using saccades as a research tool in the clinical neurosciences. Brain. 2004;127(Pt 3):460-77.

Leigh RJ, Zee DS. (2006) The Neurology of Eye Movement. Oxford University Press, New York 4th edition.

Luna B, Velanova K, Geier CF. (2008). Development of eye-movement control. Brain and Cognition 68, 293–308.

Malone SM & Iacono WG. (2002). Error rate on the antisaccade task: heritability and developmental change in performance among preadolescent and late-adolescent female twin youth. Psychophysiology 39, 664–673.

McDowell JE, Dyckman KA, Austin BP & Clementz BA. (2008). Neurophysiology and neuroanatomy of reflexive and volitional saccades: Evidence from studies of humans. Brain and Cognition 68, 255–270.

Matsuda T, Matsuura M, Ohkubo T, Ohkubo H, Matsushima E, Inoue K, et al. (2004). Functional MRI mapping of brain activation during visually guided saccades and anti-saccades: Cortical and subcortical networks. Psychiatry Research, 131(2), 147–155.

Munoz DP, Broughton JR, Goldring JE, Armstrong IT. (1998). Age-related performance of human subjects on saccadic eye movement tasks. Exp Brain Res. 121, 391–400.

Munoz DP and Everling S. (2004). Look away: the antisaccade task and the voluntary control of eye movement. Nature Rev Neurosci. 5, 218-228.

Nyffeler T, Rivaud-Pechoux S, Pierrot-Deseilligny C, Diallo R & Gaymard B. (2007). Visual vector inversion in the posterior parietal cortex. Neuroreport, 18(9), 917–920.

Quinlan DJ & Culham JC. (2007). fMRI reveals a preference for near viewing in the human parieto-occipital cortex. Neuroimage. 36(1), 167-87.

Scheiman M, Herzberg H, Frantz K, Margolies M. (1989). A normative study of step vergence in elementary schoolchildren. J Am Optom Assoc. 60(4), 276-80.

van Leeuwen AF, Westen MJ, van der Steen J, de Faber JT, Collewijn H. (1999). Gaze-shift dynamics in subjects with and without symptoms of convergence insufficiency: influence of monocular preference and the effect of training. Vision Res 39, 3095-3107.

Von Noorden GK & Campos EC. (2006). Binocular Vision and Ocular Motility. Theory and Management of Strabismus. 6th edition, Mosby.

Walker, R., Husain, M., Hodgson, T. L., Harrison, J. & Kennard, C. (1998). Saccadic eye movement and working memory deficits following damage to human prefrontal cortex. Neuropsychologia 36, 1141–1159.

Zhang M & Barash S. (2000). Neuronal switching of sensorimotor transformations for anti-saccades. Nature, 408(6815), 971–975.

6

Sequential *Versus* Simultaneous Processing Deficits in Developmental Dyslexia

Marie Lallier[1] and Sylviane Valdois[2]
[1]*Basque Center on Cognition, Brain and Language,*
[2]*Laboratoire de Psychologie et Neurocognition, CNRS UMR 5105,*
[1]*Spain*
[2]*France*

1. Introduction

Despite the large number of studies conducted on developmental dyslexia, the cause(s) of the disorder still remain(s) unclear. Researchers in this field still struggle to understand the reason why abnormal reading acquisition occurs in children who receive appropriate environmental opportunities to achieve a good education, and present normal intellectual efficiency. This introduction will focus on the presentation of the phonological hypothesis, and then move onto the presentation of the visual attention span hypothesis, which predicts at least two proximal causes to developmental dyslexia. Setting the theoretical framework for these hypotheses will help to understand why sequential and simultaneous dimensions for visual and auditory processing may have independent roles to play in typical and atypical reading development.

1.1 The phonological hypothesis: The only core deficit of the reading disorder

The phonological hypothesis (e.g., Snowling, 2000), probably the most well-known hypothesis among those formulated so far, predicts that an impairment in various phonological components (e.g., phonological short-term memory, phonological awareness, and phonological fluency) and sub-lexical processing (i.e., at the level of units smaller than the word such as graphemes, syllables or morphemes) would be detrimental for the acquisition of the skills necessary to decode new words, and acquire fluent reading (see Vellutino et al., 2004 for a review).

This hypothesis suggests that difficulties in acquiring phonological awareness and the alphabetic principle would prevent letter-to-sound mapping from developing normally. Consequently, a phonological disorder would affect reading acquisition, impairing the abilities necessary to map sub-lexical and lexical orthographic forms to their auditory counterparts. In support to the phonological deficit hypothesis, studies on typical children provided reliable evidence for a causal link between phonological skills development and reading acquisition (see however Castles & Coltheart, 2004 for a counter-argument about this causality). For example, longitudinal studies have shown that phonological skills predict later reading performance (e.g., Hulme et al., 2002). Phonology-based training programs further showed a positive impact on reading acquisition (see Ehri et al., 2001 for a review). Such data strongly suggests that the role that phonological difficulties play in the reading disorder may indeed be critical.

However, studies have questioned the restriction of the difficulties of dyslexic participants to the verbal sphere, assuming that phonological disorders would themselves result from more basic perceptual processing difficulties. Such studies propose that perceptual difficulties might affect the rapid temporal dimension of processing characterizing phonological inputs. Thus, in order to highlight a link between these difficulties and reading problems, a large number of studies have attempted to define the nature of the temporal dimension of the deficits observed in dyslexic participants. In their review of the literature, Farmer and Klein (1995) described studies showing impaired performance in dyslexic participants not only in auditory but also in visual temporal processing. The authors concluded that a temporal amodal processing deficit is associated with developmental dyslexia and that the phonological disorder would result from this temporal processing deficit. Soon after their review, Farmer and Klein were reproached for having poorly defined and circumscribed the temporal deficits found in individuals with developmental dyslexia (Rayner, Pollatsek, & Bilsky, 1995).

Starting from Farmer and Klein (1995) and from the literature published since then, the following section will present three main research axes providing coherent choices of experimental paradigms and specific interpretative frameworks regarding temporal deficits in developmental dyslexia. However, these hypotheses greatly overlap with each other, and are not mutually exclusive.

1.1.1 The rapid temporal - *sequential* - processing deficit hypothesis

Before starting to detail the rapid temporal processing deficit hypothesis, note that here, *temporal* refers to the *sequential* dimension of processing, i.e., the succession of two or more stimuli, which underlies the notion of inter-stimulus interval (ISI). ISI corresponds to the period of time separating two visual or auditory objects presented sequentially. Therefore, the shorter the ISI, the more rapid the stimuli succession speed. It is important to note that this hypothesis also accounts for another type of temporal processing, a *transient* processing (temporal change within one stimuli) which specifically relates to the magnocellular hypothesis of dyslexia (cf 1.1.2). This section more specifically focuses on *sequential* aspects of temporal processing deficits in dyslexic participants since studies testing the rapid temporal processing deficit hypothesis of dyslexia have mainly assessed this specific type (i.e., sequential) of temporal impairments.

In line with the phonological hypothesis which posits that developmental dyslexia stems from a linguistic deficit (Vellutino et al., 2004), Tallal (1980) put forward a more general hypothesis accounting for an auditory processing deficit in dyslexia. Her underlying hypothesis is that the degradation of speech temporal analysis at the phonemic level causes the reading difficulties of dyslexic participants. More specifically, Tallal reasoned that dyslexic participants could not process the fast temporal changes in the speech signal, leading to degraded and noisy representations of linguistic sounds.

The results supporting this hypothesis first came from studies of specific language impairment (SLI) children who exhibit phonological problems, like dyslexic children. The tasks used to assess the hypothesis of a general auditory disorder are temporal order and similarity judgment tasks. They involve the serial presentation of two phonological auditory stimuli and participants have to determine respectively which stimulus came first in the pair or whether the two stimuli were the same. Interestingly, deficits on these tasks were reported in SLI children only when the two stimuli were separated by a short time period; i.e., short ISI (e.g., Tallal & Piercy, 1973, 1974). Tallal's team then administered the same tasks to dyslexic children, but using non-verbal sounds such as pure tones. Deficits were reported in these children as compared to age-matched children but for ISIs shorter than 428ms (Tallal, 1980). A strong correlation was further found between dyslexic participants' performance on auditory temporal tasks and their pseudoword reading performance, thus providing first evidence for a link between rapid auditory sequential processing deficits and dyslexia.

Further evidence for a causal link between auditory and reading disorders was provided by Benasich and Tallal (1996), assessing performance of 7.5 month old infants considered "at risk" for a future language disorder on a task where participants had to distinguish various acoustic features presented at a fast rate. The performance of the infants on the task explained a significant part of variance in their later language skills and predicted a language impairment at 3 (Benasich & Tallal, 2002, see also Hood & Colon, 2004). Coupled with neuroimaging data, some training studies of auditory rapid sequential skills supported such causal link (e.g., Habib et al., 2002).

While many studies showed auditory rapid sequential processing deficits in dyslexic individuals using either verbal (e.g., De Martino, Espesser, Rey, & Habib, 2001; Heim, Freeman, Eulitz, & Elbert, 2001) or non-verbal (e.g., Laasonen, Service, & Virsu, 2001) stimuli, other results questioned the restriction of the impairment to rapid stimuli sequences. Indeed, some studies failed to reveal a deficit in dyslexic participants on the short ISI conditions only (Bretherton & Holmes, 2003; Chiappe, Stringer, Siegel, & Stanovich, 2002; Ram-Tsur, Faust, & Zivotofsky, 2006). Others found that dyslexic individuals were impaired for long intervals as well, even when using the same tasks as Tallal (Share, Jorm, Maclean, & Matthews, 2002). It follows that auditory rapid sequential deficits may not be a condition sufficient and necessary to observe dyslexia. Nevertheless, available data suggests that such rapid sequential auditory processing plays a role in normal reading (Au & Lovegrove, 2001a, 2001b) and phonological development (Walker, Hall, Klein, & Phillips, 2006).

It has also been suggested that the phoneme processing difficulties of dyslexic participants could well be part of a more general, amodal, rapid sequential processing deficit (the "rate processing deficit" hypothesis) by introducing the hypothesis of a similar impairment in the visual modality. Regarding visual *sequential* processing deficits, studies reported that as compared to controls, dyslexic individuals required longer ISIs in order to be accurate on spatial-temporal order judgment tasks, either with verbal (May, Williams, & Dunlap, 1988) or non-verbal (Hairston, Burdette, Flowers, Wood, & Wallace, 2005; Jaskowski & Russiak, 2008) visual stimuli. In these tasks – similar to those described previously in the auditory modality- participants are presented with pairs of visual stimuli appearing sequentially on a screen at different locations, and have to decide which of the two stimuli was displayed first.

As with in the auditory modality however, findings revealed that visual temporal order judgment impairments of dyslexic participants did not depend upon the ISI duration (Ram-

Tsur et al., 2006; Ram-Tsur, Faust, & Zivotofsky, 2008). Some studies even failed to show any disorder of this kind (Laasonen Tomma-Halme, Lahti-Nuuttila, Service, & Virsu., 2000, Lassonen et al., 2001). Supporting the idea of a weak link between visual sequential processing and reading, Hood and Conlon (2004) failed to show that visual temporal order judgment performance of preschoolers predicted their reading skills at Grade 1 (see also Landerl & Willburger, 2010 for similar results in both the visual and the auditory modality). However, Walker et al. (2006) showed that such performance significantly contributed to reading performance and phonological awareness abilities in a large sample of young and older adults with various reading levels.

Despite attempts to highlight an amodal rapid sequential processing deficit, very few studies have actually measured visual and auditory rapid sequential processing in the same dyslexic participants using similar paradigms (e.g., Laasonen et al., 2000, 2001; Reed, 1989). Overall, previous studies question the sequential visual impairment but the nature of the auditory processes that have been captured by the order judgment task (e.g., deciding which of two stimuli displayed sequentially appeared first) and similarity judgment task (e.g., deciding whether two stimuli presented sequentially were the same or not) still needs to be clarified (see Bailey & Snowling, 2002). Lastly, this hypothesis tends to predict a relation between visual rapid sequential processing and lexical reading, i.e., regular word or irregular word reading, but *a priori* no link with phonological processing, which is hard to reconcile with the phonological hypothesis of developmental dyslexia. Pointing out these problems, Stein and Talcott (1999) reminded that the rapid sequential processing deficit hypothesis was first grounded on temporal order and similarity judgments, which, according to them, cannot capture the temporal processing required for phonological representation build-up.

1.1.2 The magnocellular hypothesis: The "Impaired Neuronal Timing" hypothesis (Stein & Talcott, 1999)

The magnocellular hypothesis of dyslexia (Stein & Walsh, 1997; Stein & Talcott, 1999) supports the idea of visual and auditory perceptual deficits which specifically account for *transient* or *dynamic* aspects of temporal processing (i.e., rapid physical changes in real time within a stimulus). To a lesser extent, it relies to the ability to process distinct stimuli when presented serially, in sequences (see 1.1.1). Stein and Talcott (1999) claimed that sensitivity to transient events could be assessed with simple stimuli triggering the activation of neurons specifically devoted to that type of processing: the magnocellular cells. The authors assume that magnocellular cells which are part of both the visual and the auditory human systems would dysfunction in dyslexic participants (vision: Livingstone, Rosen, Drislane, & Galaburda, 1991; audition: Galaburda, Menard, & Rosen, 1994). In that sense, the magnocellular hypothesis of dyslexia differs from the rapid sequential processing deficit hypothesis because the latter does not specify any cerebral origin to the auditory and visual deficits of individuals with dyslexia.

Originally, the magnocellular hypothesis builds its foundation on the organization of the visual system and leans onto three main ideas:

1. The existence of two independent neural pathways, located deep below the surface of the brain (sub cortical structures), called the magnocellular and parvocellular pathways. Interestingly, the magnocellular system - called also *the transient system* - is tuned in to

fast temporal processing, whereas the parvocellular system is more sensitive to slower temporal processing - *sustained system*[1]);

2. The observation of these two neural pathways at the surface of the brain, (i.e., in the cerebral cortex, which plays a key role in language) via two routes called the dorsal and ventral routes respectively;
3. The dorsal route starts from the visual primary brain areas (V1) to the visual motion brain areas (MT/V5) to finish on the posterior parietal cortex, that subtends to visual selective attention and ocular movement monitoring (important in reading).

In the visual modality, the magnocellular hypothesis predicts impaired monitoring of ocular movements, leading to visual confusion, superposition and distortion during reading. In the auditory modality, a similar organization is found with the existence of two cortical routes (Clarke, Bellmann, Meuli, Assal, & Steck, 2000). Moreover, the "magnocellular" auditory neurons have been shown to be specialized in the tracking of amplitude and auditory frequency (pitch) changes within acoustic signals (Trussel, 1999). According to Stein and Talcott (1999), a phonological disorder would result from auditory transient, very fast, temporal processing difficulties. Therefore, both visual and auditory transient processing deficits would together yield a degradation of grapheme-to-phoneme mapping processes and sub-lexical reading and decoding (Pammer & Vidyasagar, 2005).

Data on behavioral tasks involving processing changes within stimuli have supported the visual transient processing deficit hypothesis of developmental dyslexia. It was indeed shown that dyslexic participants required more time to perceive the dynamic change within stimuli (McLean et al., 2011). The most commonly used tasks for revealing transient processing differences between dyslexic individuals and controls involve the detection of either a transient change in the identity of the stimulus (e.g., a single visual dot becoming two flashing dots at the same location: Edwards et al., 2004; Van Ingelghem et al., 2001), a transient change in the spatial location of the stimulus (e.g., when a visual object is moved to a different location: Jones, Branigan, & Kelly, 2008) or a transient change in the way a group of stimuli moves (e.g., when the direction of the movement of a group of visual dots changes: Cornelissen, Richardson, Mason, Fowler, & Stein, 1995). Supporting the magnocellular hypothesis deficit, visual transient processing deficits have been linked to sub-lexical reading deficits in participants with dyslexia (e.g., Cestnick & Coltheart, 1999). However, the link between visual transient processing and reading was not always established in skilled readers (e.g., Au & Lovegrove, 2001a). Moreover, strong inconsistencies have still been reported with some studies showing no such visual deficits in dyslexic participants (e.g., Amitay, Ben-Yehudah, Banai, & Ahissar, 2002; Ben-Yehudah, Sackett, Malchi-Ginzberg, & Ahissar, 2001).

In the auditory modality, a transient processing deficit has also been reported with experimental paradigms similar to the ones used in the visual modality, such as silent gap detection or segregation tasks (when participants have to detect a silence inserted within an auditory stimulus: Helenius, Salmelin, Service, & Connolly, 1999), the apparent movement task (when auditory tones moves from one hear to the other: Hari & Kiesilä, 1996 but see

---

[1] Note that the magnocellular system preferentially responds to low spatial frequencies and is very sensitive to luminance contrasts. For the purpose of the present chapter, we will specifically focus on the *temporal transient* processing deficits in relation to reading disorders and reading development.

Kronbichler, Hutzler, & Wimmer, 2002), or pitch and amplitude modulation discrimination tasks (when auditory stimuli progressively change in loudness or pitch: Witton, Stein, Stoodley, Rosner, & Talcott, 2002). Phonological skills (Talcott et al., 2000, but see Kidd & Hogben, 2007) and pseudo word reading (Au & Lovegrove, 2001a, 2001b, 2008; Walker et al., 2006; Witton et al., 2002) performance has further been linked to auditory transient (i.e., magnocellular) performance. Some data further suggests a potential causal link between auditory transient processing and phonological skills (Schäffler, Sonntag, Hartnegg, & Fischer, 2004).

However, it still remains that a phonological deficit does not always accompany difficulties in auditory or visual transient processing (Heim et al., 2008; Kronbichler et al., 2002; Ramus et al., 2003; White et al., 2006). The hypothesis of a role of these deficits in the reading disorder has been criticized particularly in the visual modality and such visual deficits have been considered as an epiphenomenon associated with reading difficulties (e.g., Hutzler, Kronbichler, Jacobs, & Wimmer, 2006; Skottun, 2000).

Interestingly, in their original proposal, Stein and Talcott (1999; Stein & Walsh, 1997) suggest that the link between magnocells dysfunction and developmental dyslexia is mediated by poor ocular movement monitoring because of the projection of magnocells to the posterior parietal cortex in charge of such visual-motor control skills. From that perspective, it has been proposed that the reading disorder may rather result from a parietal dysfunction than from the degradation of magnocells *per se* (e.g., Boden & Giaschi, 2007). Along these lines, Buchholz and MacKone (2004) concluded that phonological awareness and visual attention skills - subtended by parietal activation - are related, whereas phonology and magnocellular processing *per se* are not. This new perspective based on attentional processing will result in a new proposal explaining the cause of developmental dyslexia, favoring the role of the parietal cortex in the amodal temporal processing deficits associated with the reading disorder (Hari & Renvall, 2001).

1.1.3 The sluggish attentional shifting hypothesis

According to Hari and Renvall (2001), the magnocellular dysfunction at the cell level could lead to a variety of symptoms (including the reading disorder) which would depend on what cerebral structure is the most impaired by the magnocellular dysfunction. From that perspective, the type of temporal processing affected would not be specific to magnocell characteristics but would be supported by the cerebral structure the most affected by the magnocell dysfunction. In the sluggish attentional shifting (SAS, hereafter) hypothesis, Hari and Renvall (2001) propose the parietal cortex as the structure responsible for the reading disorder (see Figure 1 for a schematic representation of the links between the magnocellular and the SAS hypotheses in relation to reading disorders).

According to these authors, the parietal dysfunction would affect the automatic processes engaged in attentional shifting over rapid stimulus sequences in all sensory modalities (auditory, visual, and tactile). In that sense, the SAS hypothesis stands at the crossroad between the rapid sequential (perceptual) processing deficit hypothesis (see section 1.1.1) and the magnocellular deficit hypothesis of developmental dyslexia (see 1.1.2). Hari and Renvall (2001) described precisely the temporal dimension their theory accounts for and emphasized that this specific temporal processing relates, on the one hand, to the processing of *distinct successive stimuli*, and, on the other hand, to the processing of distinct changes within a *stimulus sequence* (rather than within a single stimulus).

Therefore, the SAS hypothesis does not make predictions about, for example, auditory frequency or amplitude modulation detection described by the magnocellular deficit hypothesis. Hari & Renvall (2001) propose that SAS is "*the pathophysiological link between the magnocellular deficit and the RSS* [Rapid Stimuli Sequence] *processing in dyslexic subjects*" (p.530). In this framework, a magnocellular dysfunction would not be a factor sufficient and necessary to observe dyslexia (Skoyles & Skottun, 2004) although magnocellar deficits would still potentially be associated with manifestations of reading difficulties. Rather, Hari and Renvall assume that the parietal dysfunction would be responsible for reading disabilities, via SAS skills.

The principles of the SAS hypothesis are the following: when a to-be-processed stimulus is perceived, it falls into a perceptual temporal window whose size depends upon how fast the cognitive system can integrate this stimulus. According to Hari and Renvall (2001), the time of integration would be prolonged in individuals with developmental dyslexia. When several stimuli are sequentially presented, the prolongation of the integration time would create interferences between the stimuli entering the temporal window and induce a prolonged perceptual persistence in dyslexic individuals (e.g., Slaghuis & Ryan, 1999). It is therefore inferred that dyslexic participants would show difficulties in automatically disengaging the focus of attention from one stimulus to reengage it on the next one.

In order to justify the specific attentional (and not perceptual) origin of the deficit, Hari and Renvall (2001) argue that 1) dyslexic participants do not exhibit any deficit regarding the temporal synchronization between the moment when stimulus is presented and its actual processing by the neuronal system (*phase locking*: Hari, Saaskilahti, Helenius, & Uutela, 1999a; Llinas, 1993; Witton, Richardson, Griffiths, & Rees, 1997) and 2) the SAS hypothesis can account for two attention phenomena known to be linked to reading, namely the attentional dwell time and the symptom of hemineglect. These two phenomena are explained below:

i. The attentional dwell time has been reported in all sensory modalities in paradigms where stimuli are rapidly and serially presentated (in vision: Raymond, Shapiro, & Arnell, 1992; in audition: Vachon & Tremblay, 2008). The attentional dwell time is a theoretical concept corresponding to a natural limit in attentional resources reflected by the interference induced when several stimuli fall into the same temporal integration window. Specifically, the attentional dwell time is thought to cause difficulties in processing a target falling into the same temporal integration window as a first previous target to which most attentional resources have been already allocated. This drop in performance for the second target processing would spread from 300ms to 500ms after the presentation of the first target depending on the experimental paradigm and/or the sensory modality. According to Hari and Renvall (2001), this natural limit in temporal attention resources would be stronger in individuals with developmental dyslexia because of their SAS skills. Hence, in dyslexic participants, the combination of SAS skills and attentional dwell time would lead to a prolongation of temporal input chunks falling under the attentional focus. The length of these inputs would increase their complexity, inducing poor encoding of visual or auditory sequential stimuli at higher levels (such as graphemic -letter- or phonemic -language sounds- representations).

ii. Furthermore, based on the observation that visual heminiglect patients[2] exhibit a prolongation of the attentional dwell time (Husain, Shapiro, Martin, & Kennard, 1997), Hari and Renvall (2001) proposed the left visual minineglect as a marker of developmental dyslexia, but not as a causal factor. From that perspective, this left minineglect would result from a dysfunction, and not a lesion, of the right parietal cortex (Hari, Renvall, & Tanskanen, 2001; Liddle, Jackson, Rorden, & Jackson, 2009). Supporting this idea, dyslexic children have been shown to suffer from left pseudoneglect, i.e. presenting symptoms of left hemineglect patients, in absence of any parietal lesion. The typical behavioural marker for this left pseudoneglect is the absence of the usual overestimation (facilitation for processing) of stimuli presented in the left visual hemifield (Sireteanu, Goertz, Bachert, & Wandert 2005; Sireteanu, Goebel, Goertz, & Wandert, 2006).
    Along the same lines, data collected in dyslexic individuals are in accordance with an asymmetric distribution of attention resources between right and left visual hemifields (e.g., Facoetti & Moltoni, 2001; Facoetti Paganoni, Turatto, Marzola, & Mascetti,, 2000; Facoetti & Turatto, 2000). Indeed, Facoetti's team studies show that participants with developmental dyslexia exhibit higher inhibition for the stimuli displayed in the left visual field but a facilitation of processing for those displayed in the right visual field. Moreover, it has been shown that training programs involving specific stimulation of each hemisphere individually (tachitoscopic presentation of words) improved not only the visual-spatial attentional skills of dyslexic readers in the right hemisphere/left hemifield (Facoetti, Lorusso, Paganoni, Umilta, & Mascetti, 2003; Lorusso, Facoetti, Toraldo, & Molteni, 2005) but also their reading performance (Lorusso, Facoetti, & Molteni, 2004; Lorusso et al., 2005). Note that lesions in the posterior parietal cortex can also induce auditory neglect (Marshall, 2001), the SAS hypothesis predicts similar impairment in the auditory modality.

Regarding the link between visual and auditory SAS and reading, Hari and Renvall (2001) assume that a phonological disorder would result from auditory SAS. Indeed SAS is expected to cause longer and more complex phonological input chunks, thus hindering the build-up of stable phonological representations. The link between visual SAS skills and reading is clearly explained (i.e., because the number of letters that participants have to encode during one ocular fixation during reading is increased, interferences and possible confusions in reading are observed) but their responsibility in the phonological disorder is not described. However, one can assume that both visual and auditory SAS would be linked to phonological deficits via their contribution to the acquisition of the grapheme-phoneme correspondences that are indispensable for normal reading acquisition (Pammer & Vidyasagar, 2005; Vidyasagar & Pammer, 2010).

The SAS hypothesis therefore offers an explicative framework for verbal and non-verbal auditory and visual attention sequential deficits. It furthermore specifies the

---

[2] Hemineglect patients typically suffer from a parietal lesion (interpreted as an attentional deficit at the cognitive level) which causes difficulties in encoding and processing visual object appearing in the hemifield in the opposite side of this parietal brain lesion (e.g., impairment of processing visual object appearing on the right side visual field due to a lesion in the parietal lobe of the left part of the brain).

neurophysiologic cause and specific cerebral locus of the reading disorder. In this framework, developmental dyslexia is still viewed as resulting from a phonological disorder, which however would be associated with additional visual attentional deficits whose role in reading difficulties still remains unclear.

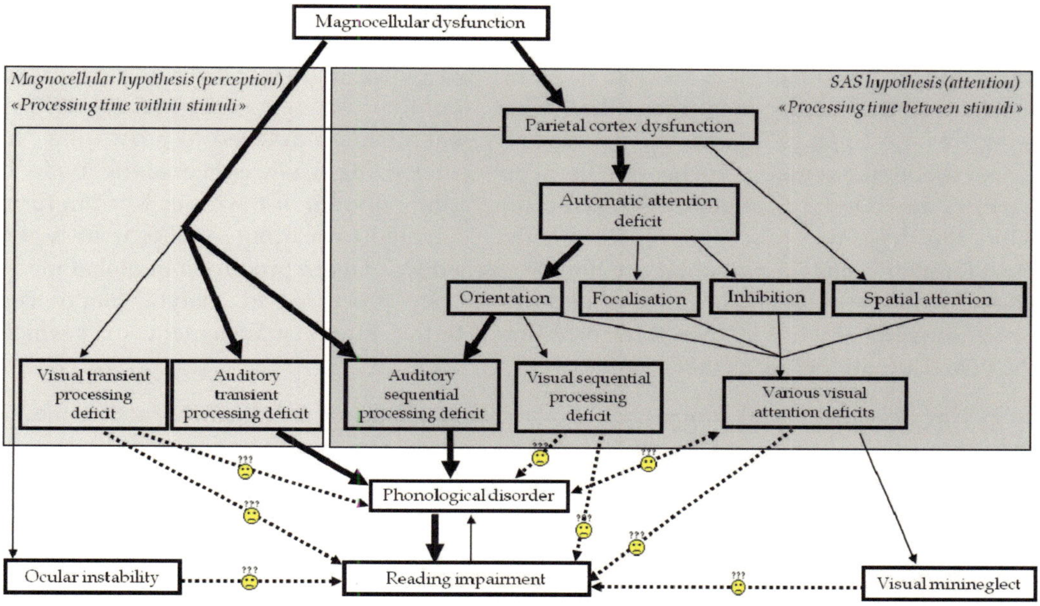

Fig. 1. Schematic syntheses of the causal cascade (plain arrows) suggested by the magnocellular and the SAS hypotheses. Dotted simple arrows represent causal links and dotted double arrows associative links as suggested in the literature but which have been questioned. Note that the SAS hypothesis explains many symptoms associated with developmental dyslexia. Adapted from Lallier (2009).

1.2 The visual attention span deficit hypothesis: Developmental dyslexia as a cognitive multifactorial disorder

So far we have reviewed hypotheses that have been put forward in order to explain developmental dyslexia as resulting from a phonological disorder. However, it appears that at least some dyslexic cases are clearly not phonological (Friedmann & Naachman-Katz, 2004; Friedmann & Rahamin, 2007; Rouse & Wilshire, 2007; Valdois et al., 2003; Valdois, Lassus-Sangosse, & Lobier, In press), thus questioning the homogeneity of developmental dyslexia. Instead, a growing body of evidence suggests that developmental dyslexia is heterogeneous (e.g., Heim et al., 2008).

The visual attention span (VA Span hereafter) hypothesis put forward by Bosse, Tainturier and Valdois (2007) is complementary to the phonological deficit hypothesis. It posits that another cause of developmental dyslexia stands in a limitation of the visual attention resources that can be allocated simultaneously to letters within words. This would in particular prevent normal encoding of whole word orthographic information. The VA Span therefore taps into parallel, simultaneous, processing, and VA Span resources are expected to be limited in at least a subgroup of dyslexic children.

The VA Span is a notion theoretically motivated by the Multi-Trace Memory model of reading (Ans, Carbonnel, & Valdois, 1998; hereafter MTM model). The MTM model was the first reading model to implement a visual attention component, called the visual attentional window (which is the counterpart of the VA Span in human participants). The VA window is a critical component of the reading system as it delineates the amount of orthographic information which is under the focus of attention at each step of the reading process. The MTM model postulates that reading relies on two global (parallel) and analytic (serial) procedures that differ regarding the visual attention window size, and therefore, regarding VA Span skills and the quantity of visual attention devoted to processing. In global mode, the window opens over the whole letter string whereas in analytic mode, it narrows down to focus attention on each orthographic sub-unit of the input word in turn. Although these two procedures are *a priori* not devoted to reading specific item types, most familiar items (in particular previously learned words) are processed in global mode whereas non-familiar items (most pseudowords) are processed in analytic mode. The visual attentional window therefore corresponds to the set of visual elements over which the visual attentional focus falls.

Following this theoretical framework, it was reasoned that a VA Span reduction (i.e., a reduction of the number of visual letters that can be processed simultaneously) should prevent normal encoding of the orthographic sequence of most words (Bosse et al., 2007). According to this idea, a reduced VA Span would be particularly detrimental when reading irregular words that cannot be accurately decoded serially.

The VA Span is typically measured using whole and partial letter report tasks which require naming all of the letters of a five-consonant string or a single post-cued letter within the string (see Fig 2). In partial as in global report, participants have to process all five consonants since the position of the letter to be reported is randomly chosen and the cue in partial report only occurs at the offset of the consonant string. Moreover, sequences are displayed for a time period short enough to avoid useful ocular saccades (<200ms), so that participants have to engage enough visual attention resources to process all five elements simultaneously (Lobier, Przybylski, & Valdois, Submitted; Peyrin, Lallier, & Valdois, 2008; Peyrin, Démonet, N'Guyen-Morel, Le Bas, & Valdois, 2011). Only consonants are used as stimuli to compose unpronounceable illegal letter strings. In random consonant strings, identification of one consonant within the string does not help identifying the other consonants, so that the number of reported letters provides a good account of the number of distinct elements that can be processed simultaneously. To avoid any potential top-down influence of orthographic knowledge on performance, the consonant strings we use do not include any multi-letter grapheme or frequent bigram (as CH or FL in French). Moreover, sequences do not correspond to the skeleton of any word (e.g., C M P T R for computer), since we know that such consonant strings activate the corresponding word orthographic information in long term memory. In the whole report task, the five elements need to be verbally reported without order constraint whereas in the partial report task the cued letter alone has to be reported. Accordingly, responses as "RHSDM", "SDHRM" or "DSRMH" are all considered as accurate (quoted 5/5) for the "RHSDM" input in global report, since all five consonants have been accurately identified in all three cases. A deficit on such tasks is reflected by a poor accuracy report score, interpreted as a reduction of the VA Span.

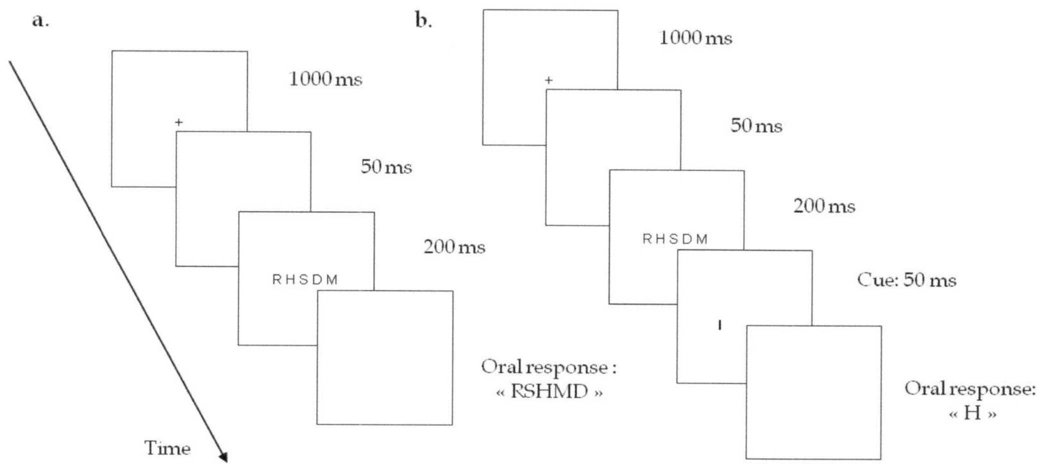

Fig. 2. Schematic illustration of the whole and partial report tasks. The whole report task requires naming as many of the 5 consonants as possible without order constraint (a.). The partial report task requires a single cued letter to be named (b.).

The link between VA Span skills and reading has been observed in a group study conducted in two populations of dyslexic children (68 French speaking dyslexic children and 29 English dyslexic children) whose performance was compared to age-matched children (Bosse et al., 2007). All children were given a screening battery comprising reading tasks, phonological awareness tasks and the whole and partial report tasks. Results showed that a large part of dyslexic children exhibited either a specific and selective phonological deficit or a specific and selective VA Span deficit. On the other hand, a smaller group of children exhibited a double deficit (i.e., on phoneme awareness *and* visual letter report tasks). Moreover, the results of the study in French speaking children revealed that both phonological and VA Span skills independently explained a significant part of variance in reading performance. The study in the English speaking children confirmed that VA Span skills contribute to reading abilities even when non verbal IQ, verbal fluency skills, vocabulary and the performance on a single letter identification task are controlled for. Bosse et al. (2007)'s findings therefore suggest that at least two independent cognitive disorders underlying developmental dyslexia can be observed. Their conclusion is furthermore supported by a case study in two French dyslexic teenagers showing that a reading disorder of the same severity could either be accompanied by a phonological disorder (rhyme judgment, sound categorization, phoneme and syllable omission, phoneme segmentation, acronyms) associated with a phonological dyslexic profile (impaired decoding skills illustrated by poor pseudoword reading and spelling skills) in the absence of any VA Span deficit on the two report tasks, *or* by a VA Span disorder associated with a surface dyslexia profile (poor lexical reading procedure illustrated by poor word reading and spelling) with no additional phonological disorder (Valdois et al., 2003).

The role of VA Span skills in normal reading development was investigated in a cross-sectional study conducted on large samples of typically developing children from 1st to 5th grade (Bosse & Valdois, 2009). Results showed that VA Span abilities contributed to reading performance from the early stages of literacy instruction even after controlling for variations in phonological performance. Indeed, the unique contribution of VA Span to reading performance was observed from the first year of literacy instruction at a time phoneme awareness skills played an important (but independent) role in reading acquisition. Furthermore, VA Span performance contributed preferentially to irregular word reading (i.e., word-specific orthographic knowledge) as compared to pseudoword reading.

Moreover regarding spelling abilities, the findings of Valdois and Bosse (Submitted) in 1st, 3rd and 5th graders strengthen the role of VA Span skills in orthographic knowledge acquisition. These authors show that VA Span skills and phonological skills independently contribute to the acquisition of orthographic knowledge. Moreover, VA Span contribution to word spelling accuracy remains even after accounting for the children's recoding skills. This suggests a role of VA Span in the acquisition of word specific orthographic knowledge. VA Span contribution to word spelling is more stable than phoneme awareness contribution over grades, suggesting a long-term influence of the VA Span on the acquisition of orthographic knowledge. In sum, a large body of data from dyslexic and typically developing children supports a role of the VA Span in reading and spelling. The overall data points to the involvement of VA Span in the acquisition of orthographic knowledge and suggests this visual attention mechanism may act as a self-teaching device process.

The VA Span hypothesis postulates that the component preventing dyslexic individuals from performing accurately a multi-element array of stimuli does not relate to any type of verbal or phonological disorder but rather, to visual attention (Bosse et al., 2007; Peyrin et al., 2011). It has however been argued that poor performance in letter report tasks might be due to verbal deficits in encoding and reporting letters, and as such reflected a visual-to-phonology code mapping disorder (Ziegler, Pech-Georgel, Dufau, & Grainger, 2010) rather than a visual attention resource limitation. Ziegler et al. (2010)'s account is based on data from a forced choice detection task in which children were shown briefly presented strings of letters, digits or symbols. At the offset of the multi-character string, participants had to choose which one of two characters previously occurred in a cued position within the string. Results showed that dyslexic children performed poorly when asked to process letter or digit strings but at the level of control children when processing symbol strings. The authors reasoned that a VA Span disorder would have predicted a deficit whenever multi-element parallel processing is required independently of the nature (alphanumeric or not) of the stimuli. Against this expectation, their data showed that the disorder was restricted to alphanumeric material. They thus concluded that their findings did not support the VA Span deficit hypothesis but rather suggested a visual-to-phonological code mapping disorder.

It is however noteworthy that the letter/digit *versus* symbol character not only differ in their phonological characteristics (pronounceable *versus* non pronounceable characters) but also in the visual ones (familiar *versus* unfamiliar visual shapes), so that differences in processing might follow from one or the other dimension.

Against the phonological account, data shows that:

- a visual-to-phonological code mapping interpretation cannot account for the whole data set;
- the VA Span disorder extends to non-verbal tasks and non-verbal material.

With respect to the first point and against the visual-to-phonological code mapping disorder interpretation, Valdois et al. (In press) showed that dyslexic children are not systematically impaired in tasks involving visual-to-phonological code mapping. Dyslexic and control children were asked to perform a 5-elements report task using letters, digits and color patches as stimuli. All three conditions required verbally reporting as many letter, digit or color names as possible at the offset of the multi-element string. Accordingly a visual-to-phonological code mapping disorder was expected to impact all three conditions. Against this expectation however, dyslexic participants were found to exhibit poor performance in letter and digit string report tasks but no disorder in the color string report task. This result goes against the visual-to-phonological code mapping disorder hypothesis.

Moreover, Valdois et al. (In press) reported a second experiment in which dyslexic children were administered two versions of the whole letter report task. Both conditions required the oral report of all five letter-names at the end of processing but the whole report task was either performed alone or together with a concurrent phonological articulation task (i.e., of counting aloud). The concurrent articulation task taxed phonological processing and verbal short-term memory and as such prevented online verbal encoding of letter names during visual processing. Dyslexic children exhibited a similar VA Span deficit in the two conditions, suggesting that performance was not modulated by on line verbal encoding. This last result suggests that difficulties of dyslexic participants on the whole report task do not result from a verbal encoding deficit.

Moreover, Lobier, Lassus-Sangosse, Zoubrinetzki, and Valdois (In press) administered a categorization task which required parallel processing of multi-elements within strings to a group of dyslexic children selected for their poor performance in visual letter report tasks. The categorization task involved the processing of verbal (digits and letters) *or* non-verbal (Japanese Hiragana characters, pseudo letters, and unknown geometrical shapes) characters. The study aimed to assess whether this group of dyslexic children exhibited similar difficulties in the processing of alphanumeric and non-alphanumeric character strings. The dyslexic participants with a VA Span deficit were found to be impaired on the visual categorization task regardless of whether the stimuli to be processed were verbal or non-verbal. They were thus impaired in a non-verbal task using non-verbal stimuli as they were found impaired in the letter report task. Taken together, these results provide strong evidence against a phonological account of poor letter string processing and VA Span skills in developmental dyslexia.

The currently available neurobiological data collected during parallel multi-element processing are well in line with the VA Span interpretation. Data from adult skilled readers showed that the letter report task elicited increased activation of the superior parietal lobules bilaterally and that activation of these regions was reduced in the dyslexic participants (Peyrin, et al., 2008). In another study carried out on dyslexic and non-dyslexic children, participants were administered a categorization task comprising two isolated and flanked conditions (inspired from Pernet, Valdois, Celsis, & Démonet, 2006) under fMRI (Peyrin et al., 2011). In both conditions, two stimuli – either two letters or two geometrical shapes or one of each – were simultaneously displayed, one stimulus was centrally presented on the fixation point, the other one was randomly presented in the right or left visual field. In the flanked condition, the peripheral stimulus was flanked with two "X"s whereas it was presented alone in the isolated condition. Participants had to decide whether the two stimuli belonged to the same category or not. Results replicated previous findings in showing that VA Span impaired dyslexic children were characterized by reduced activations within the superior parietal lobules bilaterally (Peyrin et al., 2011). Thus, multi-element parallel processing relies on brain regions that are well known for their involvement in visual attention. More recently, Lobier et al. (Submitted) investigated whether these parietal regions were sensitive to the alphanumeric or non-alphanumeric nature of the stimuli. They administered a non-verbal categorization task under fMRI using either letters or digits as targets, or pseudo-letters, shapes and hiragana characters. They found that the superior parietal lobules were involved in the processing of both alphanumeric and non-alphanumeric character strings and that activity in these regions was reduced in dyslexic individuals regardless of character type (i.e., strings composed of alphanumeric or non alphanumeric elements).

The overall results of the series of studies of Valdois'team thus support the existence in a subset of dyslexic individuals of a parallel multi-element processing disorder, i.e. a VA Span disorder, that relates to a superior parietal lobules dysfunction and dissociates from phonological problems.

2. SAS *versus* VA Span hypotheses: Sequential *versus* simultaneous processing deficits in dyslexia

We previously presented a set of hypotheses that sought to explain the cognitive origin of developmental dyslexia. The first part was devoted to the description of the phonological hypothesis which postulates that reading difficulties result from a specific impairment affecting the processing of phonological stimuli, then resulting in difficulties in mapping graphemes to phonemes during reading. Among the hypotheses presented, the SAS hypothesis postulates a deficit at the attentional level which would then lead to developmental reading disorders.

In the second part, we presented a multifactorial view of the cause of developmental dyslexia: the VA Span hypothesis. This hypothesis assumes that atypical reading development can either stem from a phonological deficit, or a visual attention deficit affecting the simultaneous processing of multiple visual stimuli. In preventing simultaneous processing of letters within the word string, the VA Span disorder is expected to prevent normal encoding of whole word forms, thus leading poor word-specific orthographic knowledge acquisition.

It is noteworthy that the type of attention processes described in the SAS and the VA Span hypotheses corresponds to what could be named "perceptual" or "automatic" attention. Such attention processes are thought to facilitate the processing of stimuli falling under the focus of attention during the first 200-250 msec after engagement of the attentional focus.

Looking at the SAS and VA Span hypotheses more carefully, we can observe that they offer complementary accounts for developmental dyslexia. While they both assume that a parietal dysfunction is the cerebral origin of the reading disorder, the two hypotheses differ in the sense that the parietal impairments described would lead to distinct, independent, cognitive deficits: a phonological deficit for the SAS hypothesis, and a visual attention deficit for the VA Span hypothesis. Moreover, it is assumed that the mechanisms underlying phonological and VA Span processing would *a priori* engage distinct dimensions of processing: one sequential, and the other simultaneous.

Interestingly, the SAS and VA Span hypotheses both predict visual attention problems in developmental dyslexia, but while the VA Span hypothesis assigns to the visual attention disorder a causal role in developmental dyslexia, the SAS hypothesis rather predicts an association between reading and sequential visual attention skills than a causal relationship, unlike what is posited in the auditory modality. Furthermore, the SAS hypothesis predicts sequential attention deficits in both the auditory and visual modalities whereas the VA Span hypothesis *a priori* predicts that the simultaneous attention deficit in dyslexic individuals is restricted to the visual modality only (see Fig 3).

The figure below provides a schematic representation of the different predictions of the SAS and VA Span hypotheses regarding visual and auditory processing deficits in developmental dyslexia.

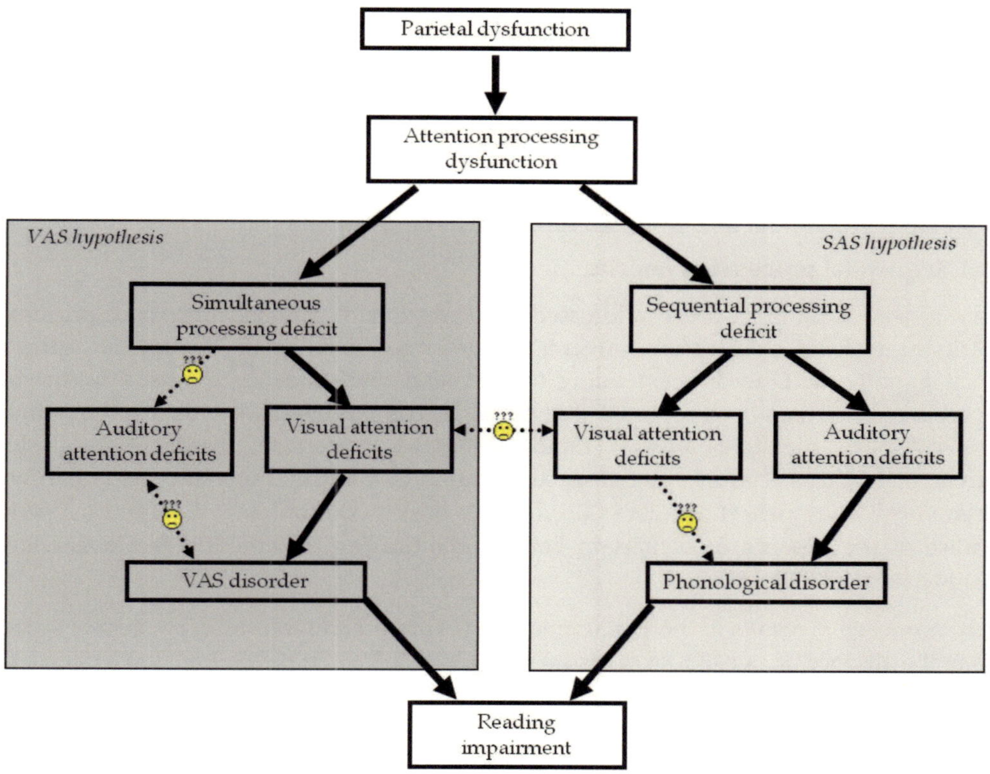

Fig. 3. Schematic representation of the VA Span and SAS hypotheses. The two hypotheses postulate that a parietal dysfunction yields the reading disorder through distinct cognitive impairments (VA Span and phonological disorders respectively). Thick arrows illustrate the causal cascade of impairments leading to developmental dyslexia for each of the two hypotheses. Dotted arrows indicate causal links (simple arrows) or associative links (double arrows) with no or weak support in the literature.

In the following section, we will present arguments in favor of a dissociation between the two hypotheses and between the expected attention impairments. The data that will be presented will address two main questions:

1. The question of amodality will be first addressed. Indeed, Hari and Renvall (2001) in their initial proposal argued for an amodal SAS in developmental dyslexia. They however reported studies that assessed SAS in either the visual or the auditory modality, but never explored the two modalities in the same dyslexic participants, therefore questioning the amodality of the sequential deficits. We will examine to what extent sequential and simultaneous attention deficits quantified on similar paradigms in both the auditory and the visual modalities can be observed in the same dyslexic participants.
2. The second question that we will address is to what extent sequential and simultaneous deficits relate respectively to the phonological and VA Span disorder in developmental dyslexia. In particular, the link between SAS and phonological disorders was never directly assessed in the previously mentioned studies, thus questioning the validity of the causal link between SAS skills and phonological deficits in dyslexia.

Based on experimental evidence, we will argue that sequential and simultaneous attention deficits may play independent roles in the reading disorder, in hindering the development of independent cognitive components which are both required for normal reading acquisition.

2.1 Amodal sequential and simultaneous processing deficits

2.1.1 Sequential processing deficits

Few studies straightforwardly addressed the question of amodal *attentional* processing deficits in dyslexia, since research interests have largely focused on the amodal *perceptual* deficit hypothesis. Disorders extending over several modalities, as expected by the SAS hypothesis, have then been reported (Meyler & Breznitz, 2005). However, a fair amount of data failed to highlight amodal rapid sequential processing disorders in dyslexic individuals, either because of the absence of deficit in the visual modality (e.g., Eddins & Green, 1995; Laasonen et al., 2001; Reed, 1989; Welch, DuttonHurt, & Warren, 1986) or because of the absence of deficits in both modalities (e.g., Bretherton & Holmes, 2003; Laasonen et al., 2000).

Such inconclusive results in the visual modality (as opposed to the auditory modality) could reflect the absence of causal role of visual sequential deficits in developmental dyslexia (see Skottun, 2000). They could also follow from the heterogeneity of the dyslexic population and lack of characterization of the cognitive deficits underlying the reading disorder of dyslexic participants at the individual level. Indeed, knowing that all cases of developmental dyslexia *are not* associated with phonological disorders (Bosse et al., 2007), performance may have been influenced by the heterogeneity of the phonological disorders in the dyslexic sample. In line with this hypothesis, Meyler and Breznitz (2005) who reported a phonological deficit in their dyslexic group did find an amodal sequential deficit in their dyslexic participants.

Differences in the choice of experimental paradigms could also have led to inconsistent results in the observation of amodal sequential deficits in dyslexia. In the original proposal of Tallal (1980), rapid temporal deficits were assessed with order or similarity judgment tasks composed of two stimuli only. Interestingly, the SAS hypothesis predicts deficits on sequences of multiple (i.e., more than two) stimuli as used in paradigms of stream segregation (Helenius et al., 1999) or attentional blink (Hari et al., 1999). These paradigms seem more appropriate to capture the nature of the auditory and visual processes engaged for the encoding of speech streams or orthographic sequences (these paradigms will be described later in this chapter).

Therefore, we propose that an assessment of SAS amodal deficit in dyslexic participants should be conducted 1) with tasks requiring the processing of long stimulus sequences (see Meyler & Breznitz, 2005, for a similar proposal) and 2) in groups of participants with developmental dyslexia diagnosed with a phonological deficit.

2.1.2 Simultaneous processing deficits

The role of amodal simultaneous processing in reading development has barely been studied. We are aware of only one study which tried to capture amodal simultaneous processing deficit in dyslexia. Geiger et al. (2008) administered to a group of dyslexic children two similar tasks, one in the visual modality, the other one in the auditory modality. In the visual modality, participants were asked to recognize letter stimuli presented in the center of a screen and ignore the letter stimuli in the periphery. In the auditory modality, they had to recognize auditory lexical stimuli presented via speakers located in front of participants (i.e., centrally) with or without the presence of auditory simultaneous peripheral lexical stimuli. Dyslexic children were found to exhibit difficulties in recognizing the central stimuli presented with external noise in both the auditory and the visual modalities. The authors concluded to a "wider perceptual mode" in the dyslexic children, which in turn may hinder their ability to focus on relevant stimuli and inhibit irrelevant information. Unfortunately, this study did not specify whether the assessed dyslexic children exhibited a phonological deficit, making impossible to determine whether such simultaneous processing deficits were found regardless of phonological deficits, as the VA Span hypothesis would predict.

2.2 Assessing visual and auditory sequential and simultaneous deficits in relation to phonological and VA Span disorders in developmental dyslexia

In the following section, we will present evidence that sequential and simultaneous disorders in developmental dyslexia can be found in the same dyslexic participants in both the visual and the auditory modalities. Moreover, we will argue that:

1. sequential and simultaneous automatic attention processes rely on different mechanisms;
2. these mechanisms relate to potentially independent literacy-related cognitive abilities, i.e., phonological (sequential) or VA Span (simultaneous), leading to different dyslexia subtypes.

We first need to emphasize the fact that when investigating auditory and visual non-verbal attention or perception abilities, the underlying cognitive deficits of the dyslexic group should be precisely defined. This is critical in order to investigate the extent to which deficits in non-verbal abilities are linked and result to specific cognitive dyslexic symptoms (i.e., phonological or VA Span disorders). Disregarding this first step may lead to highly heterogeneous performance in the dyslexic group, hence inconsistent observations between studies.

So far, most of the studies aiming to assess sequential deficits in individuals with developmental dyslexia implicitly assumed that the dyslexic participants exhibited a phonological deficit. Furthermore, other studies which explicitly reported a phonological processing deficit based their diagnosis upon pseudoword reading difficulties (i.e., decoding or sub-lexical reading difficulties), but pseudoword reading does not only require phonological abilities but also engages visual attention (Bosse et al., 2007; Bosse & Valdois, 2009; Facoetti et al., 2006; Facoetti et al., 2010; Vidyasagar & Pammer, 2010).

A number of case studies have now been reported (Dubois et al., 2010; Peyrin, Lallier, Baciu, Démonet, Le Bas, & Valdois, In press; Valdois et al., 2003; Valdois et al., In press) showing that dyslexic individuals (adults or children) with a single VA Span deficit may suffer from poor pseudoword reading abilities (reading accuracy and/or reading speed) *in spite of* any difficulties in "pure auditory" phonological processing skills.

From these considerations, it appears critical to systematically base the diagnosis of phonological disorders in dyslexic patients on measures of auditory phonological processing rather than on decoding skills. This precaution alone can ensure avoiding the impact of visual attention on performance, which would no longer reflect the "phonological disorder" primarily targeted.

We therefore will present data from a series of studies suggesting that sequential attention skills preferentially relate to phonological (and not decoding) skills rather than VA Span skills. We chose two experimental paradigms - the attentional blink and the stream segregation paradigms - that we thought had a great sensitivity to capture the rapid sequential processing abilities required for reading acquisition development (presentation of multiple stimuli in rapid sequences). These two tasks are supposed to allow the evaluation of temporal automatic attention deployment via attentional shifting, i.e., the successive engagement and disengagement of the attentional focus over a sequence of multiple stimuli.

2.2.1 Amodal sequential processing assessment: The attentional blink

Hari and Renvall (2001) predict that a prolongation of the attentional dwell time (see section 1.1.3 for a definition) in all sensory modalities would result in developmental dyslexia. The attentional dwell time has been highlighted in rapid serial presentation paradigms (10 items/sec) requiring the identification and/or detection of two targets (T1 and T2) embedded in a series of distracters. When the two targets are present in the sequence, performance on T1 is high whereas performance on T2 is lower. This drop of T2 performance (also called the attentional blink) is all the more interesting that it varies according to its temporal position as regards the presentation of T1 (Raymond et al., 1992).

In attentional blink tasks, two conditions are generally used: a dual task condition (see white dots in Fig 4.a.) where participants have to identify T1 and detect the presence or absence of T2, and a single task condition (see black squares in Fig 4.a.) which serves as a baseline, and where T1 is absent and only T2 has to be detected. Results on this task show an attentional blink, which is typically observed during a temporal window of about 300-500 ms after T1 presentation. In order to characterize the attentional blink more accurately, Cousineau,

Charbonneau, and Jolicoeur (2006) measured the phenomenon according to four parameters defining a curve fitting function (see Fig 4.b.): the duration parameter corresponds to the duration of the attentional blink, the amplitude parameter corresponds to the difference between the best and the worst performance and indicates the severity of the attentional blink, the minimum parameter corresponds to the worst performance, and lag-1 sparing parameter corresponds to the speed at which T1 processing starts to have a negative impact on T2 processing. The SAS hypothesis predicts a longer attentional blink duration in dyslexic participants with phonological disorders.

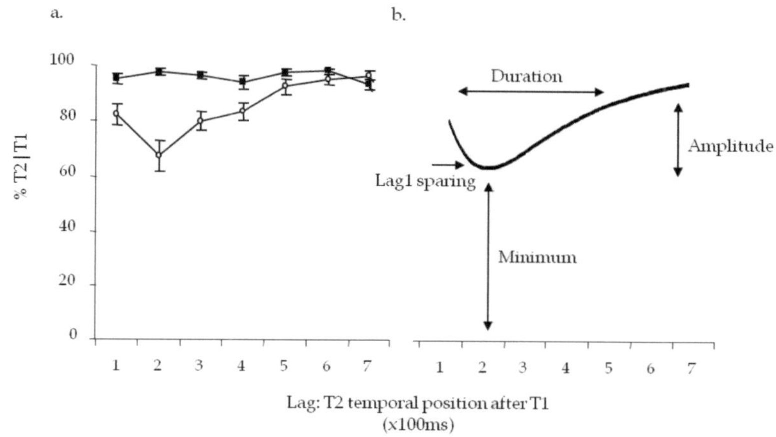

Fig. 4. Representation of the typical pattern of performance obtained in attentional blink (a). When compared to the single task condition (black squares), performance on the dual task condition (white dots) drops for the first four positions of T2 after T1. The four attentional blink parameters adapted from Cousineau et al. (2006) are presented in (b).

Several studies have shown that dyslexic individuals exhibit a prolonged visual attentional blink (lasting in average 600-800 ms) as compared to normal readers (e.g., Hari, Valta, and Uutela, 1999b; Visser, Boden, & Giaschi, 2004; Facoetti, Ruffino, Peru, Paganoni, & Chelazzi, 2008). This finding suggests that T1 captures visual attention resources for longer time in dyslexic participants than in control participants. However, research conducted on the attentional blink in impaired readers has given rise to discrepant results and has been subject to criticisms (Badcock, Hogben, & Fletcher, 2008).

Overall, previous studies conducted in dyslexic participants suffer from a lack of homogeneity regarding either the characterization of the cognitive deficit underlying dyslexia (i.e., phonological or VA Span disorder), or methodological aspects. Furthermore, although the attentional blink had been highlighted in the auditory modality (e.g., Vachon & Tremblay, 2008), no study had examined whether dyslexic participants presented an atypical attentional blink in this modality as in vision.

In a first study (Lallier, Donnadieu, Berger, & Valdois, 2010a), we assessed the amodality assumption of the SAS hypothesis by administering two similar attentional blink tasks in the visual and the auditory modalities to a French dyslexic adult participant, LL, and a group of skilled reader adults. The neuropsychological assessment of LL revealed that this patient suffered from a phonological dyslexia as characterised by slowed pseudoword reading rate and poor pseudoword spelling. LL further had poor pseudoword repetition and poor phoneme awareness skills, thus reflecting an underlying phonological disorder. On the contrary, LL showed normal simultaneous processing of letter strings on the whole and partial report tasks, thus suggesting preserved VA Span abilities.

The visual attentional blink task consisted in the rapid serial presentation of black digits. T1 was the only red digit in the stream and it was either 1 or 5. T2 was the digit 0 and was black like the distracters. The auditory attention blink task consisted in the rapid serial auditory presentation of sounds. Pure tones were used as distracters and a higher-pitched tone of 4000 Hz was used as T1 target. This tone was either a complex tone (sounding like a locust cry) or pure tone (sounding like a bird cry), giving rise to two distinct perceptions. T2 was a pure tone of 600 Hz belonging to the distracters' frequency range but it was delivered at a higher amplitude level (i.e., it was louder). In the dual task condition, participants were instructed to attend to and name T1 (1 or 5 digits; pure or complex tones) while judging whether T2 occurred or not (number 0; louder sound). For both the single and dual task conditions, we took into account eight T1-T2 lags in the analyses, i.e., from lag 1 (no intervening items, ISI = 60 ms) to lag 8 (ISI = 760 ms). For each of the visual and the auditory tasks, participants were instructed to name T1 and/or report aloud whether T2 was present or not, after each sequence was seen or heard.

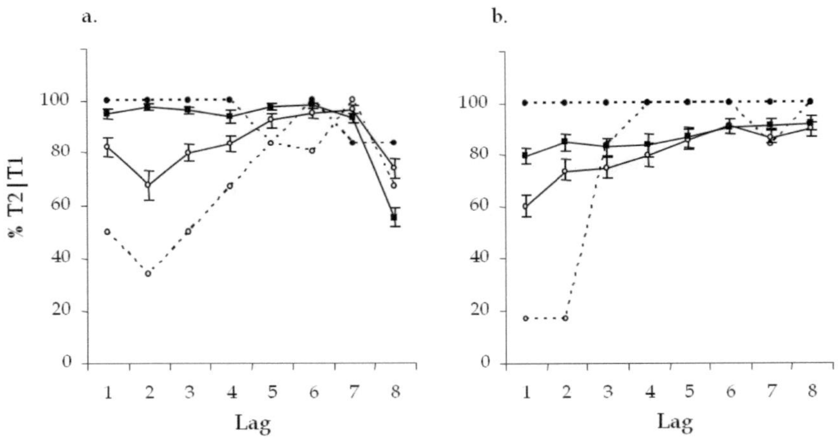

Fig. 5. Visual (a.) and auditory (b.) attentional blinks in the control group (plain lines) and in LL (dotted lines) for the single task condition (black dots) and for the dual task condition (white dots). From Lallier et al., 2010a.

When LL's performance was compared to performance of skilled readers, it revealed atypical visual attentional blink duration and atypical auditory attentional blink amplitude (see Fig 5). Both atypical attentional blinks were interpreted as reflecting prolonged attentional dwell time, thus demonstrating amodal SAS skills in LL. Interestingly, this amodal disorder was reported in a dyslexic participant with a phonological disorder, in accordance with the SAS hypothesis. Moreover, the auditory and visual attentional blink deficits were found independently of any VA Span disorder, suggesting that sequential and simultaneous attention processing could dissociate and might independently contribute to developmental dyslexia.

In a second study (Lallier, Donnadieu, & Valdois, 2010b), we used the curve fitting method of Cousineau et al. (2006) to quantify and better define the visual attentional blink deficit of dyslexic children. We further explored whether any parameter specifically related to their phonological disorder (Lallier et al., 2010b). Fourteen dyslexic children and 14 age-matched control children took part in the experiment. The dyslexic group was impaired in phonological short-term memory and showed marginally poor phoneme deletion skills but performed as well as the controls on the partial or whole report task, thus suggesting preserved VA Span skills (Lallier, 2009). All children were given the same visual attentional blink task as in Lallier et al (2010a). A group effect was revealed on the attentional blink minimum parameters, reflecting a lower minimum for the dyslexic group than the control group, but no difference regarding duration of the attentional blink. Correlation analyses on the whole sample revealed that the attentional blink minimum and amplitude parameters significantly correlated, and that attentional blink amplitude was significantly related to phonemic deletion skills.

From these findings and previous other results, it seems that deficits in several attentional blink features (see Fig 4) could occur in the same dyslexic participants. Indeed, both atypical attentional blink "duration *and* minimum" (Facoetti et al., 2008; Hari et al., 1999) and "duration *and* amplitude" (Lallier et al., 2010a) have been reported in the same participants. Such result is *a priori* not surprising given the correlation reported between all three parameters (Cousineau et al., 2006).

To sum up, our two studies assessing sequential attention processing with attentional blink tasks in dyslexic participants showed that a visual sequential attention deficit can be found in the absence of any visual simultaneous attention disorder. Moreover, both auditory and visual SAS skills were preferentially associated with phonological deficits in developmental dyslexia.

2.2.2 Amodal sequential processing assessment: Stream segregation

In another series of studies we will present in this section, we used the experimental paradigm used for the assessment of stream segregation. Interestingly, stream segregation can be observed in the two modalities. In the auditory modality (Bey & McAdams, 2003), stream segregation occurs when sequences of auditory stimuli alternate in pitch/auditory frequency (e.g. high and low pitch tones). In the visual modality (Bregman & Achim, 1973), segregation occurs when sequences of visual stimuli alternate in spatial locations (e.g. visual dots appearing above and below fixation). The resulting percept depends on both temporal and auditory frequency/visual distance intervals between two successive stimuli (Van Noorden, 1975).

For adequate auditory frequency/visual distance intervals, two perceptual temporal patterns can occur (see Fig 6):

i. When time interval is long enough, a unique auditory stream alternating high and low pitch tones (or a unique visual object composed of two dots bouncing up and down) is perceived.
ii. For short enough intervals, the participants perceive two different auditory streams, one high- and the other low-pitched (or two visual dots flickering in parallel).

Focusing on the temporal aspects of the phenomenon, auditory stream segregation has been assessed in dyslexia, showing that dyslexic individuals required longer ISIs to perceive the one unique auditory stream (i.e., the alternation of two distinct sounds) as compared to skilled readers. Hari and Renvall (2001) interpreted this result as evidence for auditory SAS skills in individuals with developmental dyslexia.

In the following series of experiments, we used the paradigms of Helenius et al. (1999) in the auditory modality, and designed a similar paradigm to assess stream segregation skills in the visual modality. For both tasks, we measured stream segregation thresholds according to an adaptive procedure that allows varying the ISI between the successive stimuli in the sequences according to the answer/perception of participants ("one stream", cf Fig 6.a., or "two streams", cf Fig 6.b.).

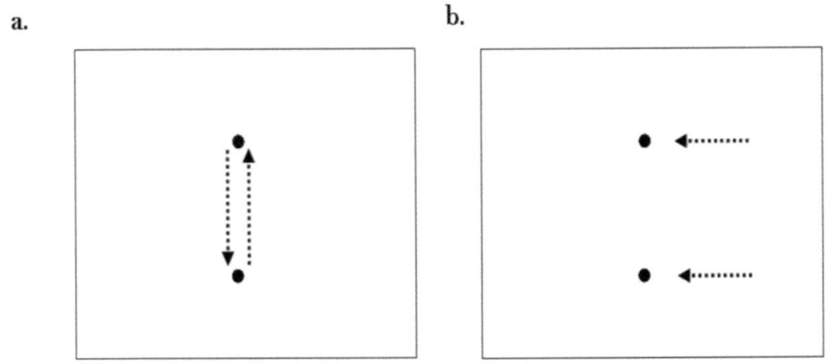

Fig. 6. Schematic representation of the stream segregation procedure. The dotted arrows symbolise the one stream (a., longer ISIs) or two streams (b., shorter ISIs) conditions. From Lallier et al. 2010c.

Stream segregation thresholds correspond to the ISI for which participants cannot straightforwardly decide if they perceive one stream or two streams of stimuli, corresponding to a response "at chance".

We interpreted stream segregation thresholds as an estimation of the fastest speed at which attention could engage and disengage automatically from one stimulus to another in order to perceive them as independent entities.

The first study (Lallier et al., 2009) combined two experiments: one with children, one with adults. In the first experiment, we tested 36 children on both the visual and the auditory stream segregation tasks. Twelve children were diagnosed as dyslexic and, as a group, showed a phonological impairment (phoneme deletion and phonological short term memory) together with a mild VA Span disorder illustrated by a deficit on the whole report task but not on the partial report task (Lallier, 2009). The other participants were either skilled readers (12 children) or poor readers (12 children). The three groups of children were matched for chronological age but significantly differed between each other on their reading skills.

Results on the segregation tasks showed that dyslexic children exhibited higher auditory thresholds than the two other groups of non dyslexic readers, suggesting SAS skills in the dyslexic group as compared to the non dyslexic groups (see Fig 7.a., top graph). Furthermore, poor readers exhibited a higher auditory threshold than skilled readers. Such results suggest a strong link between reading skills and auditory stream segregation thresholds and consequently, between reading skills and auditory automatic attention shifting, which was also supported by correlation analyses. In the visual modality no difference was reported between any of the groups (see Fig 7.a., bottom graph).

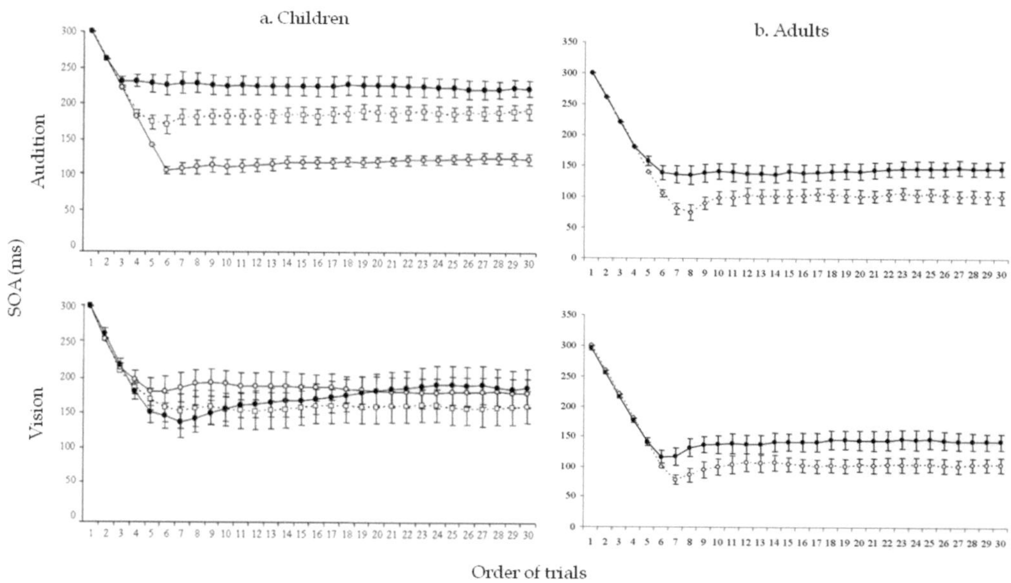

Fig. 7. Mean auditory and visual stream segregation thresholds (average ISI on the last 10 trials) together with standard error bars in children (a.; dyslexic readers, black dots; poor readers, white squares; good readers, white dots) and adults (b.; dyslexic readers, black dots; skilled readers, white dots). Adapted from Lallier et al. 2009.

The second experiment (see Fig 7.b) was carried out with 10 skilled readers and 10 dyslexic young adults. As a whole, the dyslexic group showed difficulties in performing a spoonerism task, reflecting poor phonological awareness skills. Furthermore, the group presented a VA Span disorder as compared to controls, illustrated by difficulties on both the whole and the partial report tasks (Lallier, 2009). Results on the two stream segregation tasks showed that dyslexic adults obtained auditory and visual higher stream segregation thresholds as compared to the control group: this means that they needed more time than the control individuals between successive stimuli, i.e., longer ISIs, in order to perceive them as single entities. The results on both the visual and the auditory task thus reflected amodal SAS skills in the dyslexic group. In addition, significant relationships were found in the whole group of participants (dyslexic and control individuals) between SAS, poor reading and poor phonological skills, even after controlling for non-verbal IQ and chronological age. No such relation was found between VA Span skills and visual or auditory stream segregation thresholds (Lallier, 2009).

Overall, the results of the two experiments of Lallier et al. (2009) with children and adults support the view that auditory SAS impacts on phonological abilities, and plays a role in developmental dyslexia. In addition, the comparison between children and adult results suggests that a visual sequential disorder in dyslexia might emerge at a later developmental stage, when the visual system normally becomes more expert at rapid temporal processing.

In the second study (Lallier et al., 2010c), we quantified both auditory and visual stream segregation thresholds in 13 dyslexic young adults with a phonological awareness deficit as a group (poor performance on phonemic deletion and spoonerisms) and 13 control participants, matched for cognitive abilities. Consistent with Lallier et al. (2009), we found higher auditory and visual stream segregation thresholds in the dyslexic group as compared to the controls, thus evidence for amodal SAS skills. We then used electrophysiological measures allowing us to capture the electric activity produced naturally by the brain, to determine to what extent brain responses of these dyslexic participants would reflect their atypical perception of visual and auditory stimulus sequences. For the electrophysiological experiment, the auditory and visual sequences administered to the participants varied according to different tempos that were carefully chosen based on preliminarily obtained thresholds. Participants were presented with blocks of 4 min-long sequences of either the same auditory or the same visual stimuli as those used in the stream segregation tasks, whilst their brain responses were recorded by electroencephalography (i.e., EEG). They were asked to press a button as soon as they perceived a change in the speed of stimulus alternation, and were not told or asked anything about the perception of unique or distinct streams. Electrophysiological brain responses were recorded during the task, and interpreted as an index of stimulus sequence perception. Results showed that dyslexic participants presented atypical auditory and visual brain responses to tempos variations within stimulus sequences as compared to controls.

Overall, these results strongly support the hypothesis that SAS in dyslexic participants might be responsible for their atypical perception of rapid sequential stimulus sequences in both the auditory and the visual modalities. In the auditory modality, the atypical brain response elicited by rapid stimulus sequences is likely to index the atypical perception of auditory speech streams in dyslexic participants with a phonological disorder. In the visual modality, such abnormal rapid stimulus sequences perception could well relate to difficulties encountered by dyslexic participants in rapidly shifting their attention along the orthographic sequences composing texts (Hari & Renvall, 2001). The direct links between stream segregation tasks and speech and orthographic strings processing still need to be investigated. Furthermore, our results bring new evidence supporting the link between amodal SAS and the phonological impairment in developmental dyslexia.

In our previous studies evaluating attentional blink or stream segregation performance in dyslexic individuals, links between sequential attention deficits and the phonological and VA Span disorders were studied by means of correlation analyses carried out on the whole sample of participants (i.e., including both dyslexic and skilled readers), a choice that may raise some methodological concerns. Furthermore, phonological and VA Span disorders were always defined regarding the whole group of dyslexic participants (except for Lallier et al., 2010a).

The next study conducted in adults (Lallier, Thierry, & Tainturier, Under Review b; Lallier, Thierry, Valdois & Tainturier, In progress b) was conducted in order to ascertain the relationships between amodal SAS skills and both phonological and VA Span disorders in a more stringent way. We examined performance of three groups of participants on the stream segregation tasks. These three groups included (i) a group of nine skilled reader adults, (ii) a group of nine dyslexic adults each of whom exhibited a phonological deficit at the individual level (i.e., impaired on three phonological measures out of five, among phonological working memory, phonological fluency, phonemic deletion, and spoonerism time and accuracy), and (iii) nine dyslexic adults without any phonological deficit. Regarding visual attention performance, the two dyslexic groups showed a significant VA Span deficit on the whole report task as compared to the controls. On the partial report task, the three groups of participants showed similar scores (Lallier et al., In progress b). Importantly, the three groups were matched for non-verbal IQ and chronological age, and the two dyslexic groups were matched for general reading and spelling abilities. Therefore, we were in presence of a relatively pure phonological dyslexic group, and a non-phonological dyslexic group with a VA Span disorder. In line with the hypothesis of a dissociation between phonological *versus* VA Span disorder and sequential *versus* simultaneous attention deficits in developmental dyslexia, only the dyslexic group with a phonological disorder exhibited higher auditory and marginally higher visual stream segregation thresholds as compared to the control group (see Fig 8).

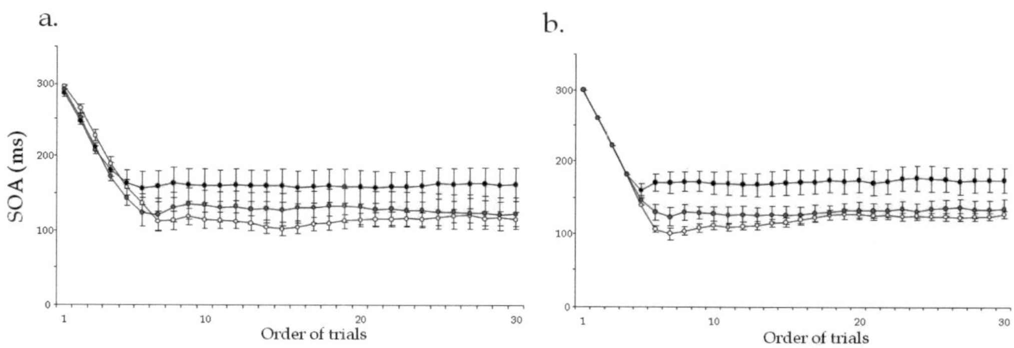

Fig. 8. Visual (a.) and auditory (b.) stream segregation thresholds together with standard error bars in the dyslexic group with a phonological disorder (black dots), the dyslexic group without phonological disorder (grey dots) and the control group (white dots). Adapted from Lallier et al., Under Review b, and Lallier et al., In progress b.

Importantly, auditory thresholds significantly differed between the two dyslexic groups. Looking at individual performance, 78% of participants with a phonological disorder (*versus* 11% without) were impaired on the auditory stream segregation task and 33% (*versus* 11%) on the visual task. These results strongly support the hypothesis of a link between auditory (and visual, but to a lesser extent) sequential deficits, impaired phonology, and reading disorders, but do not suggest any link between VA Span disorder and auditory or visual SAS in developmental dyslexia.

2.2.3 Amodal simultaneous processing assessment: Dichotic listening

In order to obtain a complete picture of the contribution of sequential and simultaneous skills to reading difficulties in the dyslexic population regarding auditory processing, we designed a task that we considered to be a reasonable auditory counterpart of the visual whole report task (Lallier, Donnadieu, & Valdois, Under Review a). That way, we aimed to assess the amodality of simultaneous attention in dyslexic children. We chose a dichotic listening paradigm (Cherry, 1953) which has broadly been used to assess simultaneous auditory attention (e.g., Asbjörnsen & Hugdahl, 1995). In dichotic tasks, different auditory sources of information are simultaneously displayed in the two ears. As opposed to the *focal* attention condition where participants have to report the stimuli presented in one ear only, the *non focal* attention reflect the performance of participants when they have to report the stimuli presented in the two ears. The latter condition makes the participants allocate their attention resources in parallel to the two ears and indexes some attention resources limitation. We measured the report scores of participants in the latter condition in order to quantify their simultaneous auditory attention abilities.

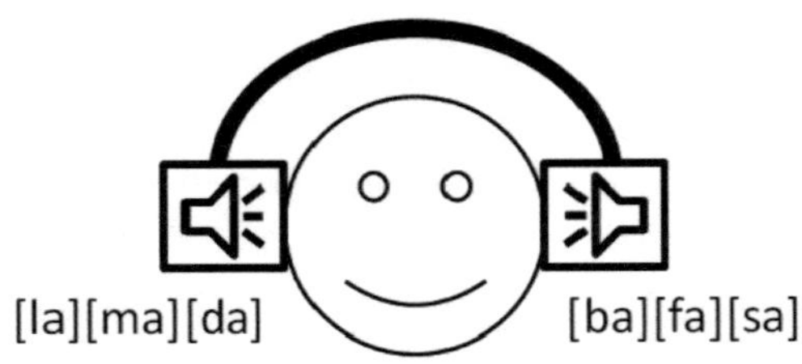

Fig. 9. Illustration of the dichotic listening task we used to assess simultaneous attention resources. From Lallier et al., Under Review a.

The dichotic sequences were composed of three syllables sequentially presented in the right ear and of three different syllables sequentially presented in the left ear (see Fig 9). More importantly, the two series of syllables were carefully synchronized so that participants had to process pairs of syllables simultaneously presented in the two ears. They were instructed to listen carefully to the syllables presented in their right ear and in their left ear and to report as many syllables as possible from both sides.

Because auditory syllables were used as stimuli, relations between dichotic performance and phonological processes were likely to be shown. We therefore assessed VA Span abilities, phoneme awareness skills and phonological short-term memory in dyslexic children together with their dichotic listening performance. We reasoned that if phonological and VA Span skills play different roles in reading acquisition and are respectively associated with sequential and simultaneous processes (Lallier et al., 2010a), performance on a task requiring a high degree of simultaneous resource allocation should fail to, or only weakly, relate to phonological skills, even when participants are presented with phonological stimuli. However, if poor dichotic listening performance is mainly driven by simultaneous processing difficulties and if the simultaneous processing disorder is amodal, then dyslexic children with a VA Span disorder should perform poorly on the dichotic listening task *whether or not* they exhibit associated phonological deficits. On the other hand, if dichotic listening poor performance is determined by difficulties in phonological/sequential processing abilities, then individuals with phonological deficits should perform poorly on the dichotic listening task regardless of their VA Span skills.

We assessed the dichotic listening performance of 17 dyslexic children and 17 skilled readers. Results showed that the dyslexic group exhibited difficulties in reporting the simultaneous syllables as compared to the controls. Moreover, in the dyslexic group, VA

Span skills correlated positively with dichotic listening scores while phonological skills did not correlate with either dichotic or VA Span measures. All the dyslexic children with a dichotic listening deficit showed a VA Span disorder, but the VA Span disorder was not systematically associated with poor dichotic listening. A high proportion of dyslexic children exhibited a phonological short-term memory or a phonemic awareness deficit whether or not they had difficulties on the dichotic listening task. Our findings suggest that processing simultaneous auditory stimuli in developmental dyslexia may be impaired regardless of any phonological deficit and be linked to similar difficulties in the visual modality.

3. Conclusion

This chapter aimed to clarify the nature of the temporal dimension of processing (sequential or simultaneous) relevant for the study of visual and auditory deficits (verbal or non-verbal) in developmental dyslexia. First, our review of the available data suggests that processes tapping into automatic attention mechanisms may be likely to highlight critical links between auditory and visual deficits and reading disorders. Second, our series of experiments provides new evidence for a potential dissociation between sequential and simultaneous processing deficits in developmental dyslexia and their respective links to distinct cognitive dyslexic profiles (VA Span and phonological disorders): when auditory automatic attentional shifting speed seems to clearly contribute to phonological processing (phonological awareness and phonological short-term memory in particular), the link between similar visual measures and reading is weaker, as previously suggested in the literature (e.g., Skottun, 2000). Our data further suggests that visual simultaneous disorders could extend over the auditory modality in participants with dyslexia regardless of their phonological skills.

3.1 The role of sequential *versus* simultaneous amodal attention processing in reading

When looking at what reading is, it seems obvious that both the auditory and visual perceptual-attentional systems have an important role to play. In their theoretical account integrating auditory and visual networks together with their role in developmental dyslexia, Pammer and Vidyasagar (2005) suggest that automatic spatial attentional orientation and focalization are the amodal mechanisms playing a fundamental role in reading acquisition. In the visual modality, such mechanisms would be in charge of screening and encoding at a pre-orthographic level the visual letter strings, such as coding letter positions within the string (e.g., Pammer, Lavis, Hansen, & Cornelissen, 2004), in order to facilitate grapheme-to-phoneme conversion rules acquisition. In the auditory modality, similar attentional mechanisms would be required to encode speech units to form adequate phonological representations (Hari & Renvall, 2001).

In the present chapter, we proposed that auditory and visual mechanisms engaged in reading acquisition require both sequential and simultaneous processes to encode phonological and orthographic inputs. The first one, a sequential attention mechanism, would lead the attentional focus to rapidly and automatically engage and disengage over speech streams and orthographic sequences, whilst being guided by salient and relevant cues (syllabic stress, Goswami, 2011; or visual syllable, Ans et al., 1998). The second one would be a simultaneous attention mechanism: because in real life situations the attended auditory and visual inputs very rarely correspond to one single small unit (such as a letter isolated on a blank page or a single phoneme presented in a quiet environment), simultaneous processing resources are required in order to integrate (VA Span hypothesis) or inhibit (noise exclusion deficit hypothesis, Sperling, Manis, & Seidenberg, 2005) all pieces of information presented at the same time (e.g., multi-letter strings or multi-speaker environments). Future studies will seek to determine to what extent these two mechanisms in charge of processing multiple inputs presented simultaneously (i.e., integrating *versus* filtering/inhibiting) contribute to literacy acquisition, and possibly independently of each other.

3.2 The hypothesis of different independent time scales auditory and visual processing and reading development?

Poeppel (2003) suggested that two types of time scales for auditory processing are relevant and important for language acquisition: one would be handled by a very high oscillatory auditory system, whereas the other would be linked to a low oscillatory auditory system. Interestingly, the latter could possibly relate to sequential processing, whereas the former could be more tightly related to the "simultaneous" dimension of processing which would in this case correspond to a sequential processing at very high rate. Future studies will aim to clarify whether these two time scales of processing could extend over the visual domain, and to what extent they would impact on reading acquisition. Moreover, it will be necessary to examine whether these two time scales of processing have different and possibly independent roles in literacy acquisition, and lead to different subtypes of developmental dyslexia.

4. Acknowledgment

The research presented in this chapter was funded by grants from the French "Ministère de l'Enseignement Supérieur et de la Recherche", the Fyssen foundation (postdoctoral fellowship) and the European commission (Marie Curie fellowship, FP7, people, BIRD project) attributed to M. Lallier. We thank all the dyslexic children and adults who took part in our studies and to Dr Catherine Billard, Andrea Reynolds, Polly Barr and Céline Prévost for their help in recruiting and testing the participants. We are very grateful to Dr Marie-Josèphe Tainturier, Prof Guillaume Thierry and Dr Sophie Donnadieu for their valuable help in this research.

5. References

Asbjornsen, A. E., & Hugdahl, K. (1995). Attentional Effects in Dichotic Listening. *Brain & Language,* Vol.49, No.3, (June 1995), pp. 189-201, **ISSN** 0093-934X.

Amitay, S., Ben-Yehudah, G., Banai, K., & Ahissar, M. (2002). Disabled readers suffer from visual and auditory impairments but not from a specific magnocellular deficit. *Brain,* Vol.125, No.10, (October 2002), pp. 2272-2285, ISSN 1460-2156.

Ans, B., Carbonnel, S., & Valdois, S. (1998). A connectionist multiple-trace memory model for polysyllabic word reading. *Psychological Review,* Vol.105, No.4, (October 1998), pp. 678-723, ISSN 0033-295X.

Au, A., & Lovegrove, B. (2001a). The role of visual and auditory temporal processing in reading irregular and nonsense words. *Perception,* Vol.30, pp. 1127-1142, ISSN 1468-4233.

Au, A., & Lovegrove, B. (2001b). Temporal processing ability in above average and average readers *Perception & Psychophysics,* Vol.63, No.1, pp. 48-55, ISSN 0031-5117.

Badcock, N. A., Hogben, J. H., & Fletcher, J. F. (2008). No differential attentional blink in dyslexia after controlling for baseline sensitivity. *Vision Research,* Vol.48, No.13, pp. 1497-1502, ISSN 0042-6989.

Bailey, P. J., & Snowling, M. J. (2002). Auditory processing and the development of language and literacy. *British Medical Bulletin,* Vol.63, pp. 135-146, ISSN 1471-8391.

Ben-Yehudah, G., Sackett, E., Malchi-Ginzberg, L., & Ahissar, M. (2001). Impaired temporal contrast sensitivity in dyslexics is specific to retain-and-compare paradigms. *Brain,* Vol.124, No.7, pp. 1381-1395, ISSN 1460-2156.

Benasich, A. A., & Tallal, P. (1996). Auditory temporal processing thresholds, habituation, and recognition memory over the 1st year. *Infant Behavior and Development,* Vol.19, No.3, pp. 339-357, ISSN 0163-6383.

Benasich, A. A., & Tallal, P. (2002). Infant discrimination of rapid auditory cues predicts later language impairment. *Behavioural Brain Research,* Vol.136, No.1, pp. 31-49, ISSN 0166-4328.

Bey, C., & McAdams, S. (2002). Schema-based processing in auditory scene analysis. *Perception & Psychophysics,* Vol.64, No.5, pp. 844-854 , SSN 0031-5117.

Boden, C., & Giaschi, D. (2007). M-stream deficits and reading-related visual processes in developmental dyslexia. *Psychological bulletin,* Vol.133, No.2, pp. 346-366, ISSN 0033-2909.

Bosse, M. L., Tainturier, M. J., & Valdois, S. (2007). Developmental dyslexia: the visual attention span deficit hypothesis. *Cognition,* Vol.104, No.2, pp. 198-230, ISSN 0010-0277.

Bosse, M. L., & Valdois, S. (2009). Influence of the visual attention span on child reading performance: a cross-sectional study. *Journal of Research in Reading,* Vol.32, pp. 230–253, ISSN 1467-9817.

Bretherton, L., & Holmes, V. M. (2003). The relationship between auditory temporal processing, phonemic awareness, and reading disability. *Journal of Experimental Child Psychology,* Vol.84, No.3, pp. 218-243, ISSN 0022-0965.

Bregman, A. S., & Achim, A. (1973). Visual stream segregation. *Perception & Psychophysics,* Vol.13, No.3, pp. 451-454, ISSN 0031-5117.

Castles, A., & Coltheart, M. (2004). Is there a causal link from phonological awarness to sucess in learning to read? *Cognition,* Vol.91, pp. 77-111, **ISSN** 0010-0277.

Cestnick, L., & Coltheart, M. (1999). The relationship between language-processing and visual-processing deficits in developmental dyslexia. *Cognition,* Vol.71, No.3, pp. 231-255, **ISSN** 0010-0277.

Cherry, E. C. (1953). Some experiments on the recognition of speech, with one and two ears. *Journal of the Acoustical Society of America,* Vol.25, pp. 975-979, ISSN 0001-4966.

Chiappe, P., Stringer, R., Siegel, L. S., & Stanovich, K. E. (2002). Why the timing deficit hypothesis does not explain reading disabilitiy in adults. *Reading and Writing: An interdisciplinary Journal,* Vol.15, pp. 73-107, ISSN 0922-4777.

Clarke, S., Bellmann, A., Meuli, R. A., Assal, G., & Steck, A. J. (2000). Auditory agnosia and auditory spatial deficits following left hemispheric lesions: evidence for distinct processing pathways. *Neuropsychologia,* Vol.38, No.6, pp. 797-807.

Cornelissen, P., Richardson, A., Mason, A., Fowler, S., & Stein, J. (1995). Contrast sensitivity and coherent motion detection measured at photopic luminance levels in dyslexics and controls. *Vision Research,* Vol.35, No.10, pp. 1483-1494, ISSN 0042-6989.

Cousineau, D., Charbonneau, D., & Jolicoeur, P. (2006). Parameterizing the attentional blink effect. *Canadian Journal of Experimental Psychology,* Vol.60, No.3, pp. 175-189, ISSN 1196-1961.

De Martino, S., Espesser, R., Rey, V., & Habib, M. (2001). The "temporal processing deficit" hypothesis in dyslexia: new experimental evidence. *Brain & Cognition,* Vol.45. No.1-2, pp. 104-108, ISSN 0278-2626.

Dubois, M., Kyllingsbæk, S., Prado, C., Musca, S.C., Peiffer, E., Lassus-Sangosse, D., et al. (2010). Fractionating the multicharacter processing deficit in developmental dyslexia: Evidence from two case studies. *Cortex,* Vol. 46, No.6, pp.717-738, ISSN 0010-9452.

Eddins, D. A., & Green, D. M. (1995). *Temporal integration and temporal resolution*. Academic Press, In M. BCJ (Ed.), Hearing. San Diego, California, U.S.A.

Edwards, V. T., Giaschi, D. E., Dougherty, R. F., Edgell, D., Bjornson, B. H., Lyons, C., et al. (2004). Psychophysical indexes of temporal processing abnormalities in children with developmental dyslexia. *Developmental Neuropsychology,* Vol.25, No.3, pp. 321-354, ISSN 0012-1649.

Ehri, L. C., Nunes, S. R., Willows, D. M., Schuster, B. V., Yaghoub-Zadeh, Z., & Shanahan, T. (2001). Phonemic awareness instruction helps children learn to read : Evidence from the National Reading panel's meta-analysis. *Reading Research Quarterly,* Vol.36, No.3, pp. 250-287, ISSN 1936-2722.

Facoetti, A., Lorusso, M. L., Paganoni, P., Umilta, C., & Mascetti, G. G. (2003). The role of visuospatial attention in developmental dyslexia: evidence from a rehabilitation study. *Brain Research Cognitive Brain Research,* Vol.15, No.2, pp. 154-164, ISSN 1872-6348.

Facoetti, A., & Molteni, M. (2001). The gradient of visual attention in developmental dyslexia. *Neuropsychologia,* Vol.39, No.4, pp. 352-357, ISSN 0028-3932.

Facoetti, A., Paganoni, P., Turatto, M., Marzola, V., & Mascetti, G. G. (2000). Visual-spatial attention in developmental dyslexia. *Cortex,* Vol.36, No.1, pp. 109-123, ISSN 0010-9452.

Facoetti, A., Ruffino, M., Peru, A., Paganoni, P., & Chelazzi, L. (2008). Sluggish engagement and disengagement of non-spatial attention in dyslexic children. *Cortex,* Vol.44, No.9, pp. 1221-1233, ISSN 0010-9452.

Facoetti, A., Trussardi, A. N., Ruffino, M., Lorusso, M. L., Cattaneo, C., Galli, R., Molteni, M., & Zorzi M. (2010). Multisensory Spatial Attention Deficits Are Predictive of Phonological Decoding Skills in Developmental Dyslexia. *Journal of Cognitive Neuroscience*. Vol.22, No.5, pp. 1011-1125, ISSN 1530-8898.

Facoetti, A., & Turatto, M. (2000). Asymmetrical visual fields distribution of attention in dyslexic children: a neuropsychological study. *Neuroscience Letters,* Vol.290, No.3, pp. 216-218, ISSN 0304-3940.

Facoetti, A., Zorzi, M., Cestnick, L., Lorusso, M. L., Molteni, M., Paganoni, P., et al. (2006). The relationship between visuo-spatial attention and nonword reading in developmental dyslexia. *Cognitive Neuropsychology,* Vol.23, No.6, pp. 841-855, ISSN 1464-0627.

Farmer, M. E., & Klein, M. R. (1995). The evidence for a temporal processing deficit linked to dyslexia: A review. *Psychonomic Bulletin & Review,* Vol.2, No.4, pp. 460-493, ISSN 1531-5320.

Friedmann N, & Nachman-Katz, I. (2004) Developmental neglect dyslexia in a Hebrew-reading child. *Cortex,* Vol.40, pp. 301-313, ISSN 0010-9452.

Friedmann, N. & Rahamim, E. (2007) Developmental letter position dyslexia. *Journal of Neuropsychology,* Vol.1, pp. 201- 236, ISSN 1748-6653.

Galaburda, A. M., Menard, M. T., & Rosen, G. D. (1994). Evidence for aberrant auditory anatomy in developmental dyslexia. *Proceedings of the National Academy of Sciences,* Vol.91, No.17, pp. 8010-8013, ISSN 0027-8424.

Geiger, G., Cattaneo, C., Galli, R., Pozzoli, U., Lorusso, M. L., Facoetti. A., and Molteni M. (2008) Wide and diffuse perceptual modes characterize dyslexics in vision and audition. *Perception.* Vol.37, No.11, pp. 1745-64, ISSN 1468-4233.

Goswami, U., (2011). A temporal sampling framework for developmental dyslexia. *Trends in Cognitive Sciences,* Vol.15, No.1, pp.3–10, ISSN 1364-6613.

Habib, M., Rey, V., Daffaure, V., Camps, R., Espesser, R., Joly-Pottuz, B., et al. (2002). Phonological training in children with dyslexia using temporally modified speech: a three-step pilot investigation. *International Journal of Language & Communication Disorders,* Vol.37, No.3, pp. 289-308, ISSN 1460-6984.

Hairston, W. D., Burdette, J. H., Flowers, D. L., Wood, F. B., & Wallace, M. T. (2005). Altered temporal profile of visual-auditory multisensory interactions in dyslexia. *Experimental Brain Research,* Vol.166, No.3-4, pp. 474-480, ISSN 1432-1106.

Hari, R., & Kiesilä, P. (1996). Deficit of temporal auditory processing in dyslexic adults. *Neuroscience Letters,* Vol.205, No.2, pp. 138-140, ISSN 0304-3940.

Hari, R., & Renvall, H. (2001). Impaired processing of rapid stimulus sequences in dyslexia. *Trends in Cognitive Sciences,* Vol.5, No.12, pp. 525-532, ISSN 1364-6613.

Hari, R., Renvall, H., & Tanskanen, T. (2001). Left minineglect in dyslexic adults. *Brain,* Vol.124, No.7, pp. 1373-1380, ISSN 1460-2156.

Hari, R., Saaskilahti, A., Helenius, P., & Uutela, K. (1999a). Non-impaired auditory phase locking in dyslexic adults. *Neuroreport,* Vo.10, No.11, pp. 2347-2348, ISSN 0959-4965.

Hari, R., Valta, M., & Uutela, K. (1999b). Prolonged attentional dwell time in dyslexic adults. *Neuroscience Letters,* Vol.271, No.3, pp. 202-204, ISSN 0304-3940.

Heim, S., Freeman, R. B., Jr., Eulitz, C., & Elbert, T. (2001). Auditory temporal processing deficit in dyslexia is associated with enhanced sensitivity in the visual modality. *Neuroreport,* Vol.12, No.3, pp. 507-510, ISSN 0959-4965.

Heim, S., Tschierse, J., Amunts, K., Wilms, M., Vossel, S., Willmes, K., et al. (2008). Cognitive subtypes of dyslexia. *Acta Neurobiologicae Experimentalis,* Vol.68, No.1, pp. 73-89

Helenius, P., Salmelin, R., Service, E., & Connolly, J. F. (1999). Semantic cortical activation in dyslexic readers. *Journal of cognitive neuroscience,* Vol.11, No.5, pp. 535-550, ISSN 1530-8898.

Hood, M., & Conlon, E. (2004). Visual and auditory temporal processing and early reading development. *Dyslexia,* Vo.10, No.3, pp. 234-252, ISSN 1099-0909.

Hulme, C., Hatcher, P. J., Nation, K., Brown, A., Adams, J., & Stuart, G. (2002). Phoneme Awareness Is a Better Predictor of Early Reading Skill Than Onset-Rime Awareness. *Journal of Experimental Child Psychology,* Vol.82, No.1, pp. 2-28, ISSN 0022-0965.

Husain, M., Shapiro, K., Martin, J., & Kennard, C. (1997). Abnormal temporal dynamics of visual attention in spatial neglect patients. *Nature,* Vol.385, No.6612, pp. 154-156, ISSN 1476-4687.

Hutzler, F., Kronbichler, M., Jacobs, A. M., & Wimmer, H. (2006). Perhaps correlational but not causal: no effect of dyslexic readers' magnocellular system on their eye movements during reading. *Neuropsychologia,* Vol.44, *No.*4, pp. 637-648.

Jaskowski, P., & Rusiak, P. (2008). Temporal order judgment in dyslexia. *Psychological Research,* Vol.72, No.1, pp. 65-73, ISSN 1430-2772.

Jones, M. W., Branigan, H. P., & Kelly, M. L. (2008). Visual deficits in developmental dyslexia: relationships between non-linguistic visual tasks and their contribution to components of reading. *Dyslexia,* Vol.14, No.2, pp. 95-115, ISSN 1099-0909.

Kidd, J. C., & Hogben, J. H. (2007). Does the auditory saltation stimulus distinguish dyslexic from competently reading adults? *Journal of Speech, Language and Hearing Research,* Vol.50, No.4, pp. 982-998, ISSN 0022-4685.

Kronbichler, M., Hutzler, F., & Wimmer, H. (2002). Dyslexia: verbal impairments in the absence of magnocellular impairments. *Neuroreport,* Vol.13, No.5, pp. 617-620, ISSN 0959-4965.

Laasonen, M., Service, E., & Virsu, V. (2001). Temporal order and processing acuity of visual, auditory, and tactile perception in developmentally dyslexic young adults. *Cognitive and Affective Behavioral Neurosciences,* Vol.1, No.4, pp. 394-410, ISSN 15307026.

Laasonen, M., Tomma-Halme, J., Lahti-Nuuttila, P., Service, E., & Virsu, V. (2000). Rate of information segregation in developmentally dyslexic children. *Brain & Language,* Vol.75, No.1, pp. 66-81, ISSN 0093-934X.

Lallier, M. (2009). Spécificités des troubles auditivo- et visuo-attentionels dans la dyslexie développementale. Doctoral dissertation, Université Pierre Mendès France, Grenoble, France.

Lallier, M., Berger, C., Donnadieu, S., & Valdois, S. (2010a). A case study of developmental phonological dyslexia: Is the attentional deficit in the perception of rapid stimuli sequences amodal? *Cortex.* Vol.43, No.2, pp. 231-241, ISSN 0010-9452.

Lallier, M., Donnadieu, S., & Valdois, S. (2010b). Visual attentional blink in dyslexic children: parameterizing the deficit. *Vision Research,* Vol.50, pp. 1855-1861, ISSN 0042-6989.

Lallier, M., Donnadieu, S., & Valdois, S. (Under Review a). How much are phonological and visual attention span disorders linked to simultaneous auditory processing deficits in developmental dyslexia? *Annals of Dyslexia,* ISSN 0736-9387

Lallier, M., Carreiras, M., Tainturier, & Thierry, G. (In progress a). Linguistic rhythm shapes auditory temporal attention: Behavioral evidence in Welsh/English bilinguals.

Lallier, M., Tainturier, M. J., Dering, R. B., Donnadieu, S., Valdois, S., & Thierry, G. (2010c). Behavioural and ERPevidence for amodal sluggish attentional shifting in dyslexic adults. *Neuropsychologia,* Vol.48, No.14, pp. 4125-4135, ISSN 0028-3932.

Lallier, M., Thierry, G., & Tainturier, M. J. (Under Review b). On the importance of considering individual profiles when investigating the role of auditory sequential deficits in dyslexia. *Cognition,* ISSN 0010-0277.

Lallier, M., Thierry, G., Valdois, S., & Tainturier, M. J. (In progress b). Is there a link between phonological processing deficits and rapid visual sequential processing deficits in developmental dyslexia?

Lallier, M., Thierry, G., Tainturier, M. J., Donnadieu, S., Peyrin, C., Billard, C., & Valdois, S. (2009). Auditory and visual stream segregation in children and adults: An assessment of the amodality assumption of the 'sluggish attentional shifting' theory. *Brain Research,* Vol.1302, pp. 132-147, ISSN 1872-6348.

Landerl, K. & Willburger, E. (2010). Temporal processing, attention, and learning disorders. *Learning and individual differences.* Vol.5, No.5. (October 2010), pp. 393-401, ISSN 1041-6080.

Livingstone, M. S., Rosen, G. D., Drislane, F. W., & Galaburda, A. M. (1991). Physiological and anatomical evidence for a magnocellular defect in developmental dyslexia. *Proceedings of the National Academy of Science,* Vol.88, pp. 7943-7947, ISSN 0027-8424.

Liddle, E. B., Jackson, J. M., Rorden, C., & Jackson S. R. (2009). Lateralized temporal order judgment in dyslexia. *Neuropsychologia,* Vol.47, No.14, (December 2009), pp. 3244-3254, ISSN 0028-3932.

Llinas, R. (1993). Is dyslexia a dysynchronia? *Annals of the New York Academy of Sciences,* Vol.682, pp. 48-56, ISSN 1749-6632.

Lobier, M., Przybylski, L., & Valdois, S. (Submitted). Letters in unrelated consonant strings are processed simultaneously.

Lobier, M., Lassus-Sangosse, D., Zoubrinetzki, R. & Valdois, S. (In press). The visual attention span is visual and not verbal. *Cortex,* ISSN 0010-9452.

Lorusso, M. L., Facoetti, A., & Molteni, M. (2004). Hemispheric, attentional, and processing speed factors in the treatment of developmental dyslexia. *Brain & Cognition,* Vol.55, No.2, pp. 341-348, ISSN 0278-2626.

Lorusso, M. L., Facoetti, A., Toraldo, A., & Molteni, M. (2005). Tachistoscopic treatment of dyslexia changes the distribution of visual-spatial attention. *Brain & Cognition,* Vol.57, No.2, pp. 135-142, ISSN 0278-2626.

May, J. G., Williams, M. C., & Dunlap, W. P. (1988). Temporal order judgements in good and poor readers. *Neuropsychologia,* Vol.26, No.6, pp. 917-924, ISSN 0028-3932.

Marshall, J. C. (2001). Auditory neglect and right parietal cortex. *Brain,* Vol.124, No.4, pp. 645-646, ISSN 1460-2156.

McLean, G. M. T., Stuart, G. W., Coltheart, V., Castles, A. (2011) Visual temporal processing in dyslexia and the magnocellular deficit theory: The need for speed? *Journal of Experimental Psychology: Human Perception and Performance,* (August 2011), ISSN 0096-1523.

Meyler, A., & Breznitz, Z. (2005). Visual, auditory and cross-modal processing of linguistic and nonlinguistic temporal patterns among adult dyslexic readers. *Dyslexia,* Vol.11, No.2, pp. 93-115, ISSN 1099-0909.

Pammer, K., Lavis, R., Hansen, P., & Cornelissen, P. L. (2004). Symbol-string sensitivity and children's reading. *Brain & Language,* Vol.89, No.3, pp. 601-610, **ISSN** 0093-934X.

Pammer, K., & Vidyasagar, T. R. (2005). Integration of the visual and auditory networks in dyslexia: a theoretical perspective. *Journal of Research in Reading,* Vol.28, No.3, pp. 320, ISSN 1467-9817.

Pernet, C. Valdois, S., Celsis, P. & Démonet, J.F. (2006). Lateral masking, levels of processing and stimulus category: A comparative study between normal and dyslexic readers, *Neuropsychologia,* 44, 2374-2385.

Peyrin, C., Démonet, J.F., N'Guyen-Morel, M. A., Le Bas, JF & Valdois, S. (2011). Superior parietal lobe dysfunction in a homogeneous group of dyslexic children with a single visual attention span disorder. *Brain and Language,* Vol.118, No.3, pp. 128-138, **ISSN:** 0093-934X

Peyrin, C., Lallier, & Valdois, S. (2008). Visual attention span brain mechanisms in normal and dyslexic readers. In M. Baciu (Ed.), Neuropsychology and cognition of language Behavioural, neuropsychological and neuroimaging studies of spoken and written language (pp. 22-4).

Peyrin, C., Lallier, M., Baciu, M., Démonet, Le Bas, J.F., & Valdois S. (In press). Dissociation of phonological and visuo-attentional processing in dyslexia: FMRI evidence from two case reports. *Brain and Language.*

Poeppel, D. (2003). The analysis of speech in different temporal integration windows: cerebral lateralization as 'asymmetric sampling in time'. *Speech Communication,* Vol.41, pp. 245–255, ISSN 0167-6393.

Ram-Tsur, R., Faust, M., & Zivotofsky, A. Z. (2006). Sequential processing deficits of reading disabled persons is independent of inter-stimulus interval. *Vision Research,* Vol.46, No.22, pp. 3949-3960, ISSN 0042-6989.

Ram-Tsur, R., Faust, M., & Zivotofsky, A. Z. (2008). Poor performance on serial visual tasks in persons with reading disabilities: impaired working memory? *Journal of Learning Disabilities,* Vol.41, No.5, pp. 437-450, ISSN 1538-4780.

Rayner, K., Pollatsek, A., & Bilsky, A. (1995). Can a temporal processing deficit account for dyslexia? *Psychonomic Bulletin & Review,* Vol.2, No.4, pp. 501–507, ISSN 1531-5320.

Ramus, F., Rosen, S., Dakin, S. C., Day, B. L., Castellote, J. M., White, S., et al. (2003). Theories of developmental dyslexia: insights from a multiple case study of dyslexic adults. *Brain,* Vol.126, No.4, pp. 841-865, ISSN 1460-2156.

Raymond, J. E., Shapiro, K. L., & Arnell, K. M. (1992). Temporary suppression of visual processing in an RSVP task: an attentional blink? *Journal of Experimantal Psychology: Human, Perception and Performance,* Vol.18, No.3, pp. 849-860, ISSN 0096-1523.

Reed, M. A. (1989). Speech perception and the discrimination of brief auditory cues in reading disabled children. *Journal of Experimental Child Psychology,* Vol.48, No.2, pp. 270-292, ISSN 0022-0965.

Robertson, E. K., Joanisse, M. F., Desroches, A. S., & Ng, S (2009). Categorical speech perception deficits distinguish language and reading impairments in children. *Developmental Science,* Vol.12, No.5, pp. 753-765, ISSN 1467-7687.

Rouse, H. J., & Wilshire, C. E. (2007). Comparison of phonological and whole-word treatments for two contrasting cases of developmental dyslexia. *Cognitive Neuropsychology,* Vol.24, No.8, pp. 817-842, ISSN 1464-0627.

Schäffler, T., Sonntag, J., Hartnegg, K., & Fischer, B. (2004). The effect of practice on low-level auditory discrimination, phonological skills, and spelling in dyslexia. *Dyslexia,* Vol.10, No.2, pp. 119-130, ISSN 1099-0909.

Share, D. L., Jorm, A. F., Maclean, N. R., & Matthews, R. (2002). Temporal processing and reading disability. *Reading and Writing: An Interdisciplinary Journal,* Vol.15, pp. 151-178, ISSN 0922-4777.

Sireteanu, R., Goebel, C., Goertz, R., & Wandert, T. (2006). Do children with developmental dyslexia show a selective visual attention deficit? *Strabismus,* Vol.14, No.2, pp. 85-93, ISSN 0927-3972.

Sireteanu, R., Goertz, R., Bachert, I., & Wandert, T. (2005). Children with developmental dyslexia show a left visual "minineglect". *Vision Research,* Vol.45, No.25-26, pp. 3075-3082, ISSN 0042-6989.

Skottun, B. C. (2000). On the conflicting support for the magnocellular-deficit theory of dyslexia: Response to Stein, Talcott and Walsh (2000). *Trends in Cognitive Sciences,* Vol.4, No.6, pp. 211-212, ISSN 1364-6613.

Skoyles, J., & Skottun, B. C. (2004). On the prevalence of magnocellular deficits in the visual system of non-dyslexic individuals. *Brain and Language,* Vol.88, No.1, pp. 79-82, **ISSN:** 0093-934X.

Slaghuis, W. L., & Ryan, J. F. (1999). Spatio-temporal contrast sensitivity, coherent motion, and visible persistence in developmental dyslexia. *Vision Research,* Vol.39, No.3, pp. 651-668, ISSN 0042-6989.

Snowling, M. J. (2000). *Dyslexia.* Oxford: Blackwell.

Sperling, A. J., Lu, Z. L., Manis, F. R., & Seidenberg, M. S. (2005). Deficits in perceptual noise exclusion in developmental dyslexia. *Nature Neuroscience,* Vol.8, pp. 862–863, ISSN 1546-1726.

Stein, J., & Talcott, J. (1999). Impaired Neuronal Timing in Developmental Dyslexia-The Magnocellular Hypothesis. *Dyslexia,* Vol.5, pp. 59–77, ISSN 1099-0909.

Stein, J., & Walsh, V. (1997). To see but not to read; the magnocellular theory of dyslexia. *Trends in Neuroscience,* Vol.20, No.4, pp. 147-152, ISSN 1364-6613.

Talcott, J. B., Hansen, P. C., Assoku, E. L., & Stein, J. F. (2000). Visual motion sensitivity in dyslexia: evidence for temporal and energy integration deficits. *Neuropsychologia,* Vol.38, No.7, pp. 935-943, ISSN 0028-3932.

Tallal, P. (1980). Auditory temporal perception, phonics, and reading disabilities in children. *Brain and Language,* Vol.9, No.2, pp. 182-198, **ISSN:** 0093-934X.

Tallal, P., & Piercy, M. (1973). Defects of non-verbal auditory perception in children with developmental aphasia. *Nature,* Vol.241, No.5390, pp. 468-469, ISSN 1476-4687.

Tallal, P., & Piercy, M. (1974). Developmental aphasia: rate of auditory processing and selective impairment of consonant perception. *Neuropsychologia,* Vol.12, No.1, pp. 83-93, ISSN 0028-3932.

Trussell, L. O. (1999). Synaptic mechanisms for coding timing in auditory neurons. *Annual Review of Physiology,* Vol.61, pp. 447-496, ISSN 00664278.

Vachon, F., & Tremblay, S. (2008). Modality-specific and amodal sources of interference in the attentional blink. *Perception & Psychophysics,* Vol.70, No.6, pp. 1000-1015, SSN 0031-5117.

Valdois. S & Bosse, M.L. (Submitted). The phonological and visual attention span bases of orthographic knowledge acquisition.

Valdois, S., Bosse, M. L., Ans, B., Carbonnel, S., Zorman, M., David, D., et al. (2003). Phonological and visual processing deficits can dissociate in developmental dyslexia: Evidence from two case studies. *Reading and Writing: An interdisciplinary Journal,* Vol.16, pp. 541-572, ISSN 0922-4777.

Valdois, S., Lassus-Sangosse, D. & Lobier, M. (in press). The visual nature of the visual attention span disorder in developmental dyslexia. In J. Stein & Z. Kapula, Visual aspects of dyslexia, Oxford University Press.

Van Ingelghem, M., Van Wieringen, A., Wouters, J., Vandenbussche, E., Onghena, P., & Ghesquière, P. (2001). Psychophysical evidence for a general temporal processing deficit in children with dyslexia. *Neuroreport,* Vol.12, No.16, pp. 3603-3607, ISSN 0959-4965.

Van Noorden, L. P. A. S. (1975). *Temporal coherence in the perception of tone sequences.* Holland, Eindhoven.

Vellutino, F. R., Fletcher, J. M., Snowling, M. J., & Scanlon, D. M. (2004). Specific reading disability (dyslexia): what have we learned in the past four decades? *Journal of Child Psychology and Psychiatry,* Vol.45, No.1, pp. 2-40, ISSN 1469-7610.

Vidyasagar, T., & Pammer, K. (2010) Dyslexia: a deficit in visuo-spatial attention, not in phonological processing. *Trends in Cognitive sciences,* Vol.14, No.2, pp. 57-63, ISSN 1364-6613.

Visser, T. A., Boden, C., & Giaschi, D. E. (2004). Children with dyslexia: evidence for visual attention deficits in perception of rapid sequences of objects. *Vision Research,* Vol.44, No.21, pp. 2521-2535, ISSN 0042-6989.

Walker, K. M., Hall, S. E., Klein, R. M., & Phillips, D. P. (2006). Development of perceptual correlates of reading performance. *Brain Research,* Vol.1124, No.1, pp. 126-141, ISSN 1872-6348.

Welch, R. B., DuttonHurt, L. D., & Warren, D. H. (1986). Contributions of audition and vision to temporal rate perception. *Perception & Psychophysics,* Vol.39, No.4, pp. 294-300, SSN 0031-5117.

White, S., Milne, E., Rosen, S., Hansen, P., Swettenham, J., Frith, U., et al. (2006). The role of sensorimotor impairments in dyslexia: a multiple case study of dyslexic children. *Developmental Science,* Vol.9, No.3, pp. 237-255, ISSN 1467-7687.

Witton, C., Richardson, A., Griffiths, T. D., & Rees, A. (1997). Temporal pattern analysis in dyslexia. *British Journal of Audiology,* Vol.31, pp. 100-101, ISSN 1708-8186.

Witton, C., Stein, J. F., Stoodley, C. J., Rosner, B. S., & Talcott, J. B. (2002). Separate influences of acoustic AM and FM sensitivity on the phonological decoding skills of impaired and normal readers. *Journal of Cognitive Neuroscience,* Vol.14, No.6, pp. 866-874, ISSN 1530-8898.

Ziegler, J. C., Pech-Georgel, C., Dufau, S., & Grainger, J. (2010). Rapid processing of letters digits and symbols: What purely visual-attentional deficit in developmental dyslexia? *Developmental Science,* Vol.13, No.4, pp.F8–F14, ISSN 1363755X.

7

The Contribution of Handwriting and Spelling Remediation to Overcoming Dyslexia

Diane Montgomery
Middlesex University, London and Learning Difficulties Research Project, Essex, UK

1. Introduction

This research details results of casework, interviews, observations and case history analysis of over 1000 dyslexics and those in schools who have not been referred. Their skills have been compared with similar numbers of control subjects.

Subjects referred to English Dyslexia Centres tend to be those with the most severe problems. Normal provision has failed with them. Remedial help within class and as an additional support has also failed. In the English system the diagnosis of need for referral for specialist tuition thus comes late, often at the transfer age of 10/11 years when the pupil is about to leave primary and enter secondary school. The delay in diagnosis is due to the Statementing system needed to gain additional resources, the specialist tuition, and lack of agreed diagnostic indicators in the early years.

In the UK up to the age of 7 or 8 years additional support within school is given. If it has not worked then a formal diagnosis is sought and expertise from a specialist tutor is applied for. What this chapter will seek to show is that:

- Diagnosis of dyslexia does not need to be delayed for several years until the child is a three time failure but can take place in the Reception class by the class teacher with a small amount of training.
- Many of the so-called 'remedial' programmes are not effective but the few that are effective need to be implemented as soon as possible to obtain the best results.
- The focus on reading throughout dyslexia research and teaching practice is possibly a mistake.
- Dyslexia may not be 'cured' but can be overcome by the right sort of tuition in primary school.
- Dyslexia is not a disorder but caused by a deficit that results in an educational delay.
- If dyslexia is remediated there can be associated improved behavioural outcomes.

2. What casework shows that experiments may not

Experimental research requires that the researcher comes to cases with a hypothesis about the condition that is then tested and accepted or rejected. The hypothesis is based upon detailed research of the relevant literature but this can mean that it is defined by that research and the prevailing paradigm or 'zeitgeist' (Snow, 1973). In case work the researcher observes the case behaviours and tries to identify patterns that might lead to a hypothesis. For example:

> James is a 6.5 year old with an IQ of 147 on the Wechsler Intelligence Scale for Children (WISC). He has failed to learn to read and does not know any of the sounds or names of the alphabet. He can read some familiar common words and appears to know some of his reading books off by heart.
>
> The school has given him extra phonics and some one-on-one tuition. Because his parents are informed about dyslexia and well-off they have had him tested privately and this has enabled him to be more rapidly referred to the specialist tuition centre. The school has supported this because James was becoming very disruptive.

What the researcher puzzles over in this case and others like it is how such a bright child who can discuss God and the universe in great detail and is an expert on prehistoric monsters can fail to learn the 26 names and / or sounds of the alphabet. He has also failed to learn the names of the days of the week and the months in order and confuses left and right. On WISC his digit span and Coding scores were typically low compared with his overall results.

We might infer from this data as many do, the popular conclusion that he has a short term or working memory problem or a sequencing and orientation deficit. It follows from this that the remedial programme would focus upon improving memory and sequencing skills. Unfortunately it would be found to have little effect (Vellutino, 1979) as the inference from fact to theory is not quite so straightforward. In addition, there is a further problem in that training on hypothesised sub skills such as working memory (McGhee, 2010) and visual sequencing does not necessarily transfer to the skills of reading (Smith and Marx, 1972). This is often because the assumed subskills are not correctly defined (Montgomery, 1997a).

Our example case, James shows that his long term memory is very good as indicated by his general knowledge of astronomy and dinosaurs. Vellutino (1987) demonstrated that dyslexics' performance on visual memory items might be good but as soon as they had to verbalise or name the items as in some digit span tests performance was significantly poorer. Koppitz (1977) had found similar results in her Aural – Visual - Digit Span (VADS) test. She also showed that as reading improved so did the performance on the digit span test. Montgomery (1997a) showed similar results. What we can conclude is that working memory, sequencing deficits and failure to learn symbol-sound-correspondence or alphabetic knowledge are associated problems in dyslexia but are not necessarily the cause of it. They could all arise from a deeper problem.

2.1 Case study patterns

The case reports of more than 1000 dyslexics were recorded and analysed for patterns.

Pattern 1: Developmental dyslexia – these cases had a severe difficulty in learning to **read and spell**. None of them had a severe reading difficulty without a severe spelling problem.

Pattern 2: Developmental dysorthographia - these had a severe difficulty in learning to **spell** in the absence of a similar difficulty with reading. Some of the pupils had learned to read, self-taught at an early age or had an earlier reading difficulty that had cleared up. In these latter cases the residual signs were slow reading and difficulties in skimming and scanning text. All had poor writing and compositional skills. Very few had been referred for remedial help in school.

Pattern 3: Developmental dysgraphia– 30% of the sample had difficulties in the area of **handwriting** as a result of a motor coordination problem in the fine skills of penmanship. This was often in the absence of reading difficulties but appeared to have caused problems in spelling development through lack of writing practice.

Pattern 4: Developmental Coordination Difficulties (DCD - dyspraxia) – these had a difficulty with motor skills, even after a reasonable period of skill acquisition. Those with gross motor difficulties usually also had fine motor coordination difficulties especially with handwriting and problems with spelling.

Pattern 5: Specific Language Impairment (SLI) – these cases had a record of early speech therapy, late speech development, articulation difficulties or stuttering. Mild speech difficulties may go undetected well into school age and in their more subtle forms have also been implicated in dyslexia (Snowling and Stackhouse et al 1985). In each of her 20 pupils the dyslexia tutor (McMahon, 1988) found a previously unrecorded history of speech therapy, subtle word finding or slight articulation difficulties.

Pattern 6: Developmental dyscalculia – in some cases there was a recorded difficulty in acquiring arithmetic skills and concepts especially in reciting tables and mental arithmetic (Miles, 1993). Many of these difficulties could be accounted for by the difficulties in reading and writing and with the dyslexic problems in establishing verbal codes (Montgomery 2011c).

Pattern 7: Complex specific learning difficulties – in some unlucky cases there were several conditions, dyslexia, dyspraxia, dyscalculia and SLI. The complex condition made their educational needs difficult to deal with in mainstream or in the remedial setting. In these cases a school that specialised in dyslexia provision was essential to meet their needs but was not always available. Severe cases are also likely to find their way to specialist clinics and research centres and it is also the case that their complex difficulties often define the way research on dyslexia is pursued and the results it obtains.

Pattern 8: Comorbidity – Dyslexia was often found associated with other specific learning difficulties such as Attention Deficit Hyperactivity Disorder (ADHD), Asperger Syndrome and dyspraxia (Kutscher 2005). Research by Montgomery, (2000); and Silverman, (2004) showed that **handwriting difficulty** is an underlying problem in underachievement and can be overlooked. It is comorbid in dyslexia (30-63% Kaplan 2000; Montgomery 2007), ADHD (50% Kaplan, 2000) and Asperger Syndrome (90% Henderson and Green, 2001).

2.2 Ratio of boys to girls with dyslexia

The ratio of boys to girls in mainstream with dyslexia (N=537) was 1.2 to 1, respectively (Montgomery, 2008). In the remedial centres it was 4 to 1 and even 5 to 1 (Montgomery 1997a) boys to girls. This data was consistent with the findings of Rutter and Caspi et al. (2004) of a ratio across Europe of 1.4 to 1 in many thousands of cases. Montgomery (1997a) found that girls were referred a year later than boys and their problems were more intractable. It was more common that boys' records revealed a history of behaviour problems as a response to their difficulties and thus it was likely that help for them would be requested sooner.

Dyslexic girls' needs appear to be overlooked in many situations and this was also borne out by 18 female teachers on a Master's programme in SpLD who had had dyslexic difficulties (personal communication, 2006). They reported that they had not received any specialist help and had been left to manage their problems and been regarded as slower learners. This helped them understand their pupils' needs and brought them to the programme. They had residual problems with spelling and composition that we could use the programme itself to remediate. This meant that as they taught strategic approaches to spelling to their pupils they could learn to apply them to their own misspellings rather than use the rote methods they had adopted from their earlier schooling.

2.3 Patterns and definition

Developing definitions of reading, literacy and dyslexia is problematic in that although we can observe outcomes we cannot see the processes that lead to them. These processes have to be inferred from performance on tasks. When it was thought that dyslexics were 'Word Blind' it was inferred that they must have visual perceptual and visual memory problems for words so visual training was important in remedial reading programmes. The teaching method that fitted with this was 'Look and Say' for whole words. Only after a sight vocabulary of 50 words was known was it thought appropriate to teach some sounds or phonics to support word attack skills. But it was this regime that appeared to cause 4 per cent of children to become dyslexic in England (Rutter and Tizard et al. 1970) and only 1.5 per cent in Scotland (Clark, 1970) where the 'Phonics First' method had been retained. In her extensive research on the effects of Phonics First versus Look and Say teaching methods, Chall (1967, 1985) found similar results. What seems surprising is that these studies had so little impact for so long in the UK until phonics was promoted in Government reports (National Literacy Strategy; DfEE, 1998; Rose Report, 2006).

Reading sub skills are not clearly defined either. The processes in the **acquisition** of reading and spelling skills may not be the same as reading and spelling **development** when basic skills have been acquired and need to be practised and extended. Most children appear to be able to learn by any method that is well-structured and sequential, dyslexics do not. Most dyslexics these days do eventually learn to read and write but the delay can cause skills deficits of 2 to 5 years (Montgomery 2007) and it could be the effects of this that is what we observe and cause what some call disordered or 'bizarre'. Although much research has concentrated on early screening, if the definitions it operates on are imprecise, the results will be equivocal and fail to predict to later problems accurately.

It is necessary to consider the effect on teaching methods for acquisition. Already differential effects of Phonics versus Look and Say have been identified (Chall, 1967, 1985; Rose 2006). This might also have a bearing on theories of literacy development some of which suggest that logographic items appear first unrelated to sound properties in children's writing (Frith,, 1980). Could this be extended as a function of a teaching method that starts with Look and Say and is this true of Phonics First systems? Can children's scribbles tell us more than a little about dyslexia, theory and practice?

Definitions, as Snow (1973) showed, can define the research, the practice and the way we think about problems and can limit our propensity for appropriate action. For example the most widely held definition that emerged in the dyslexia field was based upon the extensive surveys of Clements (1966,). He formed the view that dyslexia was a difficulty in learning to read despite conventional instruction, adequate intelligence and sociocultural opportunity. He concluded that it was a disorder that was frequently constitutional in origin.

As can be seen, there are a number of problems with this definition. It is a definition by exclusion where once we have excluded low intelligence, poor teaching, disadvantaging backgrounds and so on then the problem we have left must be dyslexia. But *'dys-lexis'* simply means a difficulty with words, particularly in their written form, a circular definition. The fact that the difficulty is defined as a problem in 'learning to read' and 'words in their written form' focuses us upon reading; not literacy skills as a whole, and in particular ignores spelling. This focus has given reading difficulties a primacy over spelling that may not have been justified. It perhaps reflects the era when the definition was formed and the emphasis on reading in education that was opposed to methods that were regarded as 'the spelling grind'. It certainly reflects the situation in the UK both then and now and it has created problems both for teaching and for research and practice. It has directed remedial provision for five decades. In the document *Excellence for All Children* (DfEE, 1997, p. 15) it firmly states:"As teachers become increasingly adept at tackling reading difficulties children with specific learning difficulties (such as dyslexia) should in all but exceptional circumstances be catered for in mainstream schools". Teachers in the UK are thus indoctrinated with this belief and target their practices accordingly.

In addition, Clements' use of the word 'disorder' carries with it another whole set of assumptions and attitudes that may not be justified. It suggests that the system from which dyslexia emanates is disordered and dysfunctional, (Regrettably some medics have prescribed drug treatments). In the end it can suggest that dyslexia is not remediable but might be patched up or be compensated for, developmental delay is not considered.

More recently, the British Psychological Society established an expert group from amongst its members researching dyslexia to advise the Society. In 1989 it offered the following definition of dyslexia: "A specific difficulty in learning, constitutional in origin, in one or more of reading, spelling and written language which may be accompanied by a difficulty in number work. It is particularly related to mastering and using written language (alphabetic, numerical and musical notation) although often affecting oral language to some degree".

This definition covered the main areas of dyslexic difficulties that research had identified since Clements and tried to give focus to the key issues. Implicitly it tells us now that dyslexia may be found across the ability range and that written language or coded symbols applies to text, number and musical scores.

My main concern with this definition is that it suggests that a dyslexic might be thought to have only **one** of the areas of difficulty i.e. reading or spelling or number and this does not fit with the case histories of dyslexics already described. They do have reading AND spelling difficulties, but rarely if ever, reading without spelling difficulties, although a significant number seem to have spelling with no reading difficulties. For example, one cohort of dyslexics (N=288; Montgomery, 2007) in the case studies referred to a Dyslexia Centre all had significant reading and spelling problems (2.8 years below chronological age).

On the waiting group of 90 pupils one third of the group appeared to have spelling problems alone.

A general guideline was in operation based on government approved SEN training that reading itself must be 20 per cent lower than the pupil's chronological age to secure specialist remedial support. This ignored the issue that if the child was well above average ability 'mental age' we could expect them to have reading that is advanced towards this level. This meant that bright children with dyslexia might be put on a waiting list for remedial help but were less likely to receive support. Moreover, those whose reading was adequate but had severe spelling problems would not be referred but remain on the waiting list.

The British Dyslexia Association's (BDA, 2004) definition was somewhat influenced by that of the BPS but went on to extend it, to cover what teachers might observe in their dyslexics and touches on the old theories of origin: "Dyslexia is best described as a combination of abilities and difficulties, which affect the learning process in one or more of reading, spelling and writing. Accompanying weaknesses may be identified in areas of speed of processing, short term memory, sequencing, auditory and or visual perception, spoken language and motor skills. It is particularly related to mastering and using written language, which may include alphabetic, numeric and musical notation. Some children have outstanding creative skills, others have strong oral skills. Dyslexia occurs despite normal teaching, and is independent of socio-economic background or intelligence. It is, however, more easily detected in those with average or above average intelligence".

2.4 British Dyslexia Association definition, 2011

> "Dyslexia is a specific learning difficulty which mainly affects the development of literacy and language related skills. It is likely to be present at birth and to be lifelong in its effects. It is characterised by difficulties with phonological processing, rapid naming, working memory, processing speed, and the automatic development of skills that may not match up to an individual's other cognitive abilities. It tends to be resistant to conventional teaching methods, but its effects can be mitigated by appropriately specific intervention, including the application of information technology and supportive counseling".

In this definition we can see a 'work in progress' and a move to include the current main definitions on the nature and possible origins of the difficulty e.g. phonological processing, rapid naming, working memory, etc. It does however now include matching against other higher cognitive abilities not just chronological age – 'may not match up to an individual's other cognitive abilities', this will help some gifted dyslexics. There is a vast body of research on phonological difficulties in dyslexia and a strong belief in it as a theory of origin and it is now the prevailing paradigm (Frederickson and Frith et al, 1998; Snowling 2000, Vellutino, 1979). The argument goes that if the underlying phonological difficulties are addressed then the dyslexia will be remediated. But is this so?

3. An examination of some contrary views of dyslexia theory and research

3.1 Speed of auditory processing hypothesis

Tallal (1980; 1994) suggested that the dyslexic problem lies in an inability to process sensory input rapidly, particularly the auditory information contained in speech (Goswami, 2008).

The deficit is in the millisecond range and could be due to cell size differences in the left language hemisphere which are smaller in dyslexics (Holmes, 1994, p. 27). But is this size a cause or a result? The processing difficulty, it is argued would create problems in 'b' and d' perception for example which last only 40 milliseconds. When the sounds were separated by 100 milliseconds dyslexics could discriminate them.

The question we need to ask is why, when pupils are taught sounds of the letters in isolation and they hear, see and write them in Reception that dyslexics fail to learn them, why is speed an issue? It appears to become an issue only if we teach by 'Look and Say' or the sentence reading methods alone. Even if methods begin with Look and Say, why is it that the introduction of symbol-sound correspondence or phonics work later does not overcome the 'dyslexic' problem? Why does dyslexia also occur in languages such as Italian, which have closer symbol-to-sound correspondence than English? Galaburda (1993) argued that this deficit does not indicate a cause of dyslexia but is a secondary effect associated with a deeper cause.

It would appear that the research has not concentrated enough upon the early acquisition processes in literacy where much time in classrooms is also spent on saying and writing single sounds using the popular 'Letterland' approach (Manson and Wendon, 1997). Although young children have better ability than adults to discriminate between sounds, what we do know according to Liberman, Shankweiler et al. (1967) is that the human ear is incapable of distinguishing the sounds in syllables. Most often the initial sound is accompanied by a stronger burst of energy and thus is easier than the rest of the syllable to become aware of (for reading) then to segment (for spelling). The rest of the letters are shingled on top of each other making them impossible to separate out. Thus teaching 'c - a - t', 'cat' is set for failure. But teaching of onset and rime makes sense 'c - at'. Especially when we have a picture clue to help us. The 'I Spy something beginning with' - game is thus a very important part of early learning in school. Dyslexics were asked which segmentation format was easiest for them to remember and said that 'c / at' was much easier for them than 'ca / t' or 'c–a–t' (Montgomery 1997a). The point this illustrates is that if early reading skills are supported by spelling skills that include segmentation, especially onset and rime methods (Bryant and Bradley 1985) then speed of processing is irrelevant in the acquisition period.

3.2 Working memory hypothesis

Working memory as already noted, appears to increase as literacy skills improve (Koppitz, 1977). Recent research by Gathercole (2008) has shown that training working memory improves concentration and attention in ADHD. However, it did not enhance the literacy skills of a group of dyslexics (McGhee, 2010). Vellutino (1987) showed that the verbal encoding required in many memory tasks produced deficits in dyslexic performance even on visual items because of attempts to sub-vocalise or name the items. This was confirmed by Montgomery, (1997a) when dyslexics were asked to tell how they remembered a set of visual symbols such as the Coding tasks on WISC and Digit Span. Giving some sort of label assisted their recall thus it is not just a visual or visuo motor recall task but a verbal-visuo-motor task.

3.3 Double deficit hypothesis

This theory (Wolf and Bowers, 1999) holds that there is a deficit in phonological processing in addition to slowness in naming and decoding fluency (Wren, 2005). The evidence used is that dyslexics even when they have learned to read and write remain slow in their reading and decoding of text. However, Rumelhart & McClelland (1995) using computer simulations, concluded that the slowness in recovered dyslexics was due to their lack of experience of print compared with normal subjects. Teacher research (Taylor, 2007) confirmed this with dyslexic cases and normal poor readers.

3.4 The phonological processing hypothesis

This is the dominant current theory in dyslexia, which postulates that in the majority of cases, dyslexia is thought to be due to an underlying **verbal processing difficulty** particularly in the **phonological area** (Brown and Ellis, 1994; Bryant and Bradley, 1985; Chomsky, 1971; Frederickson, and Frith et al 1997; Frith, 1980; Golinkoff, 1978; Liberman, 1973; Snowling, 2000; Vellutino, 1979).

According to this theory, phonological processing deficit can give rise to:

- inability to appreciate rhyme
- lack of phonemic awareness
- poor development of alphabetic knowledge
- lack of development of symbol to sound correspondence
- lack of development of phoneme segmentation skills
- lack of spelling development at the higher levels
- lack of metacognitive awareness of spelling

These phonological skills and abilities are thought to underlie the development of good spelling and reading and appear to develop incidentally in most pupils during reading and writing but not dyslexics.

Phonemic awareness and appreciation of rhyme appear to be more closely associated with reading skills and there is a strong correlation between poor phoneme awareness and later reading difficulties (Bryant and Bradley, 1985; Frederickson and Frith et al 1997). Although 'strong' is a correlation of <0.71,this is only 50 % predictive of the capacity to later literacy skill (Pole and Lampard 2002).

Alphabetic knowledge, symbol-to-sound correspondence and phoneme segmentation are more associated with spelling. Poor skills in these areas have the highest correlation or predictive power with later dyslexia (Golinkoff, 1978, Liberman, 1973, Treiman, 1993. The stronger predictive capacity of segmentation skills appears to be because even with direct teaching of phonics the dyslexic may not be able to acquire early alphabetic and segmentation skills. Thus I argued that these skills, or lack thereof, could be used as a primary indicator of dyslexia and dysorthographia in Reception classes if we were to examine children's writing. In support of this notion it can be seen that if some of the phonological skills on dyslexia tests are examined, they actually require spelling skills for success. For example, the Alliteration and Spoonerisms tests used in the Phonological Assessment Battery (PhAB; Fredrickson, Frith & Reason, 1997) can be viewed as requiring phoneme segmentation skills. The same is true for phoneme tapping tasks (e.g., Tunmer & Nesdale, 1982), whereby, dyslexics have shown poor performance, while showing normal performance on syllable tapping (Montgomery 1997a). We know that pupils will be able to decipher syllable beats by ear if they can hear and understand speech. But phoneme tapping is different since it requires segmentation of the syllable itself, which Liberman et al (1967) showed they cannot do. For example, Montgomery (1997a) has showed that when asked to tap 'seven', 'write' 'bad', dyslexics tapped 3 or 4 times, (svn or sevn) 3 times (rit), and 3 (bad) times. Matched chronological age controls tapped 5 times, 5 and 4 times and 3 times, whereas young matched reading age controls performed as poorly as the dyslexics. In a series of such experiments (Montgomery, 1997a) it became clear that phoneme tapping was only accurate if the dyslexics and controls could spell the word in the first place. Similarly, phoneme segmentation involving cutting off the initial sound c -at was facilitated by secure knowledge of the letter sound 'c'. In other words these exercises were subskills of spelling and dependent upon it.

4. Can early writing be used as an indicator of dyslexia?

Figure 1 below shows the spelling samples of three typically developing children aged 5 years 1-2 months who had not been taught to write; Yacob (top), William (middle) and Kelly (bottom). In contrast, Figure 3 shows scripts of three dyslexic children; Steven age 6.5 years (top), Caroline aged 7 years (middle) and David aged 8 years (bottom). The 5 year olds have picked up a considerable amount of phonic and orthographic information, whereas the dyslexics show some whole word knowledge for common words they will have copied many times but lack the symbol sound knowledge they need. When we look at scripts from dyslexics it is puzzling to think why they seem unable to learn a few basic phonic or phonemic skills in the infant school that would support their reading and writing. The alphabet system is elegant, efficient and simple, why can they not learn it? We need to ask what accounts for the deficits seen in the phonological processing area when stripped down to the bare essentials - a failure to learn to make symbol-to-sound connections or learn alphabetic knowledge in often very bright individuals.

'I went to bed" Yacob. 5 yr 2 mo

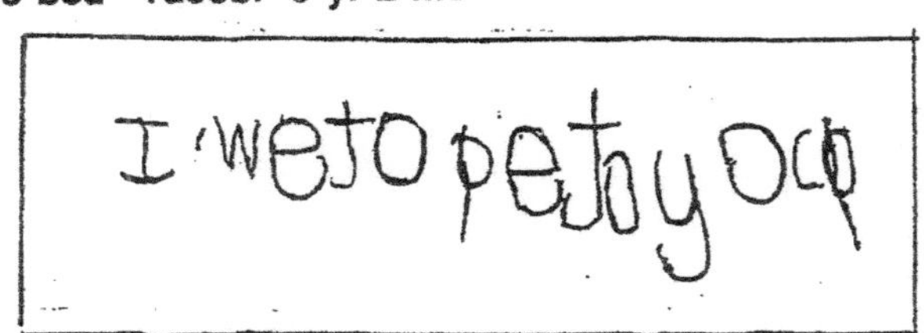

'The tree fell on top of the telephone pole wire' William 5 yr 2mo

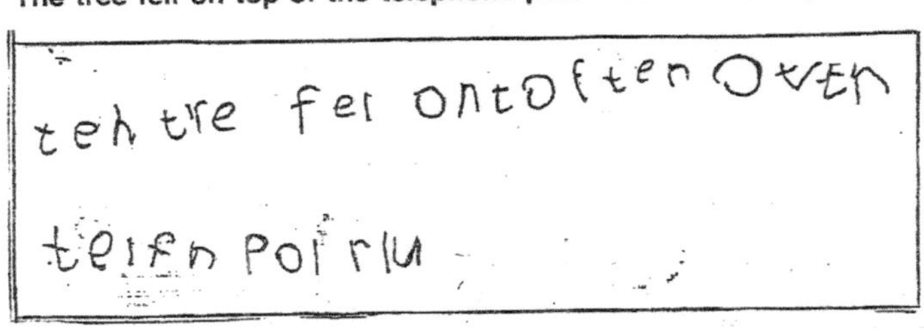

Fig. 1. The spelling of 3 non dyslexic beginning writers 5yr 1-2m Yacob and William above and Kelly below (all figures reduced by 50%)

Kelly B. 'She is in bed. She is sick. She has chickenpox.' 5 yr 1 mo

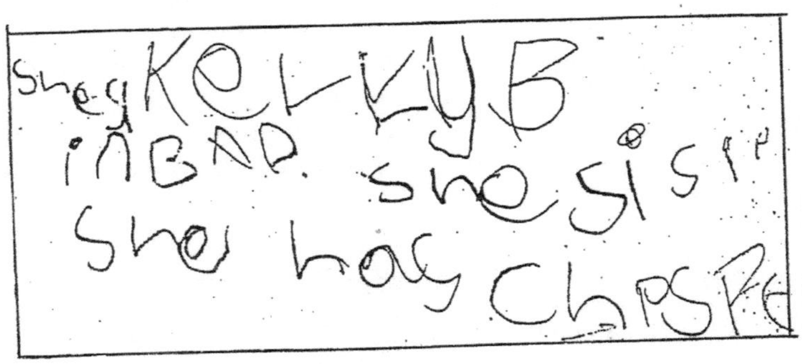

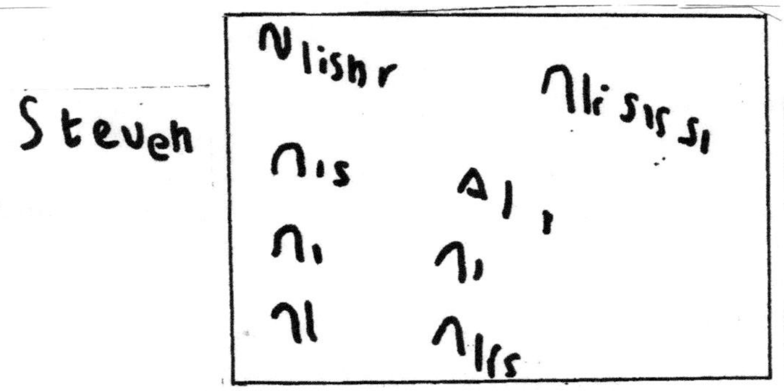

Steven, 6 years 6 months

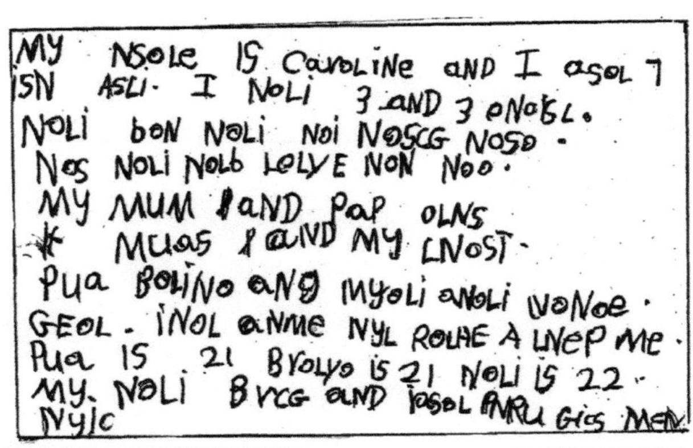

Caroline 7 years
'My name is Caroline and I am 7 years old. I have 3 brothers and 3 sisters. Some of them live at home and so do my goldfish. Paul, Breda and Mark still live at home. They are a lot older than me. Paul is 21, Breda is 21 and Mark is 22. My other —'

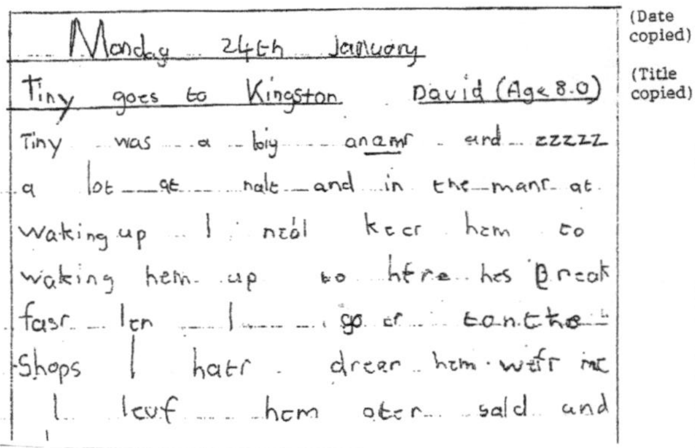

David 8 years
'Tiny was a big animal and slept a lot at night and in the morning I have to keep waking him up. I have to keep waking him up to have his breakfast. When I go to the shops I have to drag him with me —'

Fig. 2. The Writing of three dyslexics

It would seem that lack of alphabetic knowledge in early writing can be used as an early warning that dyslexia may well develop. Above, David is just beginning to crack the code.

5. An intersensory integration theory?

The core deficit in dyslexia appears to be the early failure to learn to associate sound with symbol. It requires the visual processing area of the brain (Occipital cortex) to make links between the grapheme (visual symbol) with the auditory processing area (Temporal cortex) and the sound of that grapheme (the phoneme). These linkages are found to take place in the angular gyrus (Parietal cortex; Geschwind, 1979) of the language hemisphere (left in most people). This is the intersensory integration area for sounds and symbols. But what could cause this, a dissociation problem?

The easy association between the arbitrary symbols of the alphabet and their sounds that most beginners pick up incidentally during reading is lost in dyslexics. Even in classrooms where sounds are being said slowly and the connections between them and the graphemes are made explicit, dyslexics can fail to learn them (Hurry, Silva & Riley, 1996). Even when phonics is introduced or provided in a general school based remedial programme, teachers report that they can fail to remember the connections from one day to the next (personal communication from clinical cases, 1997a, 2007)). They do not learn to segment the sound c / from 'cat' for example as other children do (Montgomery, 1997a). Ehri (1979) has suggested that this is because the sound is an **abstract perceptual unit** that has to be linked to the arbitrary graphemic unit. Could this abstract nature be the core of the problem in learning sounds and alphabetic information from which all the rest stems?

Studies of the alphabet itself lead to some significant facts. The alphabet was apparently only invented once (Gelb 1963) and was invented in the context of a Semitic language by the Phoenicians. Their Semitic language was consonantal, without vowels and consisted of 22 sounds (much like modern Hebrew). Here perhaps is the clue. If the originator had used the key cues of the articulatory pattern of each of the 22 consonants by which to assign a symbol, an alphabetic system had been invented. Anyone could learn it except perhaps dyslexics? The articulatory pattern would indeed be the only **concrete clue** between the arbitrary and abstract sound and the arbitrary and abstract visual symbol. The three of them would make a kinaesthetic multisensory triangle, to which we add the writing component, **a four-way relationship**. A more complex intersensory integration system than is overt in the term symbol-sound correspondence.

If the dyslexic does not have the awareness of the articulatory 'feel' of a particular phoneme it will make the sound - symbol association particularly problematic to acquire. As sounds with the same symbols appear in different forms (**allophones**) in syllables, this can quickly become confusing. Graphemes represent phonemes, not allophones, and so do not distinguish between different pronunciations. It is the articulatory pattern that is **concrete** and remains roughly the same and which can be used to connect the sound and the symbol. By using articulatory cues a pupil should be able to decode the consonantal structure of a syllable or a word even though vowels might be missed. This could account for the scaffold or skeletal phonics seen such as in **mstr, ws, bd** and so on when beginning spellers and dyslexics have begun to break the alphabetic code.

In a series of pilot studies and controlled experiments this articulation awareness hypothesis was developed and tested (Montgomery, 1997a). Table 1 below shows the results of the final controlled study (Montgomery, 2007) in which it was found that dyslexics in comparison with spelling age matched controls had significantly poorer articulation awareness skills even though they were two and a half years older. The higher scores on phoneme segmentation of controls and experimental group dyslexics matched their higher literacy scores compared to those in the waiting group who had made little progress in reading or spelling.

In order to assist articulation awareness and the acquisition of early phoneme segmentation to improve basic spelling skills a number of strategies termed 'multisensory mouth training' (Montgomery, 1984) for spelling were developed and used in association with the remedial programme. This involves asking the pupil to articulate a letter sound such as 'l' and then describing where in the mouth the key articulators are touching. E.g., "where is the tip of your tongue now? Are your lips open or closed? Feel your voice box, what is it doing?" and so on. Edith Norrie (1917) must have done this when she developed the Letter Case and taught herself to read and spell. Although she used a mirror to help her with her articulatory phonics this was not done in the articulatory awareness research.

Measures	Chronological Age	Reading Age	Spelling Age	Phoneme Segmentation	Articulation Awareness	IQ
Controls (N=84)	7.94	8.63	8.02	11.84	7.75	110.03
Dyslexics (N=114)	12.90	7.95	7.62	10.27	4.31	110.43
Waiting (N=30)	8.97	6.71	6.0	4.13	5.87	112.67

(Key: 15 or 10=items on tests; PS = phoneme segmentation (15 items) ; AA = articulation awareness (10 items) IQ=Intelligence Quotient,

Table 1. Results of the Main Articulation Awareness Investigations (Montgomery, 2007 p 79)

It was very surprising to discover that the dyslexics were frequently, confused about where in the mouth the key articulators were touching. Most of the dyslexic group were already started on the remedial Teaching Reading Through Spelling (TRTS; Cowdery, Montgomery et al., 1994) programme, (not those on the waiting list), but without the articulatory aspects of the phonics. Phoneme segmentation and reading /spelling abilities were strongly associated.

This leads to the questions: (1) which programmes help dyslexics crack the alphabetic code? and (2) how? Dyslexia tutors favour the 'multisensory training' method and the DfES (2010) recommends it but although many programmes include it not all are equally successful.

6. Remedial intervention patterns

Tables 2, and 3 below show the outcomes for different types of remedial programme, in particular the difference between the Orton, Gillingham, Stillman based Alphabetic-Phonic-Syllabic-Linguistic (APSL) programmes and others, non APSL that are phonics based. Reading and spelling ages are used as they tell a clearer story than percentiles and standard scores. The criterion for remedial success is for a programme to give at least two years progress in each chronological age year otherwise the dyslexic can never catch up. The researchers compared dyslexics' progress in one year on either APSL or non APSL programmes to find which programmes were effective.

Ridehalgh (1999) examined the results from teachers who had undertaken dyslexia training courses for a number of factors such as length of remediation, frequency of sessions and size of tutorial groups in dyslexic subjects taught by three different schemes: (1) Alpha to Omega (Hornsby and Shear, 1978), (2) Dyslexia Institute Language Programme (DILP/Hickey, 1977), and (3) Spelling Made Easy (SME, Brand, 1993). She found that when all the factors were held constant the only programme in which the dyslexics gained significantly in skills above their increasing age was Alpha to Omega.

Measures	Sample size	Reading Progress	Spelling Progress	Researcher
A to O	N=107	1.93	1.95	Hornsby et al (1990)
TRTS	N=38	2.45	2.01	Montgomery (1997a)
H & A to O	N=50	1.21	0.96	Ridehalgh (1999)
TRTS	N=12	3.31	1.85	Webb (2000)
TRTS	N=12	4.04	3.00	Gabor (2007)
A to O	N=10	2.4	2.4	Pawley (2007)

Table 2. Progress Made in One Year on APSL Programmes

However, in a follow up, Ridehalgh (1999) found that the users of the Hickey programme in her sample had found it more convenient to leave out the spelling pack work and the dictations! The data also showed that in **paired tuition** the dyslexics made greater gains than when working alone with the teacher. This is an important consideration in terms of the dyslexics' progress and of economics in schools. All the four tutors in the 1997 TRTS study (Table 2) worked with matched pairs of pupils.

Measures	Sample size	Reading Progress	Spelling Progress	Researcher
Eclectic mix	107	0.53	0.32	Hornsby et al (1990)
Eclectic mix	N=15	1.06	0.16	Montgomery (1997a)
SME	N=50	0.69	0.65	Ridehalgh (1999)
SME/TRTS	N=12	2.2	1.14	Webb (2000)

KEY for tables 2 and 3: TRTS – Teaching Reading Through Spelling (Cowdery et al 1994); SME Spelling Made Easy (Brand 1993);
Hickey /DILP Hickey's Dyslsexia Institute Language Programme (Hickey 1977); A to O Alpha to Omega (Hornsby et al 1976)

Table 3. Progress Made in One Year on Non APSL Programmes

Webb (2000) found that she had to cut out the dictations and some of the spellings pack work because the lessons were too short. As can be seen in Table 2 this has had an effect on the spelling results. Webb also found that in using SME (Table 3) the pupils were not making progress unless she introduced the articulatory training from TRTS to link the sound and symbol. This accounts for the better SME results than for Ridehalgh's groups.

In Gabor's (2007) study, at an international school the high progress dyslexics had supportive backgrounds and were encouraged at home to do the homework.

Pawley's (2007) study took place with 10 pupils placed in a special school for Emotional and Behavioural Difficulties (EBD). Before and after the programme the incidence of behavioural problems were recorded on the Conner's Comprehensive Rating Scale for EBD (2008) and it was found that there had been a 30.7% decrease in unwanted behaviours with all pupils' behaviour improving to a significant degree except one. The behaviour problems decreased as the literacy skills improved. Halonen and Aurola et al (2006) also established a significant correlation between reading difficulties and EBD.

These data lend support to the case observations that many pupils develop EBD as a result of their literacy problems (Edwards, 1994; Kutscher, 2005, Montgomery, 1995;). In addition, research by the BDA (Singleton, 2006) showed that 52% of young juvenile offenders were dyslexic and the Dyslexia Institute (2005) reported that the incidence in the prison population was three to four times that in the general population.

Dyslexia is thus a very serious problem for society as a whole if so many of its sufferers turn to crime. Being bright and unsuccessful in school can easily lead to alienation and even rage (Miles, 1999). Thus dyslexics may have to find other ways of being successful and using their gifts. This may mean turning to crime or becoming an independent entrepreneur. 30 per cent of highly successful entrepreneurs reported they were dyslexic (CBI, 2000).

6.1 What must a remedial programme for dyslexics include?

When a word is pronounced by a careful speaker most of its constituent phonemes can be heard and 'felt'. It is this 'citation' form that spellers need to use to support their spelling until a word is learned and can be written automatically by direct reference to the lexicon.

Learning to feel the initial sound can also give strong **concrete** support to the onset and rime strategy by helping segment the initial sound for reading as well as spelling. When

Peter, one of McMahon's (1988) dyslexic pupils aged 10, was given four twenty minute **'multisensory mouth training'** support sessions he made two years reading and spelling progress in a fortnight. It is unusual to make such an enormous gain in fortnight, none of the other 19 subjects did, but the training provided Peter the clue he needed to gain metacognitive insight into the whole process of spelling.

It will first be the consonants and consonant blends that are identified by 'feel'. The vowels do not cause the articulators to make contacts; they are open mouthed non contacting 'voiced' sounds. Vowels are varied by the position of the tongue and the shape of the lips and are particularly difficult to notice in medial positions. Beginners may often be seen mouthing their words for spelling both aloud and subvocally. Earlier researchers such as Monroe (1932) and Schonell (1942) were most insistent about the articulatory aspect of learning to spell. It is a form of metalinguistic awareness that dyslexics may fail to acquire in Reception class but may gradually do so at a later stage. Training in this area could well enable the Reception class dyslexic to overcome this phonological disability. It may then make the acquisition of the higher order aspects of the language far easier for them and some may not become disabled at all.

In cases where dyslexia goes unremediated, particularly in severe dyslexics, we find very little alphabetic knowledge, while phonemic skills are shown in the spelling (see figure 2 above). However, by about the age of 8 years many dyslexics do begin to 'crack the alphabetic code' by themselves. This is especially so where great efforts are made with multisensory phonics. By this age however, the child would be three years behind peers in literacy development and as each year goes by, the gap lengthens because the literacy teaching environment of junior schools is geared to subject teaching using already acquired literacy skills.. In addition, dyslexics would by then need to overcome errors, which cannot be unlearned. Instead, means need to be found for giving the new learning a greater propensity to be elicited.

The reason for delay in development of this refined form of propriosensitivity or integration of information above the level required not to bite the tongue is not entirely clear. What has been known for many decades is that visual, auditory and articulatory elements **must be firmly cemented in writing** (Stillman, 1940, Schonell 1942). Attention in writing is focused and helps reinforce the articulatory and kinaesthetic bridge between the visual and auditory symbols. This makes the four-way intersensory relationship **auditory - visual - articulatory and manual kinaesthetic.**

Typical of all successful remedial programmes is the focus on spelling as well as reading reinforced by writing especially in cursive for reasons discussed later. Blending and word building for spelling take place as soon as two or more letters are learned and this is followed by a steady structured and cumulative introduction to the main features of the language in its written form. This is knowledge that other children pick up automatically in the environment of print but dyslexics do not, probably because they are stuck at a pre-literate stage for so long and then on the mechanics of the process.

7. Are there levels or subtypes of dyslexia in educational terms?

Although researchers such as Boder (1973) proposed that there were subtypes in dyslexia based upon the types of errors they made in spelling and reading this is questionable. The subtypes were named dysphonetic and dyseidetic types with some having a mixture of both. These subtypes were used to describe dyslexics showing difficulties with phonics and others with problems in the images of words or correct orthography. The analysis was based upon the numbers of Good Phonetic Equivalents.

Boder's data does not support the notion of subtypes but rather it illustrates different levels of the dyslexics' knowledge. At the lower end of the learning scale with little or no phonic knowledge would be dyslexics like Steven, Caroline and David whose writing is shown in figure 2 above. This can be called Level One Skills. Yacob, William and Kelly in figure 1 above are in a transitional stage. Those who have phonic knowledge but lack a fully developed knowledge of orthography appropriate for their age and ability can be considered as at **Level Two** such as Scott in figure 3 panel 3 below.

Level 2 dyslexics have cracked the alphabetic code and are developing a knowledge of orthography but it is incomplete. As they are usually in late junior or secondary school they have little chance of ever catching up as their curricula are now geared to reading and writing to learn. However Level 2 dyslexics do need remedial intervention but it needs to be on a different level from Level 1 dyslexics.

In Figure 3 below the writing of three dyslexic pupils is shown. Chelsea's writing in the top panel of Figure 3 below, illustrates a pre-phonetic scribble stage where she has not yet cracked the alphabetic code, she has not yet been referred for remedial help. Joshua (Fig. 3 middle panel) has some knowledge of phonics and writes "I like to ride on my bike, I have fights with my brother", but his knowledge is very incomplete for a Year 5 pupil and suggests a serious earlier problem. He has been formally identified as dyslexic and referred for remedial help. Scott in Year 10 (Fig. 3 bottom panel) has knowledge of phonics and some orthographic knowledge but it is too incomplete for his age group and what he needs to be successful in the curriculum. He has had dyslexia support but it was not effective enough.

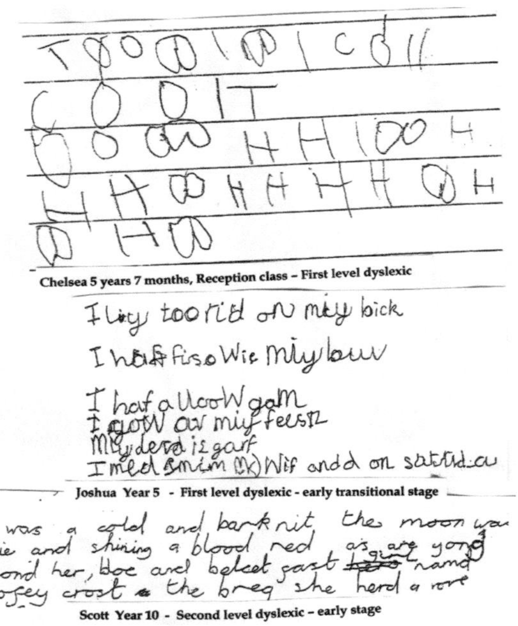

Fig. 3. Level one and level two of the dyslexic condition

Identifying these two levels is essential in the remediation process for so many of the dyslexics interviewed complained at length of forever repeating multisensory phonics work with different tutors although they already had a grasp of most of it. Their problems lay in their difficulties in building words from their phonic knowledge and arriving at the correct spelling and in correcting old misspellings. Increasing their fluency in writing however, enhanced their reading skills even when it was not the focus.

It was the tail end of this level 2 problem that was identified in a cohort of student teachers. It was for them that the **strategic approach to spelling** was developed. It was originally called the 12+1 Cognitive Process Strategies for Spelling (12 cognitive strategies plus 1 simultaneous oral spelling (Montgomery, 1997a).

7.1 Developmental stages and progress in spelling. Marsh and Friedman et al. (1980)

Marsh, among others has proposed a series of stages that most children follow in the development of writing. The basic structure has been adapted here as follows:

- Stage 1: pre-communicative / emergent stage, random scribbles and letter-like shapes, no knowledge they represent sounds
- Stage 2: semi-phonetic / alphabetic stage, pupil begins to gain an understanding of the alphabetic principle (mstr)
- Stage 3: phonetic stage, once pupil can spell consonant - vowel - consonant words progresses to other patterns; can segment speech sounds in simple words, may use rules incorrectly and over-generalise, reversal of letters in words is common until a spelling age of about 8 years, knows many common 'irregularly' spelled words. (marstr)
- Stage 4: transitional stage: pupils apply what they have learned about one-syllabled words to multisyllabled words, and have a developing knowledge of common patterns and rules. (masrtir)
- Stage 5: orthographic stage where the spelling approaches correct orthography for most common words except where new vocabulary is being learnt. (master)

These stages are helpful knowledge when working on the development of spelling in the general classroom as they can enable the teacher to monitor progress and decide how next to intervene. However it is more helpful with dyslexics to consider the barriers to their learning that occur at level one (symbol - sound knowledge) and deal with this and then at level two correcting their existing misspellings at whatever stage they present and providing strategies for generalisation to other wider vocabulary (Montgomery 1997a, 2007; author's personal observations as a clinician).

7.2 Remedial interventions at level one

Steven, aged 6.5 years (Fig. 4) was found on a visit to a student teacher who was keen to help him. He had received some phonics help already but it had not penetrated. He had been taught in a Look and Say reading teaching regime in Reception. The student was quickly taught the multisensory articulatory method of phonics work (Montgomery, in Cowdery et al. 1994 pp. 93-100). Unfortunately the joined up writing that should be part of the system was banned in this school until the children went into the junior section.

However the results are clear and after 6 x 20 minute sessions withdrawn, Steven, who originally has some word / syllable structure knowledge and uses the letters in his name repeatedly but without any phonics sense, has learned to write legibly. He has cracked the code! He was delighted with his achievement and so were his teacher and the student.

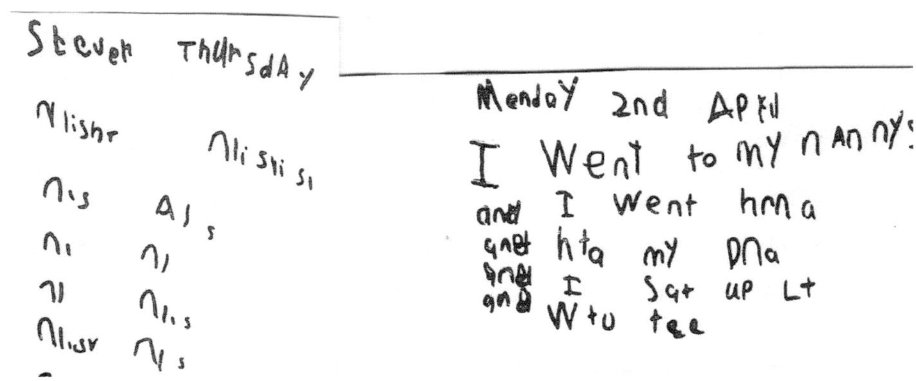

Fig. 4. Steven's spelling before and after intervention with 'articulatory phonics'

James' (aged 8.5 years) progress in figure 5 below was typical after a 50 minute lesson twice a week with his matched peer at the specialist centre. He made 3.0 years progress in reading and spelling in 1.3 years.

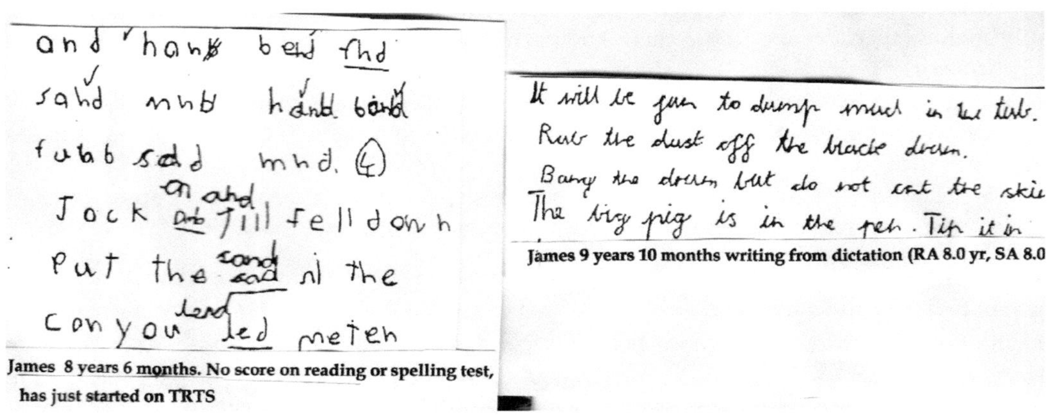

Fig. 5. James' progress on TRTS in 1.3 years

7.3 Other early screening attempts

A check of knowledge of lower case alphabet letters with 200 children in ten Reception classes in urban and suburban settings showed that after three weeks in school the majority of pupils knew between 5 to 10 names or sounds (Montgomery, 1997a). Those who knew none fell into several groups, one or two were developmentally immature and seemed unable to grasp what they needed to do, one or two were unable to concentrate on the task and had very disturbed backgrounds, the rest tried and made random associations and were unaware how they were making sounds such as: - l t d a s f in their mouths.

Forsyth (1988) followed up a cohort of pupils at age 7, who had been given a Local Education Authority (LEA) screening in three Reception classes. Forsyth found that failure to develop alphabetic knowledge was the best predictor of later reading and spelling ability at age 7 (although this was not originally included in the LEA screening inventory). Screening of this kind could be part of all teachers' Baseline Assessment procedures as well as an analysis of writing in Reception. Although Vellutino (1979) discounted the intersensory integration theory of Birch and Belmont (1964) the evidence upon which he did so was slight in comparison with his work on the other theories. This was mainly due to a problem arising from the difficulties in devising test items that would serve the purpose. Most of them were contaminated by naming or verbal processing.

Geschwind (1979) had first identified the left angular gyrus as the area where auditory, visual and kinaesthetic information is integrated. He suggested this system may not be functioning adequately due to a disconnection phenomenon. Geschwind proposed that this could cause the dyslexics' deficiency in processing and connecting graphemic symbols to their sounds. It may cause them to switch processing to the other hemisphere (Witelson 1977) which is not so well set up for verbal processing.

If there are such deficits, whatever their cause, the remedial system would need to retrain areas around the dysfunction to cause them to take over the original functions. From the experiences of stroke patients the difficulty involved in developing compensatory mechanisms, and the tremendous effort that needs to be made as soon as possible are well known (National Institute for health and Clinical Excellence NICE, 2011). It could be the reason why the system of multisensory training in writing connecting grapheme to phoneme is so essential in the first stages. In fact, experienced tutors reported that once the first few sounds and letters have been learnt the process then speeds up.

Brunswick et al. (1999) showed that young dyslexic adults, when reading aloud and using non-word recognition tests, had less activation in the left posterior cortex than controls. A deficit in the left hemisphere of the brain was said to be implicated. However, it can be argued, that this may be a **result** and not a cause of their dyslexia. Their phonological processing was not secure. In fact, when the dyslexic difficulties are given remediation and begin to clear up then the brain activation changes towards resembling that of controls (Kappers, 1990).

7.4 Remedial intervention at level two

Diagnosis of dyslexia is so often delayed for years that the pupil has developed some reading and spelling skills but they are far from automatic and errors are carried forward from earlier learning that intrude when the mind is on content rather than the basic skills of transcription. It is these pupils we can regard as having skills at Level Two. Their knowledge of sounds and symbols needs to be checked and omissions corrected but the whole multisensory training regime does not need to be set up. Instead they need interventions at the orthographic rather than the alphabetic level to supply them with the knowledge they need for word building and spelling correction and development.

7.4.1 Correcting misspellings (Montgomery, 1997a, 2007, 2011d)

The problems that have to be overcome in correcting misspellings are several. Among these, three are described:

1. The misspelling may be a creative attempt to spell an unknown word. In this case a strategy can be introduced to correct it and it may easily be learned if it is quickly understood and put to use.
2. The misspelling may have been acquired several years previously and reappears in various forms inconsistently when under pressure.
3. The misspelling may have been acquired several years ago and has defied all previous attempts.

In the first case the important feature is to lay down a new correct version in the memory. In the second and third cases the misspelling and its variants have already been learned and as they are old habits have a long track record and need **special measures** to correct them and keep them corrected. Most teachers will use Look - Cover - Write - Check to try to correct a misspelling. However, it may help lay down a new memory but it will not correct or remediate a learned misspelling. To do this two strategies are needed, these are: (1) Cursive writing and (2) Cognitive Process Strategies (CPS).

7.4.2 Why CPS and cursive writing are BOTH needed

It would appear that the incorrect spelling has already been stored in two places:

a. **In the motor control cortex for learned movements (Kimura cited in Springer et al 2003 pp 304-5)**
b. **In the word memory store or orthographic lexicon (Barry, 1994)**

Automaticity has already been established and it is this with which we have to deal. The incorrect spelling has also a memory entry in the word memory store or lexicon. We do not actually appear to lay down word memories as icons but more as rules and features and these have to be linked to the meanings of the words we learn as we learn to talk. When writing from our imaginations we think of the words we want and automatically summon the spellings we have stored and these activate the linked motor programmes. Thus we have to correct the entry in the lexicon as well as the motor programme.

A further problem is that we appear not to be easily able to forget memories in either store once we have learned them. We need therefore to lay down a new memory trace that has a higher profile than the old one so that when we summon it from the meaning linked spelling bank the correct new one emerges rather than the old incorrect one, hoping that from lack of use the old one will decay over time.

The Cognitive Process Strategies for Spelling (CPSS; described below in detail) is a strategic approach that serves the purpose of opening up the misspelling in the lexicon to intellectual scrutiny so that when we want to spell the word correctly we have given it a higher profile. As we write we can then feel it coming and can pause long enough to select the correct spelling by using the cognitive strategy. At the same time we use the cursive SOS strategy to write over the area of error.

The **Simultaneous Oral Spelling** (SOS; described below in detail) strategy used with the CPSS in the correction stage helps establish a new motor programme and pathways so that the correct word elicits the new motor programme instead of the old one. The more the new form of the word is elicited and used in writing the stronger the links become so that after a while the pause and use of the CPSS is no longer needed as the correct version comes out each time. When used with teacher education students their error rates on the third year and the final 4th year exams dropped significantly (Montgomery, 1997a). Their error types also changed from 'bizarre' to common error types and 'slips of the pen'.

7.4.3 The strategic approach to spelling – 12 Cognitive Process Strategies for Spelling (CPSS)

1. **Articulation** - The misspelt word is clearly and precisely articulated for spelling. Teachers need to encourage clear, correct speech, during classwork and in reading aloud explaining why. Mispronunciations should be corrected such as 'chimney' not 'chimley'; and 'skellington' to 'skeleton'. The point where stress comes in a word can also be noted for this will help in correcting the spellings such as harass and embarrass.
2. **Over articulation** - The word is enunciated with emphasis on each of the syllables but particularly the one normally not sounded or in which there is the schwa sound e.g. parli (a) ment, gover (n) ment, w(h)ere, ban-an-a.
3. **Cue articulation** - The word is pronounced incorrectly, e.g. Wed -nes - day, Feb - ru - ary. This points up the area of difficulty to cue the correct spelling.
4. **Syllabification** - It is easier to spell a word when we break it down into syllables, misdeanor - mis / de / mean / our, criticed crit / i / cise / d. Poor spellers and young spellers need to be taught to do this and learn to clap the beats in names and words to help them. Although the syllable division will vary, as they learn more about the structure of language they will learn to build this in to the syllabification.
5. **Phonics** - The pupil needs to learn to try to get a comprehensible skeleton of the word's sound translated into graphemic units. At first the skeletons or scaffolds will be incomplete e.g. bd for bed, and wet for went in regular words. If the words are irregular such as cum / come at least the phonic scaffold is readable and other strategies can be taught to build the correct word.
6. **Origin** - Often the word's root in another language may give clues -op / **port** / unity. the medial vowel in this word is a schwa sound and is often spelt incorrectly with 'e' or 'u'. Finding that the original meaning comes from an opening, a port or a haven means the pupil has a strong clue to the spelling.
7. **Rule** - A few well chosen rules can help unravel a range of spelling problems e.g. the l - f- s rule, that is l, f, and s are doubled in a one syllabled word after a short vowel sound - ball, puff, dress; and i before e except after c, or the two vowel rule - when two vowels go walking the first one does the talking (usually). Exceptions to these rules are saved and learned as a group e.g. pal, nil, if, gas, yes, bus, us, plus, thus.
8. **Linguistics** - The syllable types open, closed, accented and unaccented are taught as well as the 4 suffixing rules which govern most words, as well as the difference between and uses of base words and roots.
9. **Family/base word** - This notion is often helpful in revealing silent letters and the correct representation for the schwa sound e.g. Canada, Canadian; bomb, bombing, bombardier, bombardment; favour - ite, sign, signature signal. These are real families of words not common letter strings. A base word is 'form' to which we add prefixes and suffixes (reform, reforming) or make compound words back-ward.
10. **Meaning** - Separate is commonly misspelled as sep / e / rate. Looking up the meaning in a dictionary can clear this up because it will be found to mean to divide or part or even to pare. The pupil then just needs to remember 'cut or part' and 'pare' to separate.

11. **Analogy** - this is the comparison of the word or a key part of it with a word the pupil does know how to spell., e.g. 'it is like boot - hoot, root' or 'hazard' is one 'z' like in 'haze' and 'maze' . This is the closest to the letter string approach that we want to come.
12. **Funnies** - Sometimes it is not possible to find another strategy and so a 'funny' can help out e.g. 'cesspit' helped me to remember how to spell 'necessary'

7.4.4 A seven-step protocol for using CPSS

Younger pupils and those with poorer spelling will need more of the first five CPS strategies and little or no dictionary work to begin with.

1. The pupil selects **two** misspellings to learn in any one session.
2. The pupil identifies the **area of error,** usually only one letter with the help of the teacher or a dictionary.
3. The pupil puts a **ring round** the area of error and notices how much of the rest is correct.
4. The pupil is taught (later selects) a **CPSS** to correct the misspelling, a reserve strategy is also noted
5. The strategy is **talked over** with the teacher and is used to write the corrected spelling.
6. The spelling is **checked** to see if it correct - the dictionary can be used again here.
7. If correct the pupil covers up the spellings and writes the word three times from memory in **joined up / full cursive** writing using **SOS especially over the area of error if full cursive presents a problem.**

Examples: Acco(m)modate: Ac (prefix) - com/mod **(Linguistic rule - double m after the short vowel in the closed syllable)** - ate (common syllable ending) Potato(e) - tomato, 'toes are plural, o is one' ; long vowel /o/ Most modern words manage without 'es' e.g. pianos, radios, cellos, avocados

7.4.5 Simultaneous Oral Spelling (SOS)

- Look up the correct spelling in a dictionary with help if needed
- Write down the word from the dictionary **naming** the letters
- Teacher and pupil check that the spelling is correct
- Cover the spelling and then the pupil writes it from memory saying the **name** of each letter as it is written
- Check the spelling against the original to see if it is correct
- Repeat this procedure three times
- The criterion for success is that the word should be spelled correctly THREE times in a row
- Check the spelling again the next day to see if it can still be written correctly
- If an error is made build the word with wooden lower case letters then repeat SOS

This procedure was first described for remedial spelling and writing for dyslexics by Bessie Stillman (in Orton, Gillingham and Stillman,1940).

7.4.6 Casework examples with CPSS

First the lexicon entry is corrected by using CPSS and then SOS to help correct or modify the motor programme. We must do both, one or other will not work because of the inter-connectedness of thinking, writing and spelling.

13 year old Alex's work before and after 5 mini sessions of CPSS

Before:

He eat him, now I'm no exspert but **anemals** do behve **lick** that, and he did the same to the others but the had a **difrent** larws and the **PLeos cort** him eath is the most **stangest** plac I **onow Yors fafhly**hoblar

The words in bold were those chosen by Alex to tackle in the sessions.

After:

Dear Hoblar I fanck you for your letter. I've looked into your animal consirns and animals on earth have a good reputasn like Robin Hood, the Fox and Bugs Buny. I have Beny watching a lat of fims and cartoons and I disagree with you. For example police dog's save live's and guide dog's help blind people. I'll meet you at the space cafe on Wednesday 4th July

See you soon Blar

J. a Year 8 pupil (C.A. 13.6 years 9 RA 9.1 and SA 8.7 years) using CPSS - teacher's reflections

'The student and I gained a lot from this experience. The student said she thought that she'd never learn to spell words that she got wrong and she felt that now at secondary school they had given up on her. She felt by working together that she had used a lot of her own ideas when investigating words and she had enjoyed having the responsibility. She said that when we talked about things together she understood more than if she was just listening - - - She said she'd always thought that she wasn't as clever as other children and had labelled herself as 'thick' - - - I had seen a marked improvement in J's confidence, enthusiasm and spelling abilities

Casework example 1 using CPSS: Natalie was a student in Year 10, aged 15. She was somewhat impulsive and had dyslexic type difficulties (spelling age 12.4 years). She had been in the learning support class for three years. '..Her report said 'there are numerous difficulties in school as Natalie does not like to listen to criticism and does not accept help to improve her work'. Her writing was sometimes difficult to read especially when writing words she was unsure of. Her written work did not reflect her level of understanding, she wrote the minimum required, did not proof read, made many grammatical errors and was very slow at writing.

In the first CPSS session the teacher and Natalie spoke at length about the strategies and then Natalie was given a dictation. She selected the words 'edge' and 'comfortable' to tackle, put a ring round her area of error, looked them up in the dictionary, and cue articulation was suggested for ED-ge and then a 'funny' which arose when Natalie said she was reminded of a dog called 'Edger/ Edgar', then they used the phrase 'Edger has the edge'. Natalie then chose cue articulation and syllabification for the word com -FORT- able as well as the phrase which amused her 'The fort is comfortable'. She became very keen on using CPSS and over the next few weeks kept asking if she could have her spellings checked and if she could have new ones. She enjoyed identifying the word, looking it up in the dictionary and thinking of strategies to overcome it. However what she did not enjoy was the SOS and cursive writing. She was reluctant to use them despite being told why and felt they were too much like other spelling programmes she had been given before but which had failed.

A few days after the first session Natalie came in very excited because she had 'heard alarm bells ringing' when writing the word 'edge' in Food Technology and as a result of 'the bell' she had taken more time over the word and been able to correct her own writing'. Over the next three weeks they spent 10 minutes every learning support lesson reviewing spelling. Only in these sessions could Natalie be persuaded to use SOS. After a few more weeks all the words she had been learning were put into a dictation. Although Natalie complained she had not had time to review them in fact all were spelled correctly except 'thought which was given as 'though'. She said that now whenever she used the target words the alarm bells would ring although sometimes it took her a while to remember the strategy. For example she still wanted to spell the word leisure as 'leasure' but now her brain told her not to.

Other important things emerged during the mini lessons and that was Natalie became willing to share some of the stresses her problems with spelling had caused and opened a floodgate on homonyms that had troubled her for years. She was surprised that no one had thought to teach her the four suffixing rules before. As the sessions progressed she gained in confidence and was enjoying studying spelling and getting very obvious benefit that she herself could see and experience.

Her dyslexia tutor explained: 'Many of the students I work with have been following dyslexia spelling programmes with private tutors for years with little or no improvement in their ability to spell accurately when under pressure especially in a test or exam. When I first read about CPSS I was a little dubious as it seemed a time consuming way of teaching students correct spelling however I was desperate to find something which would work after years of repeatedly correcting the same errors'.

> 'It did not take long for my experimental student to feel confident about what she was doing..... it has been an extremely positive experience as it really helped raise her self esteem as well as improving the accuracy of her spelling......I have now introduced the CPSS to all the classes I teach.'

Casework example 2 using CPSS: Carl was 9 years 11 months with a spelling age of 8 years 4 months and diagnosed by an educational psychologist as 'moderately dyslexic'. He was given a 100 word dictation from his Harry Potter reading book. He misspelled 12 words and identified 5 of them: - monning (morning); itsalf (itself); bewiching (bewitching); foled (followed); turbern (turban). and :- cristmas, midde, coverd sevulal, soled punshed thay

Lesson One follows: - In the period of a fortnight they dealt with his errors

Christmas: Carl missed the 'h' in this word and said he sometimes missed the 'r' as well. Cue articulation: 'We pronounced the word 'Christ - mas'. We talked about the fact that Christmas is all about Jesus i .e. Christ. We looked up 'mass' in the dictionary and discovered that it can mean a meal or a body and that at Christmas we have a big meal to celebrate that Jesus came to earth in human body. Carl had never realised the word 'Christ' was in Christmas.

'Funny': As soon as I spelt this word correctly Carl said 'Oh look my brother's name" Carl has a brother called 'Chris' whose name he can spell quite happily so it really helped him to remember that the name 'Chris' is in 'Christmas'. SOS: He found it quite hard to make himself use the cursive writing at first but said it got a lot easier as he repeated the word. He also found it easier to remember the spelling if he shut his eyes.

Followed: Carl spelt this as 'foled' Syllabification: Carl needed help to see how the base word 'follow' can be broken down into syllables, Then he spotted the word 'low' Analogy: He was able to think of a rhyming word for 'foll' i.e. 'doll' As soon as I mentioned the past tense he remembered he needed a 'ed' ending. (Author: After analogy with 'doll' it might have been useful to introduce the l-f-s rule and/or doubling after the short vowel sound)

At the outset of lesson two Carl spelt the two words correctly and he and his teacher proceeded with the next two words. After the six sessions he was given the dictation again and Carl correctly spelled all the 12 target words. Initially he resorted to the former spelling of 'covered' and 'punishment' but in both cases he immediately realised his error and self corrected. He was quite hesitant over 'several' but got it correct after some thought. He initially put 'terban' for 'turban' but corrected it immediately. His writing in the post test was more joined.

7.4.7 When can CPSS be started?

This is a frequently occurring question and teacher researchers have found that as soon as alphabetic knowledge is established, and this does not mean learning all the sounds in alphabetical order but in use order, word building knowledge can begin. (See the *Developmental Spelling Programme* Montgomery 1997b for over 100 mini lessons and *Spelling Detective Dictionary*, (Montgomery, 2011e) for CPSS strategies. For example if a beginning speller writes 'bd' for 'bed' this is the time for basic syllable structure to be introduced - that syllables are the beats in words - practice clapping the beats in your name etc., - every syllable in English must contain a vowel. Which vowels do we know so far? etc.

Parrant (1989) introduced all her class of seven and eight year olds to CPSS strategies and compared their results with a matched class receiving Look Cover-Write-Check and the usual skills rules such as 'magic e'. The CPSS class's spelling errors decreased very significantly in comparison with the controls who went on making the same errors. The SEN group's errors in the CPSS class also decreased significantly but not by such a large amount. Since this time other teacher researchers have had similar success but have been working with small groups and individuals. Recently many teacher researchers on the MA programmes have also used CPSS with small groups and individuals and have been able to help them gain 2 years advance in spelling and reading often within six months. Interestingly enough they all report that although not directly addressed reading also improved at least to the same level. (Androsysgyn, 2002; Butt, 2003; Morley, 2001; O'Brien, 2004)

8. Why cursive writing in remedial work is important

As already indicated earlier, a significant proportion of dyslexics have accompanying difficulties in handwriting due to fine motor coordination difficulties or DCD\dyspraxia. Kaplan (2000) found this was 63 % in her sample. In the early half of the 20th century pupils in English schools learned a fully joined or cursive script from the outset 'civil service hand' with no more apparent difficulty than current print learners. It is thus a mid 20th century phenomenon that UK pupils learn print script first before converting to a joined script (Jarman, 1979). Even though ligatures are now built into the teaching system to support joining (DfEE, 1998). In many other countries cursive is still taught from the outset.

Experiments in teaching cursive from the outset again have taken place in a number of LEAs and have proved highly successful in achieving writing targets earlier and for a larger number of children (Low, 1990; Morse, 1991). It is also found to be equally readable. However custom and practice or 'teaching wisdom' is very hard to change and extremely rigid attitudes are frequently found against cursive (Montgomery, 2003).

The research of Early (1976) advocated the exclusive use of cursive from the beginning. This was because it was found that the major advantage of cursive lay in the fact that each word or syllable consists of one continuous line where all the elements flow together. This means that the child experiences more readily the total form or shape of a given word as he or she monitors the kinaesthetic feedback from the writing movements. Handwriting therefore supports spelling and this contributes to literacy development.

The cursive recommended here can be seen in figure 6 below. It is ovoid rather than upright to promote fluency and seeks to find the most efficient joining strategies. Single lower case letters and the initial lower case letters of all words begin on the line with a lead in stroke, there are loops below the line to assist flow in joining but none above, this helps reduce confusions between lines. A crucial factor of academic success at secondary level is a student's writing speed. It determines how easily and comprehensively he/she can take notes in class and can have a major influence on success in examinations. Ziviani and Watson-Will (1998) found that cursive script appeared to facilitate writing speed.

The reasons for teaching cursive writing are particularly relevant to students with handwriting coordination difficulties (developmental dysgraphia) unless their problems are severe when other strategies may need to be implemented. Specialist dyslexia programmes of Gillingham and Stillman (1956); Hickey (1977); Cowdery and Montgomery et al., (1994) all base their remediation on it in a multisensory training system. The reasons are it:

- aids left to right movement through words across the page
- stops reversals and inversions of letters
- induces greater fluency in writing so enables greater speed without loss of legibility
- more can be written in the time
- speed and fluency can make a difference of a grade at GCSE, A level or in degree programmes
- the motor programmes for spelling words, their bases and affixes are stored together (Kuczaj, 1979)
- space between letters and between words is orderly and automatic
- a more efficient fluent and personal style can be developed
- pupils with handwriting coordination difficulties experience less pain and difficulty
- legibility of writing is improved
- reinforces multisensory learning linking spelling, writing and speaking.

In addition, if taught from the outset it eliminates the need to relearn a whole new set of motor programmes after the infant stage and there is a more efficient use of movement because of cursive's flow.

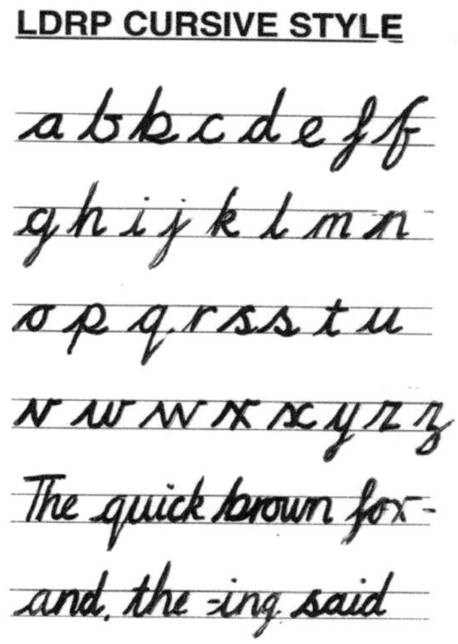

Fig. 6. Example of the recommended LDRP Cursive

This 'LDRP' ovoid form with a consistent forward (or backward) slope to aid running writing is more user-friendly for most pupils than the upright Palmer cursive used in the TRTS programme.

In the remedial setting, lines to write on and cursive have been found to be essential and Wedell (1973) had insisted that children with coordination difficulties must learn to use a continuous writing movement. Dysgraphics such as these have difficulties, once they find where to make contact with the paper in making the required shape and to the precise size and length. As soon as they lift the pen from the paper again in print script to make the next letter the directional, orientational and locational problems begin all over again. The effort involved becomes greater, the pen is seized more tightly, the knuckles go white and the whole body tenses and there is a further loss of fluency. To aid focus and concentration and stop contralateral movements the edge of the desk may be held and the tongue stuck out. It can take half an hour of formidable effort to produce a neat sentence.

Pupils with handwriting difficulties from whatever cause, whenever they can, try to avoid any written task and complain of pain and fatigue (Alston, 1993) and some even become disruptive when they are required to sit down to write. Teachers well know that, "Now write it down" can bring forth a chorus of groans. But avoidance and difficulties with writing tasks can also have a serious effect on spelling and handwriting development through consistent lack of practice. In addition lack of personalised tuition as children are learning to form their letters and monitoring on the writing task because of large classes can result in poor acquisition of writing skills as many pupils teach themselves through copying exercises.

Handwriting difficulties appear to play a much more significant role in underachievement than has often been realised (Montgomery, 2000, 2003; Silverman, 2004). Whilst estimates of developmental coordination difficulties vary between 5 to 10 per cent of the school population, ten per cent or more of pupils have mild handwriting coordination difficulties (Gubbay 1976, Laszlo, Bairstow et al 1988. Rubin and Henderson (1982) found that 12 % of pupils were considered by their teachers to have serious handwriting difficulties. Whilst in a survey carried out with 3rd year junior school pupils in Cheshire, Alston (1993) found that according to assessments made by 5 experienced remedial teachers just over 20 % of pupils were not writing well enough for the needs of the secondary school curriculum.

In a recent analysis of Year 7 scripts it was found that 30 % of pupils had some form of handwriting difficulties in form or coordination and this led to problems in legibility and speed. A speed at this age of 20 words per minute in a 20 minute essay was found to be necessary to access the school curriculum (Montgomery 2007b). The average speed of the cohorts (N=531) was 13.2 similar to that in a survey by Allcock, 2001 (N=2701). Very few primary teachers said that they regarded speed as an important feature in children's writing they focused more upon legibility and neatness (Stainthorp, et al 2001). However fluency and speed are important and this can be achieved by the majority of pupils with light training of their teachers (Christenson & Jones, 2000). Perhaps the 1 % with overt DCD should be exempt from writing and be given laptops as they find it impossible to speed up sufficiently although they invest huge effort such as in the case of David in Figure 8 below.

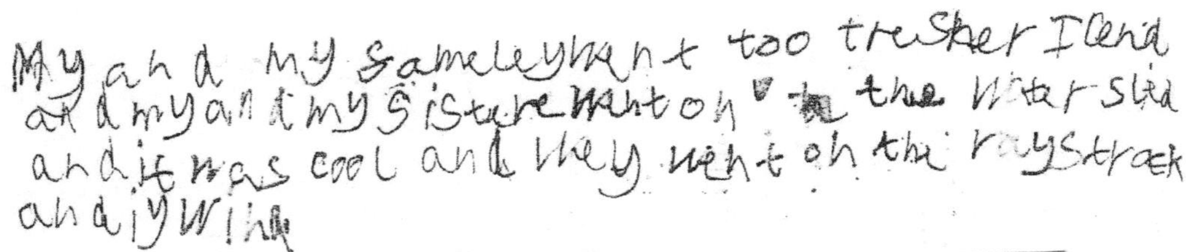

David, Year 5 Severe handwriting problem: 3.25 words per minute

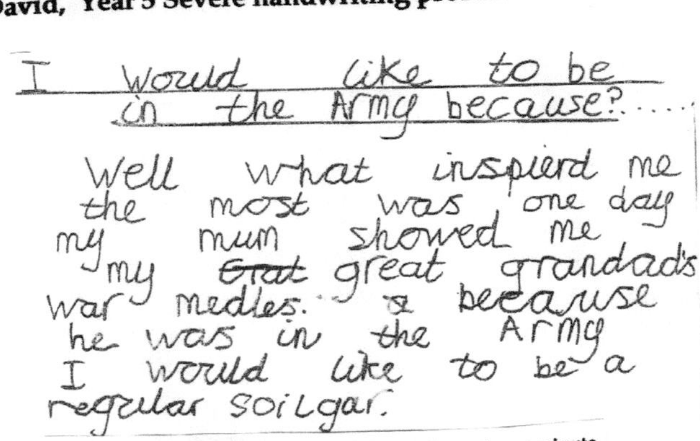

Toby, Year 5 Mild handwriting problem: 5.75 words per minute

Fig. 7. Handwriting difficulties – David above and Toby below

The checklist in Figure 9 below can be used with a pupil to get him or her to decide on the errors they make in their writing. Choose TWO features on which to intervene. The features that will give the most effect and quickly have been found to be making **the base** of the letters all the same size by using double lines to write between and trying to make **the slope** of all the letters' ascenders and descenders go in the same direction (Montgomery, 2007, 2011a).

8.1 A checklist of key indicants for diagnosing handwriting coordination difficulties

- the letters do not stay on the line
- the writing drags in from the margin towards the mid line
- wobble and shake observable on strokes in letters
- variation in 'colour' of words, lightness and dark as pressure varies or fatigue sets in
- spaces between letters are too wide
- spaces between words too are large and sometimes too small
- rivers of space run down between the words
- difficulties making complex letters so they appear large or as capital forms T, W, S, K, F
- Variations in size of other letters so they appear as large or capital forms e.g. n,m,u,h,
- a non standard pencil grip (e.g. not a tripod grip, flexible or rigid) can hamper writing and achievement,
- great pressure hampers fluency, makes holes or dents in the paper which can be felt on the reverse side
- contra lateral body and arm movements may be observed
- effort and grip causes whitening of the knuckles
- tongue may be stuck out
- fatigue rapidly sets in
- complains of aches and pains after only short periods of writing

An index of 4 or 5 such indicants would warrant further investigation and intervention.

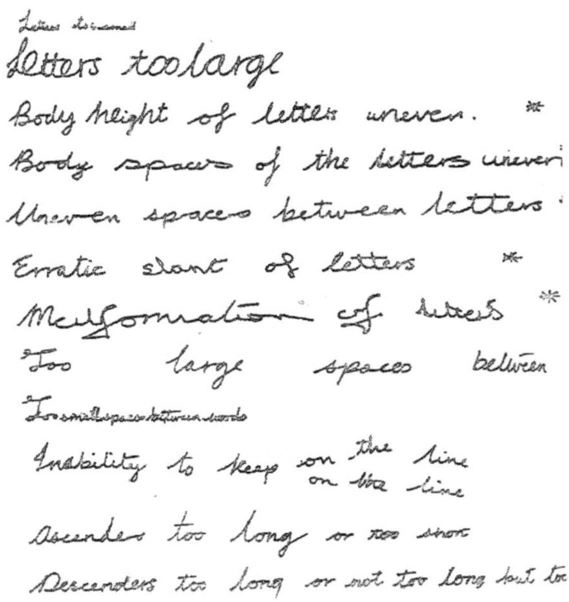

Fig. 8. A checklist to use to identify form difficulties

Some other physical characteristics – suggesting coordination difficulties

Look at the lines on the paper made by the writer, writing his or her own name and address for example.

- You can feel the writing on the reverse side of the paper, too much pressure and energy exerted.
- Is the writing variable in dark and light pressures or in being too faint and then too dark.
- Is the writing shaky and wobbly? Can suggest tremor and anxiety.
- Is the writing scribbly and or spiky? Suggests a motor co-ordination problem.

Practice in the motor movement in writing developing rhythm and flow can improve the writing patterns indicated above.

8.2 Automatic development of skills

Before the writer can become fluent in higher order compositional skills it is essential that the lower order skills of spelling and handwriting become automatic (Berninger, 2004). If a writer has to reflect on how to spell words and make up spellings or has difficulty in forming letters and words fluently in handwriting then the mental efforts required or mental resources that are committed to these processes are directed away from composition and the development of ideas, narrative and argument. The requirement is that the correct spellings should reel out from the lexicon automatically as we write just as our hands move over the keys of the piano when we have learnt to play a tune.

This means that comprehension is affected as well as the higher order skills required to write compositions and essays. If lower order skills are not automatic then the whole process of writing is slowed down and may become truncated and disrupted. Extensive researches by Berninger (2004) and her colleagues have shown that the two best early predictors of higher order compositional skills are speed of writing the letters of the alphabet and coding or spelling skills.

We know that dyslexics are poor at developing automatic levels of these skills because of their difficulties and this is not surprising for they currently acquire them late and thus have many years less practice using them. This problem persists and Connelly et al. (2001) Connelly et al. (2005) have shown this problem exists for them throughout primary and secondary schools and into higher education as they become undergraduates. At university level this can mean that they obtain degrees in the humanities and social sciences that are at least a class lower than might be predicted from their other skills. It was similar findings with teacher undergraduates that led to the investigation of handwriting problems especially of more able subjects and its contribution to underachievement (Montgomery, 2009, 2011e). It appears to be a silent disability and frequently ignored. Fortunately for dyslexics the early specialist remediators, Gillingham, Stillman and Orton (1940) were well aware of the problem and included penmanship, especially in the form of cursive writing in their programme. It is this programme and method upon which all the most successful programmes are based. For what makes a dyslexia friendly school or environment see Study Guide 4 (Montgomery 2011d)

9. Summary and conclusions

The main thrust of this chapter is that whilst the focus in education is the teaching of reading, the needs of dyslexics are different. Their core difficulty lies in the area of spelling first in 'cracking the alphabetic code'. This could be done in the Reception Year by the class teacher with some specific training. If this is not done or is not successful then remedial provision needs to be instituted in Year 1 for 'Level One' dyslexics and this should involve the use of a specialist programme such as TRTS or Hickey that systematically involve spelling, handwriting and articulatory phonics as well as reading. Older dyslexics and those with dysorthographia – 'Level Two' dyslexics, also need specific spelling help and this can be provided by the 'Strategic Approach' to spelling, CPSS already described. Both types of remedial intervention must produce 2 years uplift in skills in each year if they are to be considered successful. Addressing spelling transfers to reading whereas the reverse is not the case.

In theoretical terms it is suggested that the dyslexia is the result of a dissociation in the intersensory integration of sounds with symbols that causes early failure to learn sound and symbol correspondence. If not overcome the delay in this aspect hampers literacy development and leads to laying down many errors that in themselves become difficult to overcome. Referral in the UK may come 3 to 6 years too late and then poor literacy skills and old errors undermine achievement at all levels. In research terms it is suggested that there should be more focus on spelling and handwriting as part of literacy investigations and that a programme of early screening and intervention in Reception should be explored. In educational terms teachers in training need a better understanding that dyslexia is not just a reading problem and learn of the power and interest that can be generated by encouraging children to adopt a 'detective approach' to spelling to help lose their 'learned helplessness'. An associated benefit from overcoming literacy problems that has emerged is the decrease in problem behaviours in classrooms.

Overall this chapter has sought to present an alternative perspective to the mainline theme in dyslexia research and intervention to date. It proposes that reading is not the core difficulty and that concentration on this aspect causes confusion in diagnosis and diminishes the effectiveness of the remediation. In many instances it causes it to fail. The concept of dyslexia as an irremediable lifelong problem also needs to be challenged as does the popular notion of a sex ratio of 4 to 1 with boys more likely to have the problem than girls. A vast body or research is already available on dyslexia but it is suggested that much of it is missing the point and a closer fit needs to be made between the dyslexic's experience and the methods of meeting his or her needs.

10. References

Allcock, P. (2001) Update September 2001: 'Testing handwriting speed' *PATOSS Bulletin* November p 17

Alm, J. and Kaufman, A 2002 'The Swedish WAIS-R factor structure and cognition profiles for adults with dyslexia *Journal of Learning Disabilities* 35 (4) 321-33 ISSN

Alston, J. (1993) *Assessing and Promoting Writing Skills* Stafford, NASEN

Andrusysgen, K. 2002 'An investigation of Cognitive Process Spelling Strategies with a group of poor spellers' Unpublished MA SpLD, London: Middlesex University

Barry, C. 1994 'Spelling routes (or roots or rutes); In G.D.A. Brown, and N. C. Ellis (1994) *Handbook of Spelling: Theory, Process and Intervention* 27-49 Chichester: Wiley ISBN 0-471-94342-9

BDA (2004) htpp:// www.bda-dyslexia.org.uk/main/information/adults/ao1what.asp

Berninger, V. 2004 'Review of handwriting research and intervention' Keynote paper Annual DCD Conference, Oxford April

Birch, H. G. and Belmont, L. (1964) 'Auditory -visual integration in normal and retarded readers' *American Journal of Orthopsychiatry* 34 352-61 ISSN 0002-9432

Boder, E. (1973) 'Developmental dyslexia: A diagnostic approach based on three atypical reading patterns' *Developmental Medicine and Child Neurology* 23 663-87 Online ISSN 1469-8749

BPS (British Psychological Society) (1989) Deliberations of the Expert group on Dyslexia Leicester: BPS

Brand, V. (1993) *Spelling Made Easy 14th Edition* Baldock: Herts: Egon

Brown, G. D. A. and Ellis, N. C. (1994) *Handbook of Spelling: Theory, Process and Intervention* Chichester: Wiley ISBN 0-471-94342-9

Brunswick, N., McCrory, E., Price, C. J., Frith, C. D. and Frith, U. (1999) 'Explicit and implicit processing of words and pseudo words by adult developmental dyslexics' *Brain* 122 1901-17 Online ISSN 1460-2156

Bryant, P. and Bradley, L (1985) *Children's Reading Problems* Oxford: Blackwell

Butt, H, (2003) 'An investigation into the use of cognitive process strategies for spelling in the development of spelling skills of a group of Year 7 pupils' Unpublished MA SpLD dissertation London: Middlesex University

Calder, N. 1970 *The Mind of Man* London: BBC Publications ISBN 563-10155-5

CBI (Consortium of British Industry) (2000) CBI Survey of Entrepreneurs in Industry London: CBI

Chall, J. (1967) *Learning to Read: The Great Debate* New York: McGraw-Hill

Chall, J. (1985) *Stages in Reading Development* New York: McGraw-Hill

Chomsky, C. (1971) 'Write first, read later' *Childhood Education* 47 (6) 296-9 Online ISSN 1573-1707

Christensen, C.A and Jones, D. (2000) 'Handwriting: An underestimated skill in the development of written language' *Handwriting Today* 2 56–69 ISBN 1-982932-16-6

Clark, M. M. (1970) *Reading Difficulties in Schools* Harmondsworth: Penguin ISBN14080213-4

Clements, S.D. (1966) *National Project on Minimal Brain Dysfunction in Children - Terminology and Identification Monograph No 3 Public Health Service Publication No 1415* Washington DC: Government Printing Office

Connelly, V. and Hurst, G. (2001) 'The influence of handwriting fluency on writing quality in later primary and early secondary education' *Handwriting Today* 2 50-7 ISBN 1-872832-16-5

Connelly, V., Dockrell, J., Barnett, A. (2005) 'The slow handwriting of undergraduate students constrains the overall performance in exam essays' *Educational Psychology* 25 (1) 99-109 eISSN 1489-5820

Conners, C.K (2008) *Comprehensive Behaviour Rating Scale 3rd edit* London: Pearson ISBN 9780749148-39-3

Cowdery, L.L., Montgomery, D., Morse, P., & Prince-Bruce, M. (1994) *Teaching Reading Through Spelling Series: Foundations of the Programmes Reprint* Wrexham: TRTS Publishing ISBN 1-900283-01-8

DFEE (1997) *Excellence for All Children* London: DfEE ISBN 0-10157852-1

DfEE (1998) *NLS The National Literacy Strategy Guidance* London: DfEE

DfEE (2010) 'Multisensory approaches to learning' http://waes:elearn.waes.ac.uk/moodie-resources/Basic%Skills (Accessed 2/8/2010)

DILP (2005) *Dyslexia Institute Language Programme* (Eds) J. Walker and L Brooks Staines: Dyslexia Institute

Early, G. H. (1976) 'Cursive handwriting, reading and spelling achievement' *Academic Therapy* 12 (1) 67-74 ISSN 0001-396X

Edwards, J. (1994) *The Scars of Dyslexia* London: Cassell ISBN0-304-32944-4

Ehri, L. C. (1979) 'Linguistic insight threshold of reading acquisition' In T.G. Waller and G. E. MacKinnon, (eds) *Reading Research: Advances in Theory and Practice* New York: Academic Press

Forsyth, D. (1988) 'An evaluation of an infant school screening instrument' Unpublished SEN dissertation Kingston-upon-Thames: Kingston Polytechnic

Frederickson, N., Frith, U. and Reason, R. (1997) *Phonological Assessment Battery (PhAB)* Windsor: NFER-Nelson ISBN 9780708707081/N0078

Frith, U. (Ed) (1980) *Cognitive Processes in Spelling* London: Academic Press ISBN 0-12-268-660-8

Frostig, M. and Horn, D. (1964) *The Frostig Programme for the Development of Visual Perception* Chicago: Follett

Galaburda, A. M. (1993) *Dyslexia and Development* Cambridge MA: Harvard University Press

Gathercole, S.E. (2008) 'Working memory in the classroom' *The Psychologist* 21 (5) 382-3850 ISSN 0952-8225

Gabor, G. (2007) 'An evaluation of the process and purpose towards setting up a dyslexia programme in an international school' Unpublished MA SpLD dissertation London: Middlesex University

Gabor, G. 2009 'Follow up report of the dyslexia programme results' Personal communication

Gelb, I.J. (1963) *A Study of Writing (2nd edition)* London: University of Chicago Press

Geschwind, N. (1979) 'Specialisations of the human brain' *Scientific American* 241 (3) 156-67 ISSN 0036 8733

Gillingham, A.M., Stillman, B.U. & Orton, S.T. (1940) *Remedial Training for Children with Specific Disability in Reading, Spelling and Penmanship* New York, Sackett and Williams

Gillingham, A., Stillman, B.U and Orton, S. T. (1956) *Remedial Training for Children with Specific Disability in Reading, Spelling and Penmanship* New York: Sackett and Williams

Golinkoff, R. M. (1978) 'Phonemics awareness and reading achievement' In F.R. Murray and J.J. Pikulski (eds) *The Acquisition of Reading* Baltimore: University Park Press

Goswami, U. 2008 'Language and reading difficulties' Keynote lecture at the International Schools Council Conference London, April

Gubbay, S. S. (1976) *The Clumsy Child* London: WH Saunders ISBN 0-7216-4340-X

Halonen, A,. Aunola, K., Ahonen, T., and Nurmi, J. (2006) 'The role of learning to read in the development of problem behaviour: A cross-lagged longitudinal study' *British Journal of Educational Psychology* 76 (3) 517-534 eISSN 2044-8279

Henderson, S.E. and Green, D (2001) 'Handwriting problems in children with Asperger Syndrome' *Handwriting Today* 2 65-71 ISBN 1-8728832-16-5

Hickey, K. (1977) *Dyslexia: A Language Training Course for Teachers and Learners* Wimbledon, 19 Woodside,

Holmes, B. (1994) 'Fast words speed past dyslexia' *New Scientist* 27th August 10 ISSN 0262 4079

Hornsby, B. and Shear, F. (1976) *Alpha to Omega 2nd edition* London: Heinemann

Hornsby, B. and Farrar, M. 1990 'Some effects of a dyslexia centred teaching programme' 173-95 In P. D. Pumfrey and C. D. Elliott (eds) *Children's Difficulties in Reading, Spelling and Writing* London: Falmer Press ISBN 1-85000-691-1

Hurry, J. Sylva, K. and Riley, S. (1996) 'An evaluation of a focused literacy teaching programme in Reception and Year 1' *British Educational Research Journal* 22 (5) 617-30 ISSN 0141-1926

Jarman, C. (1979) *The Development of Handwriting Skills* Oxford: Blackwell ISBN 0-631-19230-1

Jones, D. and Christensen, C. A. (1999) 'Relationship between automaticity in handwriting and students' ability to generate written text' *Journal of Educational Psychology* 91 (1) 44-9 eISSN 1939-2176

Kaplan, B.J. (2000) 'Atypical brain development' Paper presented at the 27th International Conference on Psychology. Stockholm

Kappers, E. J. (1990) 'Neuropsychological treatment of dyslexic children' *Euronews Dyslexia* 3 9-15

Koppitz, E. M. (1977) *The Visual Aural Digit Span Test* New York: Grune and Stratton ISBN 0-8089-1032-9

Kuczaj, S. A. (1979) 'Evidence for a language learning strategy: On the relative ease of acquisition of prefixes and suffixes' *Child Development* 50 1-13

Kutscher, M. L. (2005) *Kids in the Syndrome Mix of ADHD, LD, Asperger's Tourette's and more* London: Jessica Kingsley ISBN 978-1-84310-5

Laszlo, M., Bairstow, P. and Bartrip, P. (1988) ' A new approach to perceptuomotor dysfunction, previously called clumsiness' *Support for Learning* 3 33-40 eISSN 1467-9604

Liberman, I. J. (1973) 'Segmentation of the spoken word and reading acquisition' *Bulletin of the Orton Society* 23 365-77

Liberman, A. M., Shankweiler, D.P., Cooper, F. S., Studdert-Kennedy, M. (1967) 'Perception of the speech code' *Psychological Review* 74 (6) 431-61 eISSN 1939-1471

Low, G. (1990) 'Cursive makes a comeback' *Education* 6th April p 341

Manson, J. & Wendon, L. (1997) *Letterland: Early Years Handbook* London: Collins Educational

Marsh, G., Friedman, M. P., Welch, V. and Desberg, P. (1980) 'The development of strategies in spelling' 339-54 In U. Frith (ed) *Cognitive Processes in Spelling* London: Academic Press ISBN 0-12-268-660-8

McGhee, E. 2010 'An investigation of working memory training with a group of 17 dyslexics' Unpublished MA SEN Dissertation London; Middlesex University

McMahon, J. (1988) 'An analysis of early language difficulties in a sample of dyslexics' Unpublished B Ed Dissertation Report Kingston upon Thames: Kingston Polytechnic

Miles, T.R. (1993) *Dyslexia: The Pattern Of Difficulties 2nd edition* London: Whurr ISBN1-870332-39-3

Miles, T.R. and Miles, E. (1999) *Dyslexia 100 Years on 2nd edition* Buckingham: Open University Press ISBN 0-335-20034-6

Monroe, M. (1932) *Children Who Cannot Read* Chicago: Chicago University Press

Montgomery, D. (1984) 'Multisensory mouth training' Chapter 6 in L.L Cowdery and D. Montgomery et al op cit. Reprinted 1994 ISBN 1-900283-01-8

Montgomery, D. 1989 *Managing Behaviour Problems* Sevenoaks: Hodder and Stoughton ISBN 0-340-40832-4

Montgomery, D. (1995) 'Social abilities in highly able disabled learners and the consequences for remediation' pp 226-238 In M.W. Katzko & F.J. Monks *Nurturing Talent: Individual Needs and Social Abilities* Assen, The Netherlands: Van Gorcum ISBN 90-232-3033-7

Montgomery, D. (1997a) *Spelling: Remedial Strategies* London: Cassell 0-304-32974-6

Montgomery, D. (1997b) *Developmental Spelling: A Handbook* Maldon: Learning Difficulties Research Project ISBN 1-901686-00-0

Montgomery, D. (ed) (2000) *Able Underachievers* London: Whurr ISBN 1-86156-193-8

Montgomery, D. (2003) *Reversing Lower Attainment* London: David Fulton ISBN 1-85346-561-5

Montgomery, D. (2007) *Spelling, Handwriting and Dyslexia* London: Routledge ISBN 878-0-415-40925-4

Montgomery, D. (2008) 'Cohort analysis of writing in Year 7 after 2, 4, and 7 years of the National Literacy Strategy' *Support for Learning* 23 (1) 3-11 ISSN 0268-2141

Montgomery, D. (ed) (2009) *Able, Gifted and Talented Underachievers* Oxford: Wiley-Blackwell ISBN 978-0-470-55940-8

Montgomery, D. (2011a) *M3 Study Guide: Spelling and Handwriting Difficulties* Maldon, Essex: Learning Difficulties Research Project www.ldrp.org.uk ISBN 1-901686-00-4

Montgomery, D. (2011b) *M4 Study Guide: Dyslexic Difficulties* Maldon, Essex: Learning Difficulties Research Project www.ldrp.org.uk ISBN 1-901686-00-5

Montgomery, D. (2011c) *M6 Study Guide: Mathematical Difficulties and Dyscalculia* Maldon, Essex: Learning Difficulties Research Project www.ldrp.org.uk ISBN 1-901686-00-7

Montgomery, D. (2011d*) M22 Spelling Detective CPSS Dictionary* Maldon, Essex: Learning Difficulties Research Project www.ldrp.org.uk ISBN 1-901686-00-23

Montgomery, D. (2011e) *M15 Study Guide: Able Underachievers* Maldon, Essex: Learning Difficulties Research Project www.ldrp.org.uk ISBN 1-901686-00-15

Morley, K. (2001) 'Casework with an able dyslexic in Nairobi' *Educating Able Children* 5 (1) 27–30 ISSN

Morse, P (1991) "Cursive in Kingston-upon Thames' *Handwriting Review* 5 16-21 ISBN 1-872832-16

NICE Guidelines 2011 National Institute for Health and Clinical Excellence: Stroke rehabilitation guidelines www.nice.org.uk/nicemedia/live accessed 05/11/2011

Norrie, E. (1973) *Edith Norrie Letter Case Manual* London, Helen Arkell Centre (1993)

Norrie, E. (1917) *The Edith Norrie Letter Case* London, Word Blind Institute (1946), Reprinted Helen Arkell

O'Brien, K. (2004) 'An investigation of the use of CPSS as a means of remediating or correcting spelling errors' Unpublished MA SpLD dissertation London: Middlesex University

Parrant, H. (1989) 'An investigation of remedial approaches to children's spelling difficulties' Kingston Polytechnic, unpublished SEN dissertation

Pawley, J.(2007) 'Dyslexia - the Hidden Trigger?' Unpublished MA SpLD dissertation London: Middlesex University.

Pole, C. and Lampard, R. (2002) *Practical Social Investigations: Qualitative and Quantitative Methods in Social Research* Harlow, Essex: Pearson Educational ISBN 0-136-16848-5

Ridehalgh, N. (1999) 'A comparison of remediation programmes and analysis of their effectiveness on a sample of pupils diagnosed as dyslexic' Unpublished MA SpLD dissertation London: Middlesex University.

Rose, J. (2006) *Independent Review of the Teaching of Early Reading Final Report* www.standards.dfes.gov.uk/rosereview/interimreport.doc (Accessed 12/02/06)

Rumelhart, D. E. and McClelland, R. R. (eds) (1986) *Parallel Distributed Processing Volume 1 Foundations* Cambridge MA: MIT Press

Rubin, N. and Henderson, S. (1982) 'Two sides of the same coin: variations in teaching methods and failure to learn to write' *Special Education* 9 (4) 14-18 ISSN 0305-7526

Rutter, M. L., Tizard, J., & Whitmore, K. (eds) (1970) *Education, Health and Behaviour* London: Longman

Rutter, M. L., Caspi, A., Fergussen, D., Horwood, U., Goodman, R. Maughan, B. et al (2004) 'Sex differences in developmental reading disability' *Journal of the American Medical Association* 291 9 (16) 2007-12

Schonell, F. (1942) *Backwardness in Basic Subjects* Edinburgh: Oliver and Boyd ISBN 0-05-000344

Silverman, L. K. (2004) 'Poor handwriting: A major cause of underachievement' http://www.visualspatial.org/Publications/Article%20List/Poor_Handwriting.htm Access12/03/2004

Singleton, C. (2006) 'Dyslexia and youth offending' 117-121 in S. Tresman and S. Cooke (eds) *The Dyslexia Handbook* Reading, Berks: The British Dyslexia Association

Smith, P. A. P. and Marx, R. W. (1972) ' Some cautions on the use of the Frostig test' *Journal of Learning Disabilities* 5 (6) 357-62 http://ldx.sagepub.com

Snow, R.E. (1973) 'Theory construction for research on teaching' 77-112 in R..M.W. Travers (Ed) *Second Handbook of Research on Teaching* New York: Rand McNally Library OF Congress Card No. 72-6922

Snowling, M.J. 2000 *Dyslexia 2nd edition* Oxford: Blackwell ISBN 0-631-20574-8

Snowling, M. J. and Stackhouse, J. and Rack, J. (1986) 'Phonological dyslexia and dysgraphia - a developmental analysis' *Cognitive Neuropsychology* 13 303-39 eISSN 1464-0627

Springer, S. P. and Deutsch, G. 2003 *Left Brain Right Brain: Perspectives from Neuroscience 5th edition* New York: W. H. Freeman and Co. ISBN 0-7167-3111-8

Stainthorp, R., Henderson, S., Barnett, A. and Scheib, B. (2001) Handwriting policy and practice in primary schools' Paper presented at the British Psychological Society Education and Developmental Sections Joint Annual Conference September, England: Worcester.

Stillman, B. (1940) 'On penmanship' In A. Gillingham , B. Stillman, and S.T. Orton, . op. cit

Tallal, P. (1994) 'New clue to cause of dyslexia seen in mishearing of fast sounds. An interview with Dr Tallal' by S. Blakeslee, *New York Times* 16th August 24

Tallal, P. (1980) 'Auditory temporal perception, phonics, and reading disabilities in children' *Brain and Language* 9 182-198 ISSN 0093-934X

Taylor L. (2007) 'The second core deficit. What is the effect of early intervention? Are a lack of automaticity and fluency attributable solely to dyslexic pupils? Unpublished dissertation London: Middlesex University

Treiman, R. (1993) *Beginning to Spell* Oxford: Oxford University Press

Tunmer, W. & Nesdale, A. (1982). The effects of digraphs and pseudowords on phonemic segmentation in young children. *Applied Psycholinguistics*, 3, 299-311

Vellutino, F.R. (1979) *Dyslexia: Theory and Research* London, M.I.T. Press

Vellutino, F.R. (1987) 'Dyslexia' *Scientific American* 256 (3) 20-27 ISSN 0036 8733

Webb, M. (2000) 'An evaluation of the SEN provision to improve literacy skills of Year 9 students at Nfields' Unpublished MA SpLD dissertation London: Middlesex University

Wechsler, D. (1997) *Wechsler Intelligence Scale for Children (WISC III)*. San Antonio, TX: The Psychological Corporation

Wedell, K. (1973) *Learning and Perceptuomotor Difficulties in Children* New York: Wiley

WISC - 1V (2006) *Wechsler Intelligence Scale for Children - 1V* London: Psychological Corporation ISBN 978- 0-749123-65-8

Witelson, S. F. (1977) 'Developmental dyslexia, two right hemispheres and one left' *Science* 195 309-11

Wolf, M. and Bowers, P. 1999 'The double deficit hypothesis for developmental dyslexia' *Journal of Educational Psychology* 9 (3) 1-24 eISSN 1939-2176

Wren, S. (2005) 'The double deficit hypothesis for decoding fluency' http://www.balancedreading.com/doubledeficit.html (Accessed 1/8/2010)

Ziviano, J. and Watson-Will, A. (1998) 'Writing speed and legibility of 7-14 year old school students using modern cursive script' *Australian Occupational Therapy Journal* 45 59-64 eISSN 1440-1630

8

Depression in Dyslexic Children Attending Specialized Schools: A Case of Switzerland

Tamara Leonova
University of Nancy, France

1. Introduction

Dyslexia (specific reading disability) is a common, cognitively and behaviorally heterogeneous developmental condition, characterized primarily by a severe difficulty in mastering reading despite average intelligence and adequate education (Grigorenko, 2001). A recent epidemiological study in France found 3.5% of the students in 2nd grade (CE1) were dyslexic (Billard et al., 2007).

According to an INSERM report (Expertise de l'INSERM, p. 162), even though dyslexia is the most studied of the learning disabilities, the scientific community knows relatively little about it, and most of this knowledge comes from studies done about the cognitive, social and emotional development of English-speaking dyslexics. The depressive symptoms of French-speaking children and adolescents suffering from reading disabilities have not been empirically studied.

In general, learning disabilities (LD) increase the risk of depression. According to a literature review based on research conducted between 1980 and 2003, 16 out of 24 studies (67%) found that the level of depression of those suffering from LD was significantly higher than those without LD (Sideridis, 2006). New theoretical models have been developed to explain depression in students with LD (e.g., Sideridis, 2005, 2007). In a review of publications on the links between literacy and mental disorders, Maughan and Carroll (2006) concluded "literacy problems are associated with increased risks of both externalizing and internalizing disorders in childhood" (p. 350). They also highlighted the inconsistent results found when trying to associate depression and dyslexia.

Researchers and practitioners have focused on depression[1] since it is one of the major risk factors in youth suicide. Several publications on dyslexia and schooling of dyslexic children mention that they are susceptible to developing depression (Hulme & Snowling, 1997; Reid & Fawcett, 2004; Hunter-Carsch & Herrington, 2001; Hunter-Carsch, 2001; Scott, 2004).

Researchers in the UK have been investigating depression and anxiety in children with learning disabilities for quite some time (Brumback, Dietz-Schmidt, & Weinberg, 1977;

---

[1] A single definition for depression has not been found. We use the terms depression, depressive mood, depressive disorder and depressive symptoms interchangeably. In the studies on depression and dyslexia presented in the introduction and in our study, the objective of the researchers is not to diagnose depression but rather to evaluate the level of depressive symptoms.

Stevenson & Romney, 1984), whereas in France little research on the problem has been conducted. We therefore chose to investigate the level of depressive symptoms in French speaking dyslexic students and to examine the prevalence of children with clinical symptoms of depression. After presenting the results of research on depression in dyslexic children and adolescents, we will briefly discuss the limitations of generalizing research conducted in English, dominant in this field, when extended to a sample of French-speaking dyslexic students. The second part of the chapter will present a study exploring depressive symptoms in French-speaking students.

2. Depression in children and adolescents with dyslexia

In the first decade of the 21st century, researchers have become increasingly interested in depression in children and adolescents with dyslexia (e.g. Carroll, Maughan, Goodman, & Meltzer, 2005; Maughan, Rowe, Loeber, & Stouthamer-Loeber, 2003; Miller, Hynd, & Miller, 2005; Willcutt & Pennington, 2000), as well as adults with dyslexia (Alexander-Passe, 2006). Nonetheless, the first studies on the internalized problems and depression in people with specific reading disabilities were conducted during 1980s and also at the beginning of the 1990s (e.g. Casey, Levy, Brown, & Brooksgunn, 1992; Kline, 1986). Results showed that children with dyslexia were more anxious and less happy than peers without dyslexia, despite their coming from families with high socio-economic levels, with parents having strong educational backgrounds and being well informed about dyslexia (Casey, Levy, Brown, & Brooksgunn, 1992). This study compared 28 dyslexic children with 39 children in a control group and was based of evaluations by parents.

A few years later the results of another study helped to improve our understanding of depression in people with dyslexia. By comparing depression measurements in children, adolescents and adults with dyslexia in a cross-sectional study, Boetsch, Green and Pennington (1996) showed that children and adolescents had high levels of depression compared to the control group. On the other hand, in dyslexic adults the degree of depressive symptoms was comparable to the control group. It therefore seems that people with dyslexia feel less depressed and happier as they grow up.

Willcutt and Pennington (2000) in a study comparing behavior problems in twins with and without dyslexia found that girls had higher levels of depression than boys. Reading disability and depression were specifically associated only for girls. These results support those found by Dekker, Ferdinand, van Lang, Bongers, van der Ende and Verhulst (2007) on the general population and the critical review of literature by Piccinelli and Wilkinson (2000) that found that girls suffered from higher levels of depression than boys.

Research by Maughan and al. (2003) based on results from a longitudinal study with three periods of internalized and externalized problems of dyslexic boys between 9 and 15 years old found that the percentage of boys labeled as being depressed decreased with age: 13.4% at 7 years old, 7.1% at 10 and 2.5% at 13. They suggested that reading disabilities were strongly associated with short-term depression, but that there was no increased risk of long-term depression.

In another study in the UK, Carroll, Maughan, Goodman, & Meltzer (2005) evaluated different internal and external problems in 68 girls and 221 boys from 11 to 15 years old with specific reading disabilities. Reading disabilities were associated with depressive mood in self-evaluation scores of adolescents. Although there was no association between dyslexia and depressive mood in girls, there was a strong correlation between depression and dyslexia in boys, especially younger ones. Carroll et al., thus, concluded that specific reading disabilities were associated with all the major psychiatric diagnosis except with depression where no relationship was found. No link between dyslexia and depression was found (Carroll et al., 2005).

Results from research by Miller, Hynd and Miller (2005) conducted in the USA, based on a different methodology with three sources of information, were similar to those of Carroll et al. (2005). These researchers did not test for the impact of gender due to sample size (N = 79 with 20 people with dyslexia and 59 without, from 6 to 16 years old). Instead they used three sources of information (i.e., parents, children, and teachers), and two types of diagnosis for dyslexia as well as measuring depression, anxiety and somatic symptoms. Since no significant difference in level of depressive symptoms was found between dyslexic children and the control group, when comparing depressive symptoms according to information source, type of dyslexic diagnosis or measurement, Miller et al. concluded there was no significant difference between the two groups. For dyslexic children and adolescents all the depression scores were within the norms and no age effect was found.

In a more recent study conducted by Alexander-Passe (2006), the depression scores of 19 dyslexic adolescents (12 boys and 7 girls from 14 to 16 years old) were compared with scores of different groups of subjects from other studies using the same measurements (i.e., Beck Depression Inventory-II; Beck, Steer, & Brown, 1996). These girls seemed to have a moderate level of depression, whereas boys had a low level. The overall depression scores of dyslexic adolescents were slightly higher than the norm of students without dyslexia, though not reaching clinical levels.

What conclusions can be drawn from these studies? First of all, it is difficult to compare these studies as they use different methodologies, samples and measurement tools. Secondly, when control groups were used, certain researchers found the differences significant (e.g. Casey et al., 1992), whereas others considered depression scores of dyslexic students to be similar to those of the control group (e.g. Boetsch et al., 1996; Miller et al., 2005; Alexander-Passe, 2006) or that only girls' scores were different (e.g. Willcutt & Pennington, 2000). Thirdly, only three studies namely, Alexander-Passe (2006), Miller and al. (2005) and Willcutt & Pennington (2000) refer to normal depression scores to evaluate levels of depression in the studied samples. Therefore, though problems of depression seem to be associated with reading disabilities, particularly with girls, more systematic studies using same methodologies, similar samples and same measurement protocols are needed to conclusively evaluate the risks of depression with dyslexia.

Languages' alphabetical systems differ in their degree of grapheme-phoneme correspondence transparency. Some languages have systems that are considered to be transparent as they transcribe surface phonology with relative fidelity. Others have opaque spelling; their graphic-phonologic encoding rules are inconsistent (Grigorenko, 2001; Ziegler & Montant, 2005).

Research on reading and writing acquisition in French has found that French is in between these two groups of languages. French is closer to transparent languages when being read. On the other hand, phoneme-grapheme relationships in French are much more irregular

(Peereman & Content, 1999; Sprenger-Charolles & Serniclaes, 2003; Ziegler, Jacobs, & Stone, 1996). As a result, when learning spelling, French is closer to opaque or irregular languages like English (Ziegler & Montant, 2005). Since French spelling is more regular than English, French dyslexics have less problems with reading skills than English ones do. French dyslexic reading disabilities should have less impact on other school learning than for English speakers, and thus one might argue that there should be less symptoms of depression. English-speaking dyslexics seem be the most linguistically and thus socially disadvantaged. Applying generalized findings about the psychological well-being of this group to other groups with linguistic advantages would be unjustified. We can conclude that in the case of dyslexia, the language spoken by a dyslexic person must be taken into consideration when evaluating their difficulties.

Language regularity is not the only factor limiting the external validity of findings with English-speakers. Other factors, part of cultural context, are also pertinent as they affect the quality and quantity of difficulties that dyslexics confront. Some studies have highlighted the effect of school choice on dyslexic child self-esteem (Burden, 2005; Humphrey, 2002; Thomson, 1990) and on general psychological functioning of children with learning disabilities (Wiener & Tardif, 2004). Even if the findings of these studies are sometimes contradictory or difficult to interpret due to methodology (e.g., no control group or inadequate sample selection) they still suggest that school choice influences the psychological well-being of dyslexic children.

We hypothesize therefore both that language characteristics (opaque verses transparent spelling) influence the visibility of dyslexia in a person and that educational systems, in particular specialized ones, affect a student's psychological well-being. Since educational systems in different countries, attitudes towards dyslexia and knowledge about this specific learning disability in different cultures are quite different, generalizing findings from research on English-speakers or other countries or languages would be unjustifiable.

3. Objectives

Our study has two objectives: 1) examine the level of depressive symptoms in French-speaking dyslexic children in a specialized school in French-speaking Switzerland and compare them with children without dyslexia, and 2) evaluate the level of depressive symptoms in the two populations. Little international research has been conducted on this type of specialized schooling for dyslexic children.

4. Method

4.1 Participants

Sixty-six children participated in the study: 35 dyslexic children in a specialized school and 31 children without dyslexia. All were from Fribourg canton in Switzerland and had French as their maternal and only language spoken at home. They all had started school at age 5 to 6[2], had traditional schooling, no serious neurological, sight or hearing problems, took no regular medication, nor had any oral language problems, anxiety or depressive disorders.

[2] In Fribourg canton, school is not obligatory for children when they are 5 years old. Most children start primary school at age 6.

This information was obtained from parents' responses to a questionnaire designed for this study. The socio-demographic characteristics of the families are presented in Table 1. Informed and written consent was obtained from subjects' parents.

4.1.1 Selection of the dyslexic children

35 (13 female and 22 male) dyslexic children (M = 10 years 7 months, SD = 1.49, from 8 years 2 months to 14 years 10 months) took part in the study. All had been diagnosed as dyslexic by age 8 - 9 years by the canton school system. All had global IQs greater than 80 (IQ scores were indicated in their school files). All the children had remedial speech therapy three times per week during the school year (average weekly duration: one and half hours) and their reading skills were between 1 year 8 months and 4 years 9 months behind, according to Test de l'Alouette. Their hyperactivity scores in SDQ (Goodman, 2001) were less than 6 (within the normal range).

Age chosen for the sample is justified since obligatory schooling in Switzerland is from 6 to 15 years old. As a result, one of dyslexia's known characteristics, being 2 years behind in reading skills, can be found in 8 year old children.

4.1.2 Selection of children in the control group

The children in the control group were all recruited from French-speaking schools in Fribourg canton. 31 (16 female and 15 male) children (M = 11 years 2 months, SD = 2.46, from 8 years 4 months to 15 years 1 month) participated in the study. All children had their parents' consent. To collect information about families and their child's development, parents also completed a questionnaire identical to the one completed for dyslexic children. Dyslexic and control groups were matched for age and gender as best possible. The socio-demographic characteristics of the families are presented in Table 1.

Data analysis suggests that more mothers finished secondary school in the control group than did mothers of dyslexic children. More mothers of dyslexic children have manual professions. Significantly more mothers of the control group are housewives. Overall, mothers of children without dyslexia had higher levels of schooling, and as housewives, they had more opportunity to take care of the children and better help them with their schoolwork.

We were not allowed to give IQ tests to the control group: according to the school, all children in the normal school system had normal IQs. The children in the control group took a reading test (i.e. Test de l'Alouette) to test the reading skills, as well as Children's Depression Inventory by Kovacs (2001). The Test de l'Alouette results confirmed that children in the control group had normal reading skills for their age. Since students' schedules were already quite busy, the school did not authorize us to diagnose for dyslexia using ODEDYS (*Outil de Dépistage des Dyslexies*) tests.

4.2 Procedure

During the first step, we tested to confirm that the children in the dyslexic group were properly diagnosed as dyslexic. Reading level was assessed using Test de l'Alouette (Lefevrais, 1967), a standard reading achievement test widely used with French children. A meaningful passage was presented, and the participant had to read it aloud (within a 3-min time limit). Time (in sec/syllable) and accuracy (number of errors, adjusted for the amount of text read) were measured.

We used ODEDYS (2002), which offers a number of tasks designed to evaluate skills that are frequently limited or deficient in dyslexic children. The scores for each task in ODEDYS are presented in Table 2.

		Dyslexic children (n = 35)	**Control group** (n = 31)
Age		M = 10.7 years SD = 1.49	M = 11.2 years SD = 2.46
Sex	*Girls*	37[a]	52
	Boys	63	48
Mother's level of studies	*Primary*	5.4	3.2
	Secondary	43.3[b]	58.1[b]
	Higher education	45.9	38.7
	No response	5.4	-
Mother's profession	*Manual*	24.3[c]	12.9[c]
	Non manual	64.9	67.7
	Housewife	5.4[d]	19.4[d]
	No response	5.4	-
Father's profession	*Manual*	48.7	41.9
	Non manual	45.9	58.1
	No response	5.4	-

[a] %
[b] $p < .001$ (χ^2 (2, N = 62) = 17.94
[c] $p < .05$ (χ^2 (2, N = 62) = 3.90
[d] $p < .001$ (χ^2 (2, N = 62) = 23.09

Table 1. Demographic characteristics of the sample

The second step was to evaluate children's depression.

All of the evaluations took place individually in a room set aside by the corresponding school for the researchers. To insure that dyslexic students' reading difficulties did not interfere with their understanding the questionnaire, each item of the CDI (*Children's Depression Inventory*, Kovacs, 2001) was read aloud to the dyslexic child, after which the child indicated the sentence that best described himself/herself. The same procedure was followed with the control group.

At the end of the session each student was thanked and received a candy.

ODEDYS tasks	*M*	*SD*
Number of irregular words correctly read	6.61 (20)[a]	4.66
Time taken for task (sec)	51.52	25.85
Number of regular words correctly read	14.39 (20)	4.42
Time taken for task (sec)	44.85	24.32
Number of pseudo words correctly read	12.06 (20)	4.38
Time taken for task (sec)	46.76	22.95
Number of correct responses in suppression task	6.67 (10)	2.47
Number of correct responses in fusion task	6.91 (10)	2.55
Short term memory		
- right span	5.91 (8)	1.91
- wrong span	2.73 (8)	1.13
Number of irregular words correctly written	2.36 (10)	3.00
Number of regular words correctly written	6.06 (10)	2.81
Number of pseudo words correctly written	5.61 (10)	3.07

[a] Number in parentheses is maximal score for each task.

Table 2. Means and standard deviations of the ODEDYS tests

4.3 Measurements

Children's Depression Inventory (CDI) (Kovacs, 2001)

CDI is a self-evaluation scale of depression for children and adolescents, 7 to 17 years old, elaborated by Kovacs in 1981. It has 27 items to specifically evaluate the different aspects of depression. Each item has three phrases , rated 0 to 2, to describe the increasing intensity of the depressive symptom. The child chooses the phrase that corresponds best to his state during the last 15 days (Bouvard et al., 2002). The global depression score is the sum of the scores of the 27 items. Global scores run from 0 to 54, higher scores representing more severe depression. CDI scores above 13 correspond to a moderate-severe depression (Greenham, 1999).

We chose this test for three reasons. First, it is often used in research about depression in children and adolescents. It may be the optimal measurement of depression in children and adolescents (Vella, Heath, & Miezitis, 1992). Secondly, it is relatively short (27 items compared with 79 in MDI-C (*Multiscore Depression Inventory for Children,* Berndt & Kaiser, 1999), which is also validated in French); as a result it is particularly well adapted for students with learning disabilities whose attention and concentration spans are quite limited. Finally, it has good psychometric characteristics (see Table 3 for comparison with alphas of Cronbach) and good retest reproducibility ($r = .82$) after a period of one month (Finch, Saylor, Edwards, & McIntosh, 1987). The validity of CDI has been confirmed by significant correlations with other methods of depression self-evaluation (Asarnow &

Carlson, 1985; Shain, Naylor, & Alessi, 1990) and with ranking of depressive symptoms by clinical psychologists (Hodges & Craighead, 1990; Shain and al., 1990).

Subcategories	Our study	Kovacs (2001)	French version of Lise Saint-Laurent
Pleasure	.60	.66	-
Negative mood	.48	.62	-
Feeling of inefficiency	.52	.63	-
Interpersonal problems	.71	.59	-
Negative self-esteem	.64	.68	-
Global CDI	.85	.71-.89	.92 [a]

[a] after Cuillerier (2004)

Table 3. Cronbach's alphas of CDI by Kovacs (2001) from different studies

5. Results

5.1 Level of depressive symptoms

To compare the level of depression between dyslexic students and those in the control group, we performed an analysis of variance (ANOVA), using 2 (Group: dyslexics vs control) x 2 (Sex: girls vs boys) x 2 (Age: 8-10 vs 11-15 years old) as between-subjects variables with variable Group introduced as a fixed variable and the variables Sex and Age as covariates. The results show that there was no significant main effect of the variable Group ($F(1, 62) = 1.23$, $p > .05$). There was no main effect of the variable Sex ($F < 1$) and the variable Age ($F < 1$). The means and standard deviations are presented in Table 4.

5.2 Prevalence of depressive symptoms in dyslexic children and adolescents

Do dyslexic children and the control group have the same risk of depression? To answer this question, we analyzed the two groups by comparing the dimension of the severity of depression. One of the advantages of CDI scale is that it has normative references used by professionals to establish the clinical level of depression. Global CDI scores above 13 correspond to a moderate to severe depression. Table 4 shows means and SD of CDI scores for dyslexic and non-dyslexic children.

To evaluate the severity of depression in children, we reassigned the global score of depression a categorical value of 1 for CDI scores between 0 and 13, and 2 for scores over 13. We thereby distinguished between weak and clinical cases of depression (i.e. moderate and severe). We then calculated percentages of children with weak and clinical levels of depression for each group. The results presented in Table 5 clearly show that in the group of dyslexic children 80% have weak levels of depression and 20% have moderate to severe levels. Results from the control group revealed that in children without dyslexia 97% had weak levels of depression and only 3% had clinical levels. Separate chi-square tests for each group showed significant differences in the number of students with weak vs clinical levels of depression ($p < .01$).

	M	*SD*
Children with dyslexia (*n* = 35)	8.74	7.24
Children without dyslexia (*n* = 31)	6.77	3.99
Girls (*n* = 29)	7.14	5.19
Boys (*n* = 37)	8.35	6.55
8-10 year-olds (*n* = 34)	8.44	6.80
11-15 year-olds (*n* = 32)	7.16	4.98

Table 4. Means and standard deviations of depression scores as a function of group, sex and age.

	Dyslexics (*n* = 35)		Control group (*n* = 31)	
	Low level of depression	High level of depression	Low level of depression	High level of depression
Global CDI	80^{ac}	20^{ad}	97^{bc}	3^{bd}

^{a,b} $p < .001$
^{c} $p < .05$
^{d} $p < .05$

Table 5. Percentage of students with low vs high levels of depression as a function of group

6. Discussion

The objective of our study was to compare the levels of depressive symptoms in dyslexic French-speaking students in specialized schools with students without dyslexia and to establish the prevalence of depressive symptoms in these dyslexic students. As mentioned in the introduction, relatively little research has been conducted to investigate depression in people with dyslexia. Their results are inconsistent. In addition, most of these studies have been carried out with English speakers. Nonetheless, educational systems and specialized educational structures differ from one country to the next. Furthermore, different languages offer intrinsically different levels of difficulty for people with dyslexia. The extremely irregular grapheme-to-phoneme correspondence (GPC) of English is quite an obstacle for students learning to read, and particularly so for dyslexic children (Seymour, Aro, & Erskine, 2003). Even though French is classified as a language with irregular GPC, as noted earlier, it is more regular for reading than English.

The findings in this study suggest that global scores of depression appear to be the same for dyslexic children and the control group. These results are consistent with those found by Miller et al. (2005), who used CDI with children and adolescents from 6 to 16 years old.

Their results are also similar to those found by Alexander-Passe (2006), who found no difference between dyslexic adolescents (14-16 years old) and those without dyslexia though using a different research methodology. The study by Willcutt and Pennington (2000) based on the comparison of twins with and without dyslexia revealed the same results. This last study is all the more valuable since Willcutt and Pennington used CDI to measure depression. Our study found no difference due to gender or age. As such, our results agree with those of Carroll et al. (2005) and de Miller and al. (2005).

In our study, no difference was found when average global scores of depressive symptoms were compared between student groups with and without dyslexia. Nonetheless, evaluation of the prevalence of those having clinical levels of depression showed that dyslexic students were much more susceptible to develop depression than students without dyslexia. Twenty percent of the dyslexic children and adolescents in our study had clinical levels of depression whereas 3% did in the control group. As 10% of the general population is considered to have clinical levels of depression (Greenham, 1999), this leads us to conclude that dyslexic students are more at risk of developing depression.

6.1 Limitations and research perspective

The first limitation of this study is its limited generalization. We have investigated depression level in dyslexic students going to a specialized school in French-speaking Switzerland. While these children may have severe levels of dyslexia (which justify their placement in this school), they are in a school environment that is well adapted for their disabilities. Scholastic expectations, rhythm and individual assistance are appropriate to meet their specific needs. In this school a medico-pedagogical team of specialized teachers, psychologists, and speech therapists accompanies each child and offers effective social support to both the student and parents.

When we consider the favorable context of the dyslexic students in our study, we are concerned about the psychological well-being, especially depression, of dyslexic students in integrated in traditional classes. Different systems of school integration for dyslexic students may offer different levels of support. A recent study of parents of Irish dyslexic children (Nugent, 2007) found that when schooling began these parents preferred integrating their children in traditional classes. Nonetheless, Nugent (2007) argued that their children would benefit from better schooling conditions in specialized schools. In Sweden, mothers of dyslexic students integrated in traditional classes emphasized that schools did not offer appropriate support for the needs of their children (Roll-Pettersson & Mattson, 2007). Another study suggested that dyslexic students integrated in traditional classes in the Netherlands considered teachers and peers as threatening their self-esteem (Singer, 2007). Empirical evidence also supports specialized schooling. Butler and Marinov-Glassman (1994) concluded that with LD students' self-perception in specialized schools was more positive than that of students with LD in special classes or low-achieving students without LD. Burden (2005) found that specialized schools promote the psychological well-being of dyslexic students.

The conclusions of these studies lead us to be extremely prudent when making generalizations about dyslexic students from our findings. This limitation opens the perspective of intercultural research on the psychological well-being of dyslexic children as a function of different systems of school integration of these children in countries such France, Switzerland, Canada and Belgium. Research in this field until now has been limited to investigating self-esteem.

6.2 Pedagogical and educational implications

What recommendations and warnings can be drawn from the results of this study?

First, dyslexic children in a specialized school do not show more signs of emotional distress than students without dyslexia. As a group, regardless of age or sex, they are no more at risk of becoming depressed than peers without dyslexia.

Secondly, though as a group dyslexic students had a relatively low level of depression, the percentage of dyslexic students with clinical depression is significantly higher than that of the control group. This implies that parents and teachers must be attentive to these children's psychological well-being and wary of their slightest signs of distress. Adults must constantly be aware of the considerable individual differences within a group of dyslexic students. As risk factors and protection have not been studied much in dyslexic students, we can only conclude that these students are not all the same when facing psychological problems they may develop during their years of schooling. Though the current results showing no difference between dyslexic and non-dyslexic children may be reassuring, they must not be generalized for all dyslexic students, regardless of system of integration in school, nor even within a group of dyslexic students in the same system.

7. Acknowledgments

We would like to extend our gratitude to the direction of Institut Saint-Joseph in Fribourg (Switzerland), Mr. Noël and Ms. Savoy, as well as the medico-pedagogical team, whose open-minded and helpful attitude allowed us to complete this research. We would also like to sincerely thank the parents and children who participated in this study.

8. References

Alexander-Passe, N. (2006). How dyslexic teenagers cope: an investigation of self-esteem, coping and depression. *Dyslexia*, 12, pp. 256-275

Arnold, E.M., Goldston, D.B., & Walsh, A.K. (2005). Severity of emotional and behavioural problems among poor and typical readers. *Journal of Abnormal Child Psychology*, 33, pp. 205-217

Asarnow, J.R., & Carlson, G.A. (1985). Depression self-relating scale: Utility with child psychiatric inpatients. *Journal of Consulting and Clinical Psychology*, 53, pp. 491-499.

Beck, A.T., Steer, R.A., & Brown, G.K. (1996). *Beck Depression Inventory*, The Psychological Corp: San Antonio

Bender, W.N., Rosenkrans, C.B., & Crane, M. (1999). Stress, depression, and suicide among students with learning disabilities: Assessing the risk. *Learning Disability Quarterly*, 22, pp. 143-156

Billard, C., Fluss, J., Richard, G., Ziegler, J., Ecaille, J., Magnan, A. et al. (2007). *Résultats préliminaires d'une étude épidémiologique transversale des apprentissages en lecture, orthographe et calcul au CE 1. Dyslexie, dysorthographie, dyscalculie : bilan des données scientifiques*, Publications INSERM, Paris

Boetsch, E.A., Green, P.A., & Pennington, B.F. (1996). Psychosocial correlates of dyslexia across the life-span. *Development and Psychopathology*, 8, pp. 539-562

Bouvard, M., Le Heuzey, M-F, Mouren-Simeoni, M-C, Abbou, H., Bange, F., Martin, C., Reneric, J-P, Saiag, M-C., & Touzin, M. (2002). *L'hyperactivité de l'enfance à l'âge adulte*, Doin éditeurs, Rueil-Malmaison

Bruck, M., Genesee, F., & Caravolas, M. (1997). A cross-linguistic study of early literacy acquisition. In : *Foundations of reading acquisition and dyslexia: Implications for early intervention*, Blachman, pp. 145-162, Erlbaum, Mahwah, NJ

Brumback, R.A., Dietz-Schmidt, S.G., & Weinberg, W.A. (1977). Depression in children referred to an educational diagnostic center: Diagnosis and treatment and analysis of criteria and literature review. *Disturbances of the Nervous System*, 38, pp. 529-535

Burden, R. (2005). *Dyslexia and self-concept*, Whurr Publishers, London

Butler, R., & Marinov-Glassman, D. (1994). The effects of educational placement and grade level on the self-perceptions of low achievers and students with learning disabilities. *Journal of Learning Disabilities*, 27, pp. 325-334

Carroll, J.M., Maughan, B., Goodman, R., & Meltzer, H. (2005). Literacy difficulties and psychiatric disorders: Evidence for comorbidity. *Journal of Child Psychology and Psychiatry*, 46, pp. 524-532

Casey, R., Levy, S.E., Brown, K., & Brooks-Gunn, J. (1992). Impaired emotional health in children with mild reading disability. *Developmental and Behavioural Paediatrics*, 13, pp. 256-260

Chaix, Y., Trabanino, M., Taylor, M., & Demonet, J.F. (2005). La dyslexie développementale: Apports récents de la génétique et de la neuro-imagerie, In *Neuropsychologie de l'enfant et troubles du développement*: Hommet, Jambaqué, Billard, & Gillet, pp. 73-101, SOLAL, Marseille

Colbert, P., Newman, B., Ney, P., & Young, X. (1982). Learning disabilities as a symptom of depression in children. *Journal of Learning Disabilities*, 15, pp. 333-336

Cuillerier, L.M. (2004). Fiche sur l'inventaire de dépression pour enfant de Kovacs version candienne-française. Site sur les instruments psychométriques par l'Université McGill de Montréal. Vu le 20 décembre 2006

Dekker, M.C., Ferdinand, R.F., van Lang N., Bongers, I., van der Ende, J., & Verhulst, F. (2007). Developmental trajectories of depressive symptoms from early childhood to late adolescence: gender differences and adult outcome. *Journal of Child Psychology and Psychiatry*, 48, pp. 657-666

Finch, A.J., Saylor, C.F., Edwards, G.L., & McIntosh, J.A. (1987). Children's Depression Inventory: Reliability over repeated administrations. *Journal of Clinical Child Psychology*, 16, pp. 339-341

Frith, U. (1999). Paradoxes in the definition of dyslexia. *Dyslexia*, 5, pp. 192-214

Frith, U., Wimmer, H., & Landerl, K. (1998). Differences in phonological recoding in German- and English-speaking children. *Scientific Studies of Reading*, 2, pp. 31-54

Goldstein, D., Paul, G.G., & Sanfilippo-Cohen, S. (1985). Depression and achievement in subgroups of children with learning disabilities. *Journal of Applied Developmental Psychology*, 6, pp. 263-275

Goldston, D. B., Walsch, A., Mayfield Arnold, E., Reboussion, B., Sergent Daniel, S., Erkanli, A., Nutter, D., Hickman, E., Palmes, G., Snider, E., & Wood, F. B. (2007). Reading problems, psychiatric disorders, and functional impairment from mid- to late adolescence. *Journal of American Academy of Child And Adolescent Psychiatry*, 46, pp. 25-32

Goodman, R. (2001). Psychometric properties of the Strengths and Difficulties Questionnaire (SDQ). *Journal of the American Academy of Child and Adolescent Psychiatry*, 40, pp. 1337-1345

Goswami, U. (2000). Phonological representations, reading development and dyslexia: Towards a cross-linguistic theoretical framework. *Dyslexia*, 6, pp. 133-151

Goswami, U., Gombert, J.E., & Barrera, L.F. (1998). Children's orthographic representations and linguistic transparency: Nonsense word reading in English, French, and Spanish. *Applied Psycholinguistics*, 19, pp. 19-52

Greenham, S. L. (1999). Learning disabilities and psychosocial adjustment: A critical review. *Child Neuropsychology*, 5, pp. 171-196

Grigorenko, E. (2001). Developmental dyslexia: An update on genes, brains, and environments. *Journal of Child Psychology and Psychiatry*, 42, pp. 91-125

Hall, C.E., & Haws, D. (1989). Depressive symptomatology in learning-disabled and nonlearning-disabled students. *Psychology in the Schools*, 26, pp. 263-275

Hasher, L., & Zacks, R.T. (1979). Automatic and effortful processes in memory. *Journal of Experimental Psychology: General*, 108, pp. 356-388

Heiervang, E., Stevenson, J., Lund, A., & Hugdahl, A. (2001). Behaviour problems in children with dyslexia. *Nord Journal of Psychiatry*, 55, pp. 251-256

Hinshaw, S.P. (1992). Externalizing behavior problems and academic underachievement in childhood and adolescence: causal relationships and underlying mechanisms. *Psychological Bulletin*, 111, pp. 127-155

Hodges, K., & Craighead, W.E. (1990). Relationship of Children's Depression Inventory factors to diagnosed depression. *Psychological Assessment*, 2, pp. 489-492

Hoy, C., Gregg, N., Wisenbaker, J., Manglitz, E., King, M., & Moreland, C. (1997). Depression and anxiety in two groups of adults with learning disabilities. *Learning Disability Quarterly*, 20, pp. 280-291

Hulme, C., & Snowling, M. (1997). *Dyslexia: Biology, cognition and intervention*, Whurr Publishers, London.

Humphrey, N. (2002). Teacher and pupil ratings of self-esteem in developmental dyslexia. *British Journal of Special Education*, 29, pp. 29-36

Hunter-Carsch, M. (2001). *Dyslexia. A psychosocial perspective*. Whurr Publishers, London.

Hunter-Carsch, M., & Herrington, M. (2001). *Dyslexia and effective learning in secondary and tertiary education*. Whurr Publishers, London.

Huntington, D.D., & Bender, W.N. (1993). Adolescents with learning disabilities at risk? Emotional well-being, depression, suicide. *Journal of Learning Disabilities*, 26, pp. 159-166

Kline, C.L. (1986). The dyslexia-emotional dyad: implications for diagnosis and treatment. *Canadian Journal of Psychiatry*, 31, pp. 517-520

Kovacs, M. (2001). *Children's depression inventory*, Multi-Heath System, New York.

Lefavrais, P. (1967). *Test de l'Alouette: Manuel*, ECPA, Paris.

Maag, J.W., & Behrens, J.T. (1989). Depression and cognitive self-statements of learning disabled and seriously emotionally disturbed adolescents. *The Journal of Special Education*, 23, pp. 17-27

Maag, J.W., & Reid, R. (2006). Depression among students with learning disabilities: Assessing the risk. *Journal of Learning Disabilities*, 39, pp. 3-10

Maughan, B., & Carroll, J. (2006). Literacy and mental disorders. *Current Opinion in Psychiatry*, 19, pp. 350-354

Maughan, B., Rowe, R., Loeber, R., & Stouthamer-Loeber, M. (2003). Reading problems and depressed mood. *Journal of Abnormal Child Psychology*, 31, pp. 219-229

Mayes, S., & Calhoun, S. L. (2006). Frequency of reading, math, and writing disabilities children with clinical disorders. *Learning and Individual Differences*, 16, pp. 147-157

McNulty, M.A. (2003). Dyslexia and the life course. *Journal of Learning Disabilities*, 36, pp. 363-381

Miles, E. (2000). Dyslexia may show a different face in different languages. *Dyslexia*, 6, pp. 193-201

Miller, C. J., Hynd, G. W., & Miller, S. R. (2005). Children with dyslexia : Not necessarily at risk for elevated internalizing symptoms. *Reading and Writing*, 18, pp. 425-436

Nugent, M. (2007). Comparing inclusive and segregated settings for children with dyslexia - parental perspectives from Ireland. *Support for Learning*, 22, pp. 52-59

ODEDYS (2002). Laboratoire Cogni-Sciences IUFM de Grenoble. Web: http://www.grenoble.iufm.fr/recherch/cognisciences

Peck, M. (1985). Crisis intervention treatment with chronically and acutely suicidal adolescents. In *Youth suicide*, Peck, Farberow, & Litman, pp. 112-122, Springer, New York.

Peereman, R., & Content, A. (1999). LEXOP: A lexical database providing orthography-phonology statistics for French monosyllabic words. *Behavior Research Methods, Instruments, and Computers*, 31, pp. 376-379

Piccinelli, M., & Wilkinson, G. (2000). Gender differences in depression. Critical review. *British Journal of Psychiatry*, 177, pp. 486-492

Prior, M., Smart, D., Sanson, A., & Oberklaid, F. (1999). Relationships between learning difficulties and psychological problems in preadolescent children from a longitudinal sample. *Journal of the American Academy of Child and Adolescent Psychiatry*, 38, pp. 429-436

Reid, G., & Fawcett, A. (2004). *Dyslexia in context. Research, policy and practice*, Whurr Publishers, London.

Reynolds, W.M. (1984). Depression in children and adolescents : Phenomenology, evaluation, and treatment. *School Psychology Review*, 13, pp. 171-182

Riddick, B. (1996). *Living with dyslexia. The social and emotional consequences of special learning difficulties*, Routledge, London.

Riddick, B., Sterling, C., Farmer, M., & Morgan, S. (1999). Self-esteem and anxiety in the educational histories of adult dyslexic students. *Dyslexia*, 5, pp. 227-248

Rie, H.E. (1966). Depression in childhood: A survey of some pertinent contributions. *Journal of the American Academy of Child Psychiatry*, 5, pp. 653-685

Roll-Pettersson, L., & Mattson, E. (2007). Perspectives of mothers of children with dyslectic difficulties concerning their encounters with school: a Swedish example. *European Journal of Special Needs Education*, 22, pp. 409-423

Rourke, B.P. (1988). Socioemotional disturbances of learning disabled children. *Journal of Consulting and Clinical Psychology*, 56, pp. 801-810

Sanson, A., Prior, M., & Smart, D. (1996). Reading disabilities with and without behaviour problems at 7-8 years: predicting from longitudinal data from infancy to 6 years. *Journal of Child Psychology and Psychiatry*, 37, pp. 529-541

Scott, R. (2004). *Dyslexia and counselling*, Whurr Publishers, London.

Seymour, P., Aro, M., & Erskine, J. (2003). Foundation literacy acquisition in European orthographies. *British Journal of Psychology*, 94, pp. 143-174

Shain, B.N., Naylor, M., & Alessi, N. (1990). Comparison of self-rated and clinician-rated measures of depression in adolescents. *American Journal of Psychiatry*, 147, pp. 793-795

Sideridis, G., D. (2005). Goal orientation, academic achievement, and depression: Evidence in favour of a revised goal theory framework. *Journal of Educational Psychology, 97,* pp. 366-375

Sideridis, G.D. (2006). Understanding low achievement and depression in children with learning disabilities: A goal orientation approach. *International Review of Research in Mental Retardation*, 31, pp. 163-203

Sideridis, G., D. (2007). Why are students with LD depressed? A goal orientation model of depression vulnerability. *Journal of Learning Disabilities*, 40, pp. 526-539

Singer, E. (2007). Coping with academic failure, a study of Dutch children with dyslexia. *Dyslexia*, 14, pp. 314-333.

Sprenger-Charolles, L., & Colé, P. (2003). *Lecture et dyslexie : Approche cognitive*, Dunod, Paris

Sprenger-Charolles, L., & Serniclaes, W. (2003). Acquisition de la lecture et de l'écriture et dyslexie : revue de la littérature. *Revue Française de Linguistique Appliquée*, 1, pp. 63-90

Stevenson, D.T., & Romney, D.M. (1984). Depression in learning disabled children. *Journal of Learning Disabilities*, 17, pp. 579-582

Thomson, M. (1990). *Dyslexia and Development*. Whurr Publishers, London

Vella, D.D., Heath, N.L., & Miezitis, S. (1992). Childhood depression assessment issues. In: *Creating alternatives to depression in our schools: Assessment, intervention, prevention*, Miezitis, pp. 95-106, Hogrefe and Huber, Toronto, ON

Wiener, J., & Harris, P.J. (1993). Les relations sociales des sous-groupes d'enfants ayant des troubles d'apprentissage. *Enfance*, 47, pp. 295–316

Wiener, J., & Tardif, C. (2004). Social and emotional functioning of children with learning disabilities: Does special education placement make a difference? *Learning Disabilities: Research and Practice*, 19, pp. 20-32

Willcutt, E.G., & Pennington, B.F. (2000). Psychiatric comorbidity in children and adolescents with reading disability. *Journal of Child Psychology and Psychiatry*, 41, pp. 1039-1048

Wimmer, H., & Goswami, U. (1994). The influence of orthographic consistency on reading development word recognition in English and German children. *Cognition*, 51, pp. 91-103

Wong, B. (Ed.) (2004). *Learning about learning disabilities*, Elsevier Academic Press, New York

Wong, B., & Donahue, M. (2002). *The social dimensions of learning disabilities*, Lawrence Erlbaum Associates, Publishers, Mahwah, NJ

Wong, D.A. (1985). The relationship between learning disabilities and depression in children. Unpublished doctoral dissertation, California School of Professional Psychology, Los Angeles

Wright-Strawderman, C., & Watson, B.L. (1992). The prevalence of depressive symptoms in children with learning disabilities. *Journal of Learning Disabilities*, 25, pp. 258-264

Ziegler, J.C., & Montant, M. (2005). L'apprentissage de la lecture dans différentes langues: un problème de taille. *Le Langage et l'Homme*, 12, pp. 149-160

Ziegler, J.C., Jacobs, A.M., & Stone, G.O. (1996). Statistical analysis of the bidirectional inconsistency of spelling and sound in French. *Behavior Research Methods, Instruments, and Computers*, 28, pp. 504-515

Ziegler, J.C., Perry, C., Ma-Wyatt, A., Ladner, D., & Schulte-Körne, G. (2003). Developmental dyslexia in different languages: Language-specific or universal? *Journal of Experimental Child Psychology*, 86, pp. 169-193

9

Dyslexia and Self-Esteem: Stories of Resilience

Jonathan Glazzard
University of Huddersfield
United Kingdom

1. Introduction

This study investigates stories of resilience in people with dyslexia. It provides a brief overview of some of the key literature in this area and draws on earlier research which I conducted (Glazzard, 2010). Data was collected using narrative genre. Four informants volunteered to tell their stories. The study considers ways in which dyslexia has shaped the self-esteem, self-concepts and identities of the informants. The stories provide powerful insights into the lives of people with dyslexia and the reader is invited to draw their own interpretations from the narratives. The study concludes that an early diagnosis of dyslexia is essential for creating a positive self-image and recommends that further narrative research is necessary to explore the significant impact that dyslexia has on people's sense of self.

2. Theoretical framework

2.1 Summary of key literature

According to Humphrey:

> Despite a barrage of anecdotal evidence from teachers and practitioners, there is a paucity of published research in self-concept and self-esteem in children with dyslexia.
> (Humphrey 2002: 30)

Much of the research into dyslexia has focused on causation and remediation. Consequently this study examines the effects of dyslexia on people's lives in general and on their self-concepts and self-esteem more specifically. Gurney defines 'self-concept' as 'the image or picture that we have of ourselves which we carry around and use to define ourselves as well as to categorise our behaviour' (Gurney, 1988: 4). In contrast, self-esteem is defined as 'the relative degree of worthiness, or acceptability, which people perceive their self-concept to possess' (Gurney, 1988, p.13)

According to Lawrence:

> One of the most exciting discoveries in educational psychology in recent times has been the finding that people's levels of achievement are influenced by how they feel about themselves (and vice-versa)'.
> (Lawrence, 1996, p.x1)

Key research findings indicate that learners with dyslexia experience teasing and bullying and feelings of exclusion (Edwards, 1994; Riddick, 1995; Riddick, 1996; Humphrey, 2001;

Humphrey, 2002; Humphrey, 2003). Unfair treatment by teachers has also been a consistent theme in the literature (Edwards, 1990; Osmond, 1996; Humphrey, 2001; Humphrey and Mullins, 2002; Humphrey, 2003) as well as teacher resistance to the existence of dyslexia (Riddick, 1996).

Osmond (1996) presented case studies with children and adults with dyslexia. According to Osmond 'the worst problem any dyslexic has to face is not reading, writing or even spelling, but a lack of understanding' (1996: 21). Osmond's case study descriptions show evidence of pupils experiencing feelings of anger and frustration with their own difficulties. The reader is provided with vivid descriptions of life experiences using the participants' own words. There is evidence of pupils' efforts being destroyed by teachers and persecution from other pupils (Osmond, 1996, p.21). There is evidence in this research of pupils experiencing anxiety when placed in situations where their difficulties were exposed. Examples of this include forcing pupils to read out in class and being made to leave their regular class for special lessons. Osmond's interviews with the pupils' parents provide evidence of schools and local education authorities adopting dismissive attitudes towards dyslexia. He quotes one parent who said:

> I think they regarded us as middle-class pushy parents, probably making too much fuss over a problem that would come right of its own accord…
>
> (Osmond, 1996, p.75)

The case studies which Osmond (1996) describes, provide rich detail of pupils' experiences of living with dyslexia. This detail is essential in order for the reader to develop understanding of what it is truly like to have dyslexia or be a parent of someone with dyslexia.

Edwards (1994) carried out case studies on a sample of eight adolescent boys from a special school for dyslexics where she worked. During her interviews with the students, it became evident that the majority of the participants had suffered extremely bad experiences as a result of having dyslexia. Many of these experiences were related to their education prior to coming to the special school. Indeed, Edwards was deeply shocked by the severity, extent and multiplicity of unpleasant experiences, which the pupils in her study had suffered. She found that five out of the eight boys had been on the receiving end of violence from their teachers, the cause of which they attributed to them having dyslexia. This is alarming. Edwards (1994) also found that seven out of the eight students had been humiliated and 'shown-up' by their teachers and incidents ranged from work being torn up, 'put-downs' and low teacher expectations. Additionally, Edwards (1994) found evidence of teasing and persecution from other students. This was in the form of verbal abuse and tormenting about their dyslexia. Seven of the students registered an extreme lack of confidence and all the students developed behaviour problems at some point.

Edwards' (1994) research provides an insight into the lives of students with dyslexia. Whilst both studies are now dated, they make an important contribution to the knowledge base within this field. Interestingly more recent studies have demonstrated similar findings.

Humphrey's (2002) study into teacher and pupil ratings of self-esteem of pupils with developmental dyslexia also makes an important contribution to the knowledge base on the relationship between dyslexia and self-esteem. Humphrey (2002) gathered data from three groups of pupils. In this study, the pupils ranged in ages between the ages of eight years to fifteen years. One group of pupils with dyslexia were taught in mainstream settings, a second group attended specialist units for specific learning difficulties and a third group formed a control group of pupils who did not have learning difficulties. Teachers' ratings of their pupils' levels of self-esteem were assessed using an adaptation of Lawrence's (1996) self-esteem checklist. Humphrey (2002) used a Likert scale to assess the behavioural manifestations of self-esteem. The teachers who were involved in the research were asked to assess the frequency of each behaviour trait on a four-point scale: 'Never', 'Sometimes', 'Most of the time' and 'Always'. An example of this is that the teacher was asked '*Does he/she make excuses to avoid situations which may be stressful?*' The teacher responded by circling one of the four words. In addition to the teacher ratings of pupil's self-esteem, Humphrey (2002) measured pupils' ratings of self-esteem using the 'semantic differential' method adopted by Richmond (1984). The pupil participants were required to place themselves on a seven-point scale between two opposite adjectives to represent their perception themselves. This relates to Lawrence's (1987) concept of 'self-image'. Humphrey (2002, p.31) provides an example to illustrate this: The pupils were asked for example, to place themselves on a scale of popularity ranging from popular to unpopular with a score of one representing 'extremely popular' to a score of seven indicating 'extremely unpopular'. The scale consisted of ten items. On completion of the initial scale, the pupils were asked to repeat the task but on the second scale, the pupils were required to indicate where they would like to be on the scale. This relates to Lawrence's (1987) concept of 'ideal self'. Humphrey (2002) then calculated the discrepancy scores between the pupils' self-image and ideal image for each item and mean discrepancy scores were then calculated for each group. The results of Humphrey's (2002) teacher ratings indicated that the pupils with dyslexia in mainstream settings and in units were significantly more likely to ask continually for help and reassurance than the pupils in the control group were (Humphrey, 2002, p.32). His findings also indicated that both dyslexic groups were more likely to display timid behaviour and avoid situations of possible stress compared with the pupils in the control group (Humphrey, 2002, p.32). The results of the pupil ratings of self-esteem also produced interesting findings. According to Humphrey (2002), the dyslexic-mainstream group had significantly lower levels of self-esteem than the other two groups in reading ability and writing ability. Humphrey (2002) also found that there was a significant difference in self-esteem related to spelling, intelligence and popularity between the dyslexic mainstream group and the control group, with the mainstream group having significantly lower levels of self-esteem in these three areas. Interestingly, Humphrey (2002) found no significant differences in pupils' ratings of self-esteem between the control group and the group from the specialist units in the areas of reading, spelling, writing, perceptions of intelligence and popularity. Humphrey argues that his results 'support the notion that dyslexia has an effect on the self-esteem of children' (Humphrey 2002, p.34). He argues that his results show differences in the self-concept and self-esteem levels between pupils with dyslexia who are placed in mainstream settings and pupils without learning difficulties. However, he also argues that his research shows that dyslexic pupils who are placed in separate units 'develop more positive self-concepts and levels of self-esteem than those left in mainstream education' (Humphrey 2002, p.34). This could be due to teachers in units having specialist training, more knowledge about self-esteem and smaller class sizes which enable them to spend more time talking to their pupils than their mainstream colleagues. The validity of the findings depends on whether self-esteem remains stable or changes over time and this has been debated in the literature.

Humphrey and Mullins (2002) collected rich qualitative data relating to pupils' individual experiences of dyslexia. They interviewed the pupils about their general self-concept and self-esteem, peer relations, teacher-pupil relations and academic self. This allowed the pupils to have a 'voice' and gave them the opportunity to provide richer information relating to their experiences of being dyslexic than quantitative data was able to supply. They found that around half of the pupils with dyslexia in mainstream settings and special units were regularly bullied or teased about their dyslexia. This is in line with the findings of Edwards (1994) and Riddick (1996). They also found that almost half of the dyslexic pupils in mainstream settings and in special units, prior to their placement, had been 'persecuted' (Humphrey and Mullins 2002, p.7) by their teachers. Indeed, they state that '...many of the participants had been called lazy, stupid or thick by teachers' (Humphrey and Mullins 2002, p.7). This is in line with Dewhirst's finding (1995) who quotes an extract from an interview with a teacher:

> **Teacher:** Well...I mean, it's one of those things that has been conjured up by 'pushy parents' for their thick or lazy children; quite often both.
>
> (Dewhirst, 1995 in Riddick, 1996 p.94)

Humphrey and Mullins (2002) found that around one third of the dyslexic mainstream group felt they were 'stupid', 'lazy' or 'thick' (p.8). They also found that one quarter of the dyslexic mainstream group and one third of the dyslexic pupils in special units felt that they were less intelligent than their peers. In addition, they found that in both groups, the pupils felt least confident in situations where their dyslexic tendencies were on display, such as reading out in front of the class. Another interesting finding was that around half of the pupils in both groups indicated a desire to swap places with someone else. The data provides evidence that the pupils with dyslexia in the special units have had negative experiences prior to their placement in the units. According to Humphrey and Mullins (2002) this has left them with 'emotional baggage' (p.10), or what Edwards (1994) refers to as the 'scars' of dyslexia.

The research by Humphrey and Mullins (2002) indicates that the experience of dyslexia can have a negative impact on pupils' self-concept and self-esteem. In addition, they found that pupils with dyslexia tended to attribute success to external factors rather than internal factors (Humphrey and Mullins, 2002), thus illustrating the theory of 'learned helplessness' (Peterson, Maier and Seligman, 1993). Research has indicated that learners with dyslexia attribute success to factors such as teacher quality rather than to their own intelligence (Humphrey and Mullins, 2002). Success is therefore blamed on external factors rather than being perceived as something which can be controlled (Humphrey and Mullins, 2002). This suggests that learners with dyslexia have a very poor internal locus of control. They feel that they are not in control of their own success in relation to learning, due to their own perceived inadequacies. Research has pointed to the link between learned helplessness, attributional style and low self-concept (Butkowsky and Willows, 1980; Humphrey, 2001). In contrast learners without dyslexia blame failure on internal factors such as lack of effort or lack of interest in a subject but not lack of ability, thus protecting their self-concept (Humphrey and Mullins, 2002). This suggests that learners without dyslexia have a very strong locus of control.

Burden and Burdett (2005) focused on pupils' attitudes towards learning and their sense of agency in an independent residential school for pupils with dyslexia. The researchers use their data to challenge the findings by Humphrey and Mullins into the relationship between dyslexia, self-esteem and locus of control. In contrast, Burden and Burdett (2005) found that the pupils with dyslexia had 'highly positive attitudes towards learning' (p.103) and had a strong sense of being in control of their own destinies. The study found that the participants felt in control of their own learning and they felt capable of achieving their ambitions. Thus, the participants had not generally internalised feelings of learned helplessness (Burden and Burdett, 2005).

> It is just feasible that similar results might be forthcoming from a comparison group of pupils with dyslexia attending mainstream secondary schools, but we very much doubt it.
>
> (Burden and Burdett, 2005:103)

My own research (Glazzard, 2010) challenges this hypothesis. The mainstream pupils with dyslexia whom I interviewed were all very confident and they attributed this to the diagnosis and ownership of the label. For these pupils the label helped them to explain their difficulties. They realised that they had a specific difficulty and that this was unrelated to intelligence. Prior to the diagnosis their self-esteem was significantly lower than it appeared to be after diagnosis, in part due to negative interactions with peers or teachers. Their self-esteem had been damaged as a result of negative interactions with teachers and peers, although in all cases the parents had worked hard to preserve their self-image (Glazzard, 2010). Research has also indicated that peers are an important source of self-esteem (Kirchner and Vondraek, 1975). My data suggests that the negative influences from both teachers and peers negated the positive support provided by parents (Glazzard, 2010). The diagnosis was a turning point in terms of building up confidence, self-concept and self-esteem and consequently its significance should not be under-estimated. Thus, I concluded that the need for an early diagnosis is therefore crucial in order to stop children from developing learned helplessness.

3. Methodology

I have chosen to use narrative as a methodological tool to explore the effects of dyslexia on self-esteem. In adopting a narrative genre I have used the life history specifically to tell the stories of four people who were diagnosed with dyslexia. I had personal and professional connections with the informants and this is a common thread in life history research. Through my connections with the informants it became evident that dyslexia had had a profound impact on their lives. The stories they tell illustrate the powerful effects of dyslexia on self-esteem and personal identity and what emerged throughout all the stories was the theme of resilience. This theme united all the informants and this formed the basis for selecting the sample.

The life history method emerged in the early part of the twentieth century and was further popularized by the emergence of feminism and the growth of sociology as a discipline. I have chosen to dedicate most of this chapter to telling the stories of my informants and in doing so, I make no apologies. My intention is to privilege the stories that people have told me, to let their voices speak and consequently to allow the reader to make their own sense of the stories they have been told. Clough (2003: 448) believes that narratives should 'challenge their readers to create their own meanings from them'. He believes that the narrative should 'lead the reader to a place where they might begin to search for the meanings and issues that lie behind and surround the story' (Clough, 2003: 448). In keeping my analysis relatively brief, my intention is to allow the reader to make their own sense of the stories that they have been told.

Drawing on Goodson and Sikes (2001) I view a life stories as as stories as told. In contrast my analysis essentially transforms the stories into life histories by exploring the wider contextual discourses which have shaped the lives of my informants. I believe that life histories can expose suffering, pain, misfortune, and injustice in order to 'speak to the heart of social consciousness' (Clough, 2002: 8). According to Goodson and Sikes (2001: 42), 'as social beings we are constantly storying our lives'. People enjoy telling and listening to stories and this renders this approach dynamic in that it has the potential to expose pain and suffering and illuminate the wider political, social and cultural discourses which have shaped people's lives. For my informants this approach can be empowering and emancipatory(Goodson and Sikes, 2001). Bowker (1993) has argued that an age of biography is upon us.

It has been argued that:

> …in their nature, already removed from life experiences: they are lives interpreted and made textual. They represent a partial, selective commentary on lived experience.
>
> (Goodson and Sikes, 2001: 16)

In presenting my stories I accept that I have presented partial and edited lives. In choosing specific storylines, I have effectively rejected others (Goodson and Sikes, 2001). This inevitably raises ethical issues around researcher neutrality. However I reject assertions that any research can be objective, neutral or value free (Greenbank, 2003). I am mindful that some critics question the value of approaches that are value-laden, subjective, non-generalisable (see for example Tooley's critique of educational research, 1998). I am not concerned with such criticisms. In my view stories can serve as powerful research tools by casting lights onto the lived experiences of those whose voices have been silenced and consequently marginalized. I argue that certain criteria used to judge the credibility of a piece of research (for example, objectivity, reliability, validity) are inappropriate indicators for judging the credibility of narrative research. I do not claim that my stories are generalisable but they are stories that others might relate to and consequently for some readers, the stories might ring true to them. In evaluating the quality of this research I hope that my readers choose to evaluate the extent to which the events of the stories engage them, and seem to be true. My intention is for the readers to bring their own interpretations to the stories. Several authors have emphasised that criteria other than objectivity, validity and reliability should be used to judge literary work. For example, Denzin (2003) cites Ellis (2000) who argues that texts should be engaging and have the capacity to evoke thoughts and feelings. Ellis (ibid) argues that texts should include authentic and life-like experiences woven into a good dramatic plot. Two other authors are cited by Denzin (2003), namely, Bochner (2000) and Richardson (2000a and b). Bochner (ibid) wishes to read a story that 'moves me, my heart and belly as well as my head' (cited in Denzin, 2003: 255). Richardson (2000a) is concerned with stories that contribute substantially to our understanding of social life, which are 'a credible account of a cultural, social, individual or communal sense of the "real"' (Richardson, 2000b in Denzin, 2003: 255). Hitchcock and Hughes (2003) refer to the criteria of 'authenticity' or the extent to which the events in the story ring true to life. I share these positions and hope that my readers can take something away from the stories I have chosen to present.

4. The stories

4.1 Rich

Context:

The 1944 Education Act in England emphasised the importance of segregated education for children who were deemed to be 'uneducable'. The term 'educationally subnormal' was used to describe children who had learning difficulties. During the 1960s the disability rights movement emphasised the rights of children with disabilities to a mainstream education. The comprehensive system of education was introduced and the 1970 Education Act facilitated the development of special education units within mainstream schools. There was an increasing acceptance during this time that children with learning difficulties had rights to a good education within mainstream provision.

Rich was born in 1959 to a middle class family in South Yorkshire, England. His father was a relatively successful engineer. His mother, whose background was from a working class family in Barnsley, England, had great ambitions for both of her children. She had achieved little in her own life and was seemingly intent on rectifying the situation by driving her children to success at all costs. Rich was, as a young child, placid and somewhat withdrawn. He lacked confidence when faced with social interactions with his peers and in such situations, whenever possible, would stay by the side of his older sibling for comfort and reassurance. In more familiar situations he appeared comfortable. He generally conformed to the expectations of the household, that he should be seen and not heard and other than an occasional confrontation with his sister was in general a very easy going child. Shortly after his birth his mother suffered from severe post natal depression and for the first 18 months of his life Rich and his sister were brought up by their elderly grandparents.

In 1964, 3 months before his 5th birthday, Rich began full time education in a local primary school. From the outset he found this new experience distressing. He spent much of each day choosing to isolate himself from his peers and in tears. His teachers would frequently call upon his older sibling to visit him in his classroom to offer him reassurance. However this only provided temporary consolation, and as soon as she left, the traumas of school life quickly enveloped him again. Rich would stand alone anxiously searching for his older sister during playtimes. His distress was so great that he was unable to develop relationships with his peers. Within only a few months of starting school life it became evident that Rich was struggling with early reading and writing skills. This in turn caused his mother great distress. Her anxieties were evident and these must have been transmitted to her son. However it cannot be doubted that all subsequent events retold in this story were intended to be in his best interests.

Rich seemed unable to grasp the rudiments of the alphabetic code. As children in his class began to make progress and develop a basic knowledge of phoneme/grapheme correspondence, Rich sat in a wilderness, seemingly unable to make sense of it all. His mother set to work cutting graphemes from sticky backed paper and adhering them to his bedroom wall in an attempt to support him. Relentlessly his mother subjected him to several coaching sessions each day. These had little or no effect and the alphabetic code continued to remain inaccessible to him. The obvious anxiety and desperation exhibited by his mother, without doubt, was absorbed by Rich who became more withdrawn. Unsurprisingly his behaviour also became more challenging. He would become very uncooperative, refusing to comply with even the most trivial expectations. He would begin to undertake tasks but would rarely complete them. The household became a battle ground and Rich became more and more unhappy and challenging, resulting in his mother becoming increasingly anxious. The downward spiral had begun.

Within a year of Rich starting school his mother contacted a local teacher and weekly private tuition was arranged. Rich was offered exactly the same diet as he was being given at school. There was simply more of it. His private tutor found him difficult to motivate and it was equally difficult to keep him focused on a task. He much preferred to engage with her dog or to engage her in discussions which in her view had little relevance to given tasks and were simply a means of distracting her from the role she had been given. She suggested to Rich's mother that private tuition was not supporting Rich and even indicated that they had so little value that the tuition was of no value and should cease. Rich's mother did not appear to hear such comments and the private tuition continued for a further two years while Rich made very little headway. When he was 7 his private tutor withdrew her services. This was apparently due to her retirement although this is questionable and may have been a means of dismissing her challenging pupil and his equally persistent mother.

Rich continued to display challenging behaviour at home. By now he had begun to feel a failure in many aspects of his life. His initial difficulties were in reading and writing as well as some aspects of maths. He was now perceived by his mother as badly behaved, uncooperative and as having an inability to concentrate. Their relationship was deteriorating rapidly.

The school which Rich attended became the next target. The classes were too big and in the eyes of his mother Rich was simply not receiving enough attention. A private education became the next perceived solution to his difficulties. Smaller class sizes would surely result in more attention being given to Rich and he would quickly make progress. A private school in the city was chosen where Rich would continue his education. He was only 8 years old. The school clearly had reservations about Rich joining their role. These were ignored by Rich's mother and a transfer to this fee paying school was swiftly arranged. Rich hated every day of every week that he attended the school. There were frequent communications from the school in regard to Rich relating to his lack of academic ability. He continued to struggle in school and after only a year he returned to the primary school where he had initially begun his education. He was certainly happy to return there despite the fact that he continued to find reading and writing, particularly difficult.

His secondary education did little to improve the situation. Reports from school consistently made reference to his 'poor' work, lack of concentration and inability to organise the daily demands of school life. Another private tutor was employed to support him but this tutor also quickly expressed concerns and declined to support him further.

The comments made by Rich's teachers poerfully illustrate the medical model of disability that prevailed during this time. Within-child factors were blamed for Rich's problems. There was no onus on the school to reflect on its policies or practices and make adaptations to cater for Rich's needs. Consequently Rich was labelled as a failure by a schooling system that failed to accept that it played a significant part in the problems that Rich was experiencing.

As a teenager, he was reminded on a daily basis of his 'failings'. Homework, which must have already been a challenge for him, heralded a daily battle ground. He was, by now, extremely de-motivated and frequently failed to complete homework. He often denied that any homework had been set. Communication between home and school all those years ago was sadly lacking and this enabled Rich to dodge the bullets until the annual parent's evening when his lies were usually unearthed. He began to truant from school. Everyday tasks were a challenge for him. His mother no longer blamed schools for Rich's difficulties. On a very personal basis his failure was now totally levelled at him. She perceived him as 'difficult' and uncooperative and their relationship was at an all time low. Rich took exams but his grades were poor and he left school at the age of 16. It is only thanks to his father that he managed to acquire a job in the mining industry as a fitter. Within 5 years he was, unfortunately made redundant and for the next ten years did not work again.

Redundancy resulted in Rich living at home with his parents. They were thrust together for 24 hours each day. The relationship between Rich and his mother was one of total conflict. His father was now retired and disabled and such conflicts caused him great stress. The stress placed upon him now resulted in a rapid decline in the relationship between Rich and his father. There were tranquil moments but these would be short lived. The inevitable conflict between Rich and his mother resulted in a snowball effect and would quickly lead to conflict between Rich and his father, who simply wanted peace and quiet.

Over the next 10 years Rich was perceived as the centre and cause of all conflicts within the household. He applied for several new jobs which would inevitably lead to renewed conflicts as he struggled to complete applications forms. His father would write them for him but he found it difficult to copy what had been written. Time and again a new form had to be sent for before yet another error was made as he tried to copy onto the form. Arguments and verbal abuse would follow.

Life continued in the vain for several years. How the family existed on a day to day basis under the same roof is nothing short of miraculous. In 1991 Rich's father suffered his final illness. It was a surprise to his family that although his father's death was imminent Rich made no attempts to visit him in the hospital. This was in fact to be the turning point in Rich's life. He was informed of his father's death. He chose not to be present at the funeral. Rich made one last visit to his home several weeks after his father's funeral. There was another dispute with his mother who ordered Rich out of the house. Twenty years later Rich has never been seen by any members of his family since that day. No-one has any idea of his whereabouts. He has simply vanished without trace. His mother is left distraught by the absence of her son, seemingly confused by his ability to cut himself off from his family. Rich, however, is happy and well. In 1959 there was seemingly little support or understanding of children with dyslexia. For Rich there was additionally little support or comfort offered by his parents. He simply made his escape to begin a new life. There is a plethora of support which he can now access to overcome his difficulties. Rich was never diagnosed as having dyslexia. This could well have remained the case today. He did, however, encounter severe difficulties in both reading and writing. He faced an uphill struggle, but, having left his old life behind him, he has successfully made a transition to a life in which he has managed to overcome his difficulties in peace and without judgement.

At the time when Rich went to school in the 1960s and 1970s there was no assumption that a child's learning difficulties could be the product of a schooling system that has failed to meet the needs of a child. The medical discourse located the problems firmly within the child. Had Rich attended school in the late 1990s rather than in the 1960s his story could have had a very different ending. Rich was ultimately failed by a system of education that assumed he was responsible for his own problems. The inclusion agenda, in contrast, places an onus on schools to be practive in meeting children's individual learning needs.

4.2 James

Context:

The Warnock Report (Warnock, 1978) examined the education of handicapped pupils and recommended the concept of 'handicap' be replaced by the term 'special educational needs'. The report recommended the integration of pupils with special educational needs into mainstream schools and classes and it emphasised the importance of parent partnership and an expansion in the role of local authority support services to support the needs of children with specific needs. The 1981 Education Act established the concept of integration and the statementing process. This process (which still exists today in the UK) involves local education authorities in conducting an assessment of the child to identify their specific needs. If the needs are severe, local authorities issue statements of special educational needs which set out the statutory educational entitlements that the school and Local Authority must provide to ensure that a child's needs are met. The 1988 Education Act saw the introduction of a National Curriculum which became an entitlement for all children, irrespective of the type of school that a child attended. In 1989 the United Nations Rights of the Child emphasised the social and educational inclusion of children with special educational needs and disabilities. The 1994 UNESCO Salamanca Statement emphasised the rights of all children to an education and the important role that mainstreaming can play in combating discriminatory attitudes. The 1993 Education Act resulted in the first Code of Practice. This led to the introduction of a named person within schools who was responsible for the education of children with special educational needs, the special educational needs coordinator (SENCO).

James is 28 years old. He is the eldest child from a marriage between 2 teachers. James views his life today as happy and secure and he eagerly looks towards the future with great optimism. He is no different in many respects to thousands of people of the same age. Life is good and the future looks bright. So what makes James and his enthusiasm for life different? In reality James has travelled a very long and often turbulent journey. It is that journey that has made James the young man he is today. His journey has paved the way to what he now believes to be a future abounding with renewed optimism.

James was born in Sheffield, England in 1983. He was the first child of a middle class couple and his arrival in the world was welcomed and celebrated by both his parents and their extended families.

James was not the easiest baby. He was born at 36 weeks and spent the first month of his life in intensive care. He rapidly made progress and was discharged from the hospital to return home with his parents. In terms of sleeping he was a challenge for his young parents and from the early weeks of his life would sleep for only three hours before waking. This continued until James began full time education shortly prior to his 5th birthday. The school he attended was placed in a very middle class catchment area and systems in the school can only be described as traditional. James had always been an extremely active child. His energy levels seemingly had no bounds. He was inquisitive, the world was exciting and every waking moment was a journey of exploration and intrigue. Life was full of questions. He had a genuine love of books and the times he frequently shared these with his parents were undoubtedly the only occasions on which he ever sat still. School life was not the easiest of transitions for James. Suddenly there was an expectation that he would sit still and listen for extended periods of time. He asked copious questions and within weeks he was already labeled as difficult to motivate. The questions he asked were viewed a challenge to authority. On one occasion he had spent an entire Friday afternoon immersed in developing a model. As the school day drew to a close he was asked to disassemble his creation. He enquired as to whether or not he could leave his construction and complete it the following week. This was viewed as challenging behaviour and communications with his mother quickly followed. His teacher was clearly none too impressed. James was happy when engaged in practical tasks. Such opportunities rarely presented themselves and he quickly developed a reputation for being a disruptive influence on his peers. His parents endeavored to offer James additional support at home. They would concede to this day that James much preferred situations in which learning was active and as teachers made every effort to capitalize on this need to engage him in his learning. James enjoyed a degree of success although he was clearly falling behind his peers in terms of his attainment in school. Life was for living, life was fun and quickly James became the class clown. He was by no means a naughty child. He could best be described as a rogue and both at home and at school he would often test the boundaries and needed to know exactly where those boundaries were. His antics gained him huge popularity with his male peers and he loved the attention. In retrospect it was clear that James was a square peg in a round hole. The educational establishment chosen for him did not effectively meet either his needs or his preferred learning style. He spent many play times completing unfinished work. James clearly found acquiring both early reading and writing skills challenging. He worked slowly and was made to complete one task set by his teachers before beginning and completing the next. To enable him to do so he often missed the elements of the curriculum that he so enjoyed such as physical education. and technology. Consequently he spent the most part of each day tied to a desk, trudging through endless reading and writing tasks that he clearly hated and found very challenging. There were few opportunities for him to express himself or to engage in physical activities which he clearly needed. James gravitated towards children with similar personalities. They often came from backgrounds which were very dissimilar to his own and such children did not enjoy the support of parents like those of James. He found a common ground with these children and was thrilled by their antics and freedoms in life. His parents continued to work with James and also to work alongside the school to support him. James at the very least raised a few eyebrows amongst his teachers. By the age of 8 he encountered one very severe teacher who was prepared to make absolutely no adjustments to her 30 years of practice to accommodate the likes of James. Her systems and approaches were extraordinarily rigid and there was absolutely no room for manoevre. His mother later recalled the ways in which she had attempted to work in collaboration with this same teacher. She accepted, as a teacher herself, that James may not be the easiest or most willing child to educate. To some degree this teacher did enjoy a modicum of success with James. He was indeed terrified of her and would make every effort to complete written tasks. She required a written product at the end of every lesson and was perhaps the first teacher to ever successfully extract this from James. James spent much of his days in school seated alone. By now he was clearly operating at a level below that of the majority of his peers. He was however increasingly sharing, what he perceived to be, his current new found success with his mother. At the end of the academic year there was an annual parents' evening and with a new found optimism James' mother attended a meeting with the teacher. James' mother, although dubious about the teaching styles of the class teacher, did acknowledge the change in her son who by his accounts was seemingly more focused in his work and making progress. The meeting began. A torrent of negative attitudes in relation to James was all that his mother was offered. Yes he was completing writing tasks but, but, but….his writing was untidy, he could not spell words correctly even though they had been learned by him a month before. His reading was not fluent; he was only really focused when he was making things or 'playing' on a computer. The result of this conversation was an unexpected and unrehearsed outburst from James' mother. She had listened to a torrent of negative comments about her son from the very beginning of the conversation; she had not heard one positive comment. As if from no where James' mother halted the conversation and enquired as to whether the teacher had any positive comment whatsoever to make in relation to James. Stunned the teacher confirmed that James was both a polite and kind child. He was able to share and always carefully considered the needs of others. 'Thank you' his mother replied before explaining that she felt that James indeed needed to be aware of the ways in which he could make improvements to his work but that he must also be made aware of his strengths. She wished to communicate both to him on her return home. She then terminated the meeting thanking the teacher for advising her of the areas in which James needed to focus but most importantly for identifying some positive aspects of his nature.

For the next 2 years James slowly built on his progress in reading and writing. His reading was slow and he often read 'new' words using an over reliance on a phonological approach. Indeed when writing phonics was the prime approach he used to aid spelling. His mother continued to engage James in exciting first hand experiences at home in a continuing effort to both support and motivate him. She was now convinced that James, although very distractible, was also facing a genuine difficulty in acquiring skills in both reading and writing.

James' experiences at primary school illustrate the dominant discourse of integration that was prevalent in the 1980s following the publication of the Warnock Report and the 1981 Education Act. Integration placed an onus on James to assimilate into a system of education that did not address his specific needs. The result was that James became demotivated and began to disengage with education. Within the discourse of integration there was no onus on the teacher or school to make any adaptation to practices and the medical model dominated traditional thinking around special educational needs

As James began his final year in primary school he was to meet a teacher who he recalls with total admiration to this day. For the first time in his relatively young life James was made acutely aware of his strengths. As with other teachers she identified his interests and strengths. Unlike previous teachers she capitalized on his strengths and interests. This same teacher embraced his enthusiasm for computers. James was no longer expected to record all of his work through pen and paper. He was encouraged to record much of it through word processing. This was of course well received by James. Writing was no longer a chore and became more enjoyable. This new approach however clearly began to identify that James did indeed experience genuine difficulties in spelling and writing. He was now happy to engage in the process and it became easier to identify his difficulties. James had without doubt mastered the basics of the alphabetic code, however as he was now approaching his 11th birthday his work clearly identified his over reliance on phonics as the prime approach to spelling new words. The teacher was fascinated by what she had discovered and in discussions with James' mother expressed her concerns that James was showing all the signs of having surface dyslexia. This year in school was, for James, the happiest to date. He worked with enthusiasm as his teacher celebrated his achievements but he was now also able to acknowledge his difficulties and worked tirelessly to overcome these by sharing them with a supportive mentor. As the time to move to secondary education quickly approached this information was shared with the receiving school. James' future suddenly took on a whole new and positive meaning.

The final year in primary school quickly became a distant memory of a successful and motivating time in James' life. The days of despair returned on his transfer to secondary school. His difficulties with both reading and writing were rapidly identified again. This of course was a positive beginning to his life in a new school. Surely James would continue to receive the support he needed. The reality was to the contrary. He was once again perceived to be failing and there were few support systems in place. Within only a few weeks James was again in the role of the class clown. He lacked focus in most lessons and failed to complete tasks that involved written work. Homework was rarely completed and again he gravitated towards other disruptive influences. During one parents' evening he was described by one teacher as the most stupid child she had ever met. His efforts now focused on having fun, taking risks and he came under the spell of peer pressure. James was excluded from school for taking alcohol onto the premises to drink with friends during the dinner time break. A watch with an alarm was deliberately set by him to coincide with the middle of a mathematics lesson. He was cautioned but repeated the prank the following week At home, despite the best efforts of his parents, he refused to complete homework. He had given up on school and was now relishing the excitement of testing and breaking rules and boundaries. A significant act of defiance is often recalled by his parents. They had negotiated a contract with him as vital examinations approached. He was to focus on revision during the day and could then enjoy time with friends in the evening. One night James prepared to leave the house to meet friends. He had not revised for his exams during the day. He was now 15 years old. His departure was stalled by his father. James had broken their contract and would not be allowed to meet his friends that night. In an act of total defiance James left the house. He never returned that night and it was only on the afternoon of the following day that he came home. His parents felt that this one incident was a turning point. James had realized that he was ultimately in control of his own life. He coped with the confrontations that followed his challenges to authority and when they were over he challenged it again. When he was just 14 his mother noticed a dramatic change in his behaviour and his personality. Intuitively she knew that such changes could well be the result of James experimenting with drugs. His father was far from receptive to this suggestion. James quickly identified and capitalized on such opposing opinions and skillfully used them to his advantage. He portrayed his mother as a crazed individual which compounded his father's view that indeed she was paranoid. The marriage did not survive this ordeal and James' parents separated. James and his sister stayed with their mother whilst their father moved on to pastures new. Indeed only two months after the separation James was 'outed' as a drug addict. Family life became very turbulent and strained. His younger sister also suffered as a result of his habit which now revolved around heroine. She was arrested when police forced entry into the house. She lived the nightmare of police knocking on the door in the middle of the night. He fraudulently took several thousand pounds from his mother's account. Eventually his mother was faced with the dilemma of meeting the needs of both of her children. Her decision was difficult but unavoidable and James moved out to live with his father.

James' experiences at secondary school in the early 1990s illustrate the dominant discourse of integration. James was perceived by his teachers to be a failure. There was no onus on the school to be proactive by making adaptations to meet James' educational needs. Consequently James was stigmatised and marginalised by an education system that was based on a medical model of disability. This had disastrous consequences for James and his parents, as illustrated in the events below.

The years that followed were turbulent years in so many different respects for the different members of James' family. James divorced himself from his mother for much of the next 7 years. There were meetings and telephone conversations. James was admitted to hospitals on several occasions with life threatening conditions and his mother was always present and James was glad to see her. His parents recalled the stresses felt by both themselves and James during his admittance to hospital. In the main the system was supportive. James would be prescribed methadone. It was rarely administered 'on time' and James would quickly begin to suffer from withdrawal symptoms, threatening to discharge himself from the hospital. Frequently hospital staff refused to communicate with James' parents in relation to his drug addiction. In attempts to ensure that James remained in hospital to receive treatment for life threatening conditions they found themselves in the unthinkable position of collecting heroine for him. Once discharged from hospital he went back to his chosen lifestyle which was financially supported by his father in an attempt to prevent James from thieving to finance his habit. To a certain extent such financial support did minimize the number of occasions on which James became involved with the police although there were several occasions on which he was arrested and he was, on one occasion charged with shop lifting.

During this time James entered into a relationship and within 18 months his son was born. On the day his son was born James was himself in hospital awaiting major surgery and was unable to be present at his son's birth. The relationship floundered. James gave little emotional and no financial support to the mother of his child and the couple separated. James made a few attempts to see his son but has now lost contact with him. Another relationship began and a second child, a daughter, was born two years later. This relationship was with a woman who also had a police record and seemed to prefer to live life on the wrong side of the law. It was an extremely volatile relationship and disagreements between the couple often resulted in James making his escape to return to his father only to be beaten up by gangs. His ribs were broken on several occasions and during one such incident James was stabbed.

Finally, James admitted to wanting to escape from the horrific lifestyle he had chosen. With the continued support of his family he finally sought help. An initial appointment with the family doctor was made by James. He attended with his father. There was to be no lifeline. Many medical practices had a policy that drug addicts were not treated. Eventually James was accepted by a medical practice several miles away and began a methadone program. The distance between his home and the fact that he no longer resided with his father, meant that James rarely attended appointments with his doctor or missed appointments at the chemists where he was given methadone. Time and again the doctors began a methadone program for James ensuring that he also had access to human resources to support him. Time and again the program failed.

In 2009 James' mother and his father financed a program in a rehabilitation centre. James was admitted for a week and placed under heavy sedations. On discharge from the centre he convalesced with his mother. He was weak, emaciated and 'on his own.' During the ensuing two years James continued to meet his needs for heroine from time to time. He never fully returned to the days of being an addict. Today James is finally 'clean'. He ensures that he attends all follow up appointments and is reunited with his family. James is 'high' on life. He finds casual work whenever and wherever he can, and looks forward to the day when he can find full time employment. His relationship with the mother of his daughter ended and currently he is engaged in a legal battle to ensure that he is able to be involved in his daughter's life. James and his family are indeed positive about the future. James frequently suffers periods of remorse and he still has a need to discuss those lost years. It is all part of the healing process for both James and his family. Without the support of a loving family James may well still be wandering the streets in search of his next heroine fix. In reality he is now well on the road to recovery and a 'new' life. James is eternally grateful for the support given by his family and the medical profession. His family is eternally grateful for his determination to battle through the hell of withdrawing from heroine. James and his family have lost over 10 years of his life to heroine. It is an experience that they will never forget. James' parents never stopped loving their son. Today, they watch proudly, as James boldly takes steps towards the future.

4.3 Alex

Context:

Alex is slightly older than James. He was born in 1979 just after the publication of the Warnock report and during his early schooling in the 1980s the dominant discourse was one of integration. The medical model of disability prevailed at this time and 'within-child' factors were blamed for the cause of children's difficulties.

Alex began primary school in 1984. He attended a large school with approximately 400 pupils on roll in a two form entry system. Alex had good memories relating to school in general until he reached the age of 9. The year was 1989 and his clear memory was of being summoned, with no prior warning, to the Head Teacher's office. His initial reaction was one of concern and he made the immediate assumption that this was a result of a misdemeanor on his part even though he was unable to identify what this could have been. On entering the office Alex was greeted by the Head Teacher (Mrs. P), his parents and his class teacher (Mrs. E).

It was at this meeting that, for the first in his life, Alex was made aware that he was considered to be a 'slow learner.' This was a totally new revelation to Alex who until this point in time was completely unaware that either his teacher, his, parents or the school held any concerns relating to his progress. Mrs. E explained that Alex had found it challenging to complete given tasks, in reading and writing, within a given time constraint. Mrs. P's solution to this problem was to suggest that Alex would benefit from a transfer to a special school. It was evident that Alex had absolutely no control or influence in the matter. The decision regarding his future education had already clearly been made. From the outset Alex had reservations about leaving a school where he was, happy settled, and had form strong friendships with his peers. The term 'special school' did not bode well with Alex either. Despite his anxieties Alex did not express his feelings. His mother insisted that Alex would indeed transfer to the 'special school.' Within three weeks of this meeting taking place Alex was attending his new school on a part time basis. Within half a term his placement was on a full time basis.

Under the dominant discourse of integration the school had not been proactive in making changes to its practices to meet Alex's needs. Alex had been integrated into a school that was designed to educate the masses and no specialist provision had been made availalable to enable him to make progress. He had been labelled as a slow learner and no attempt had been made to differentiate the learning to cater for his needs. He was ultimately blamed for his difficulties, illustrating a dominant medical model of disability which prevailed in the post-Warnock period.

There swiftly followed a series of assessments, resulting in a diagnosis, for Alex, of moderate learning difficulties. Alex had been placed in a special school which supported pupils facing a multitude of differing special educational needs. He was educated in a class of approximately six other children. He witnessed events that are emblazoned on his memory to this day. Events that, until this point in his life, he had never witnessed before. Many of his peers frequently displayed aggression. Chairs were flung across the classroom, rulers were used as weapons, children were frequently restrained and teachers were verbally abused and assaulted. School reports for Alex changed significantly. They frequently made reference to his immature, irresponsible and unacceptable behaviour. His friendships were with those who had been placed in the school to support them in overcoming challenging behaviour. This disruptive behaviour was however, quickly halted following a severe verbal reprimand from and educational psychologist, witnessed by his parents. Thereafter his behaviour improved and he was frequently rewarded for meeting behavioural expectations.

At the age of 12 Alex was offered the option of returning to mainstream secondary education. He embraced this opportunity but quickly struggled to be educated alongside his main stream peers in larger classes. His entry to secondary school had already been delayed by one year. The transition was difficult for him and he faced it with neither peer support nor carefully considered transition planning in place. Consequently Alex made a decision to move to the 'secondary special needs school' and was reunited with his peers and the challenging behaviours they displayed.

Alex has a clear recollection of facing National Curriculum test papers in mathematics and writing. The outcomes of these tests were never communicated to him. He does however recall, again, struggling to complete the writing of a story within the time constraints. Spelling also remained a challenge for him. There was never an opportunity for Alex to work towards GCSE examinations. He did, however, have the opportunity to undertake focused work placements.

As Alex completed year 11 in secondary school he had gained no qualifications. To the amazement of his parents, however, Alex made the decision to pursue his education at the local further education college. He had not enjoyed school life in more recent years but was able to identify the reasons for this. The challenging behaviour and constant disruptions effected by his peers had been central to his unhappiness. Alex however had never lost sight of the importance and value of education.

At college Alex enrolled on a Health and Social Care course. He still did not perceive that he had encountered any difficulties in learning despite attending two special schools. On being asked if he had any learning difficulties Alex responded in the negative. Alex had a desire to reinvent himself and this seemed to be an appropriate time to do so. He wished to eradicate any associations with the special schools and wished to remove the label of 'the boy with special needs.' During his first year at college his tutor suggested that he should be assessed to determine whether he had dyslexia. Alex agreed to this and subsequently he was given a diagnosis of dyslexia. Following his diagnosis Alex encountered many other students, some of whom were mature, who also shared diagnoses of dyslexia. He listened to their personal recounts of school life which often mirrored his own experiences. Additionally students recalled incidents when they had been the recipients of verbal and physical abuse from teachers. Many had been excluded from lessons. For Alex this was a defining moment in his life. From these frank and open discussions he acquired a true sense of belonging and his sense of isolation was quickly dispersed. Alex was now being educated with like minded people who had similar aspirations for their future but who had all shared similar experiences in their formative years in education.

A diagnosis of dyslexia for Alex opened the doors to additional focused support. He was able to access additional tutor support; computer aided dictionaries and electronic spell checkers as well as being able to readily access laptops during lessons. Through such support Alex achieved a distinction in his Health and Social Care course and further progressed onto vocational qualifications which led into a career in the health sector. Currently Alex is studying towards a science degree.

The impact of Alex's experiences continues, to some degree, to affect his life today. Attending courses to further enhance his own professional development are daunting experiences for him. He worries that on such occasions there may be an expectation for him to read or write in front of others. Alex continues to struggle with spelling, reading and writing and displays a strong preference for using a computer rather than writing by hand. In many aspects of his work he is required to hand write commentaries and notes, such situations are unavoidable and remain a source of stress to Alex.

Alex's later educational experiences at Further Education College powerfully illustrate a shift in thinking from a medical to a social model of disability. Ajustments were made to enable Alex to achieve his full educational potential and resources were provided which helped to break down barriers to learning and participation. Alex's experiences at college demonstrate the shift from a dominant discourse of integration to the discourse of inclusion, post Salamanca. Alex was no longer blamed for his difficulties and the proactive response demonstrated by the college is synonymous with inclusion which was advanced as a policy agenda under the Labour government post 1997.

4.4 Sophie

Context:

The 1994 UNESCO Salamanca Statement emphasised the rights of all children to an education and the important role that mainstreaming can play in combating discriminatory attitudes. The 1993 Education Act resulted in the Code of Practice for special educational needs. This led to the introduction of a named person within schools who was responsible for the education of children with special educational needs, the special educational needs coordinator (SENCO). Differentiated educational provision became more common during the 1990s and teachers became skilled in planning learning activities to meet the diverse needs of a range of learners as the social model of disability began to dominate thinking around disability. . The Labour government advanced the inclusion agenda post 1997 and this placed an onus on all educational institutions to be proactive in meeting children's individual needs by making adaptations to policies and practices. Disability Discrimination legislation in the 1990s placed a duty on teachers to make 'reasonable adjustments' to cater for the needs of children with special educational needs.

Sophie was almost 5 years old when she went to school in a small village in England. Before this time in her life Sophie had enjoyed the continual love and support of her family. She had spent her young life enjoying the love and affection of her parents and grandparents and was never far away from either of them. Sophie found the transition from the securities of home life to the new experiences of school life traumatic. She struggled to cope when her mother left her at school each morning. Each experience was a new experience for Sophie and she yearned to be with her mother for support and comfort. Two weeks late, Sophie continued to find the transition difficult. Her teacher instigated a meeting with Sophie's mother in an attempt to work collaboratively to ease Sophie's distress. This was the prime purpose of the meeting and it was assumed by Sophie's teacher that the reasons would be totally transparent.

On the day of the meeting Sophie's mother arrived, already clearly distressed. She was in fact convinced that Sophie's teacher was poised to reveal her greatest fear. That Sophie was dyslexic. Sophie's mother explained in minute detail her reasoning. She had obviously held this fear for a long time. Well before Sophie had begun her full time education. Schools in England are usually unable to secure such a diagnosis until a child reaches the age of 7 and at this moment in time Sophie's teacher had no evidence to suggest that Sophie was dyslexic. She did not however dismiss the concerns of Sophie's mother. In two weeks she had no evidence to suggest that Sophie was encountering such difficulties. The main areas of concern were Sophie's social and emotional needs.

As the weeks went by the events of this meeting remained fresh in the teacher's mind. Why had Sophie's mother seemed so certain that Sophie was dyslexic? She had spent almost 5 years with Sophie and although the evidence she presented could have related to most children of a similar age she was convinced of her findings. Indeed throughout the following year Sophie did begin to find it immensely difficult to acquire early reading and writing skills. She would appear to master a new skill but quickly lost the skill only needing to be supported again to address it. This vicious circle continued and Sophie's overall attainment, in these areas of her learning, became a cause for concern. She became very distressed when she anticipated the need to complete a reading or writing activity. Frequently her fears were unfounded but if she predicted that she would be asked to read or write she would become inconsolable. Her teachers were supportive and compassionate and Sophie consistently enjoyed praise for her achievements. This was to no avail. Sophie had already developed an innate fear of applying these skills. When engaged in other activities Sophie was confident and during discussions she was extremely articulate.

During the ensuing 2 years the school worked in collaboration with Sophie's mother, never denying that there was now a possibility that Sophie was dyslexic. There was access to little support for the school to support Sophie. Any enquiries were quickly and abruptly dismissed. There was an age barrier to accessing further support for Sophie. Her mother and now her teachers were convinced that Sophie needed additional support to overcome her difficulties. Sophie finally reached that mile stone 7th birthday and the process of screening for dyslexia could finally begin.

In reality the process was slow. External agencies were involved and there was doubt that Sophie was dyslexic. Her mother and the school remained convinced. The specific diagnosis was not a concern. Their shared mission was to receive additional advice relating to supporting Sophie. It was in fact almost 3 years later before Sophie was officially diagnosed as having dyslexia. Until that time the school had worked tirelessly to support Sophie. Sophie in turn had begun to use her difficulties as a crutch. She approached all aspects of reading and writing with a dyslexic barrier firmly placed between herself and the teacher. She was difficult to motivate and had a plethora of excuses. She was able to support her negative attitudes with a multitude of reasons as to why she could not attempt them. The staff in school found her attitudes challenging and on occasions she was confronted by their frustrations. They made every effort to remain clam but the barrage of information relating to 'my dyslexia' aimed at them by Sophie became a huge challenge. Sophie's views were acknowledged and much was done in an attempt to meet her needs. One practitioner recalled the day when Sophie was using a computer to word process her work. She was particularly difficult to engage on this occasion and finally explained that she found it difficult to work when the screen background was white. The screen was in fact yellow and had already been changed to meet her needs as Sophie had previously requested.

During the final year of Sophie's primary school education she finally received the diagnosis she and her mother had sought. Additional support was now readily available for Sophie, her mother and the school. Much of what was offered had already been provided by the school in the years before her diagnosis. However the difference in Sophie's attitudes towards her learning was swift and positive. No one had ever doubted her difficulties with reading and writing, she had been supported by every teacher and yet it was her diagnosis that was the key to opening the door to engaging Sophie in working towards overcoming the challenges she faced. It was as if, in Sophie's mind, everyone now believed her.

Sophie's experiences illustrate that the process of formally recognising a child's specific needs in England can be a long drawn-out process. The statementing process that was introduced following the 1981 Education Act is complex and in reality children may not receive a diagnosis until the end of their primary education.

Sophie enjoyed her final year in primary school. She and her mother were now more relaxed and at ease. She was frequently visited by specialist and her diagnosis indeed did much to develop her confidence and self esteem.

Sophie's battle was briefly revisited when she began her secondary school education. It is thanks to her mother, who worked tirelessly for 6 months to ensure that Sophie received the support she was entitled to, that Sophie again began to make progress. Sophie enjoyed her success and left the secondary school with 6 GCSE s before continuing her education and also gaining 3 'A' levels. This was followed by a course in which she successfully qualified to become a nursery nurse.

Sophie eventially managed to recieve the support she needed at secondary school to enable her to make good progress. This demonstrates the shift from integration to inclusion during the 1990s. The discourse of inclusion reflected a social model of disability which placed an onus on all educational institutions to make changes to their policies and practices to enable learners to make progress. Consequently Sophie was able to thrive during the final years of her school career due to the support that she received.

Sophie secured a position as a nursery nurse where she enjoyed every moment of the next 4 years. Her work was consistently praised and acknowledged. Sophie worked with a range of children with widely differing needs. She effectively supported them all. Over time, working under the direction of someone else became a frustration for Sophie. She had ideas and strategies of her own, which she wished to implement, but was unable to do so in the position she held. Her ideas of a new and different future began to form. In September 2008 Sophie applied to begin a teacher training course and was accepted.

Sophie was thrilled to have secured the opportunity to train as a teacher. Her difficulties with reading and writing had by no means disappeared and throughout her teacher training course she accessed a great deal of readily available additional support to aid her with the many assignments she was required to complete. She learned how to overcome her difficulties and spent far more time completing assignments than her contemporaries. Her grades began to improve. By now Sophie was married and the dedication to succeed she demonstrated was met with anger and aggression from her husband. He understood neither her drive nor her determination. The short marriage ended and Sophie was left devastated but still held onto a belief that she could succeed. In the practical aspects of her course Sophie excelled. She was truly committed to her chosen career path. She was creative and would spend hours carefully considering the ways in which she could engage her pupils whilst meeting their many individual needs. Committing her plans to paper was time consuming for Sophie but was deemed time well spent as she was highly motivated to ensure that her pupils enjoyed success. Sophie had been well supported throughout her life to overcome her difficulties. Her mother knew that from an early age Sophie was dyslexic. Could this possibly be because she recognized a mirror image of her own difficulties?

Whatever the reasons she worked tirelessly to ensure that Sophie could access the support she required. Throughout her life in school Sophie's difficulties, even before she gained an official diagnosis of dyslexia, were acknowledged and she eventually gained the specialist support that she needed. The greatest contribution to Sophie's success must be Sophie herself. She has shown great determination and ambition which culminated in Sophie now being poised to begin her first year in teaching as a newly qualified teacher. The future looks bright for Sophie and her dreams have finally become a reality

5. Discussion

The stories illustrate the powerful discourses which have influenced children with learning difficulties at various times. Rich's story illustrates schooling in England in the 1960s which failed to recognise individual needs and emphasised perceived deficits: *'There were frequent communications from the school in regard to Rich relating to his lack of academic ability' .... 'Reports from school consistently made reference to his 'poor' work, lack of concentration and inability to organise the daily demands of school life'.* A powerful normalising discourse pervaded at the time. Children were expected to keep up with the rest of the class and deviations from the norm were treated as failures.

Interestingly, the stories of James and Alex illustrate that two decades later, in the 1980s, little had changed despite policy rhetoric which emphasised the necessity for schools to meet children's individual needs. The influential Warnock Report (DES, 1978) had introduced the language of special educational needs and emphasised the capacity of mainstream schools to meet a diverse range of needs. However, under this discourse of integration, James' story powerfully illustrates that no attempts were made to meet his specific needs. Throughout his primary education teachers focused on his deficits and rather than the deficits in their own teaching, which may have contributed to James' disengagement. Within this normalising discourse, James was simply expected to assimilate into a largely unchanged system. Alex's story also illustrates a normalising discourse. The school failed to meet his diverse needs and consequently he was marginalized and excluded. He was viewed in terms of his deficits and punished by not being allowed to attend his mainstream primary school. This story powerfully illustrates the extent to which integration placed the onus on the child to adapt to the schooling system and how not adapting led to punishment. Both Alex and James' story illustrate how integration could be perceived as a normalising discourse which emphasised children's deficits. No attempts were made by Alex's and James' teachers to identify deficit aspects of their practices which could have contributed to their disengagement.

The connecting theme for Rich, James, Sophie and Alex is a theme of discrimination. The consequences of this discrimination were severe in James' case and his subsequent decision to engage in a life of crime could have been the consequence of his low self-concept. For Alex and Sophie discrimination was evident through a late diagnosis of dyslexia and, for Alex, his exclusion from mainstream education.

Sophie's story illustrates powerfully the impact of dyslexia on her self-concept. She approached tasks anxiously and with fear and often used made excuses to avoid certain tasks. Both Sophie's story and Alex's story illustrate the benefits of the diagnosis. In both cases the diagnosis was delayed but following the diagnosis both enjoyed additional support. It is pertinent to note that in both cases, the diagnosis came in the 1990s when

England was moving towards an agenda for inclusion. This discourse placed more of an onus on the schools to proactively meet the needs of the child rather than adopting a deficit perspective.

In all the stories there is an emerging theme of parental support but in some stories it is evident that parents had to fight to get support and worked tirelessly to achieve help for their child. Sophie's mother, for example, worked tirelessly to obtain a diagnosis of dyslexia. In Rich's story it is evident that parental support can be a negative factor: *'On a very personal basis his failure was now totally levelled at him. She perceived him as 'difficult' and uncooperative and their relationship was at an all time low'.* In Alex's case his parents were supportive but were clearly influenced by the views of more powerful professionals when the decision was made by the school for Alex to attend a special school. It was interesting that, at this time, the views of both Alex and his parents were seemingly irrelevant. This was a time before the dominant discourse which exists currently which emphasises the rights of parents and children to be involved in all decision making. This is now clearly articulated in the Code of Practice for Special Educational Needs (DFEE, 2000).

A connecting theme for all stories relates to the impact that dyslexia has had on the informants as adults. Sophie continually has to address her literacy difficulties every day whilst working as a teacher and he has to find strategies to overcome these. Form filling and note taking is problematic for Alex in his current job. Rich struggled to fill in job applications and needed support from his father. James continues to struggle with day-to-day writing tasks. However, despite this, a theme of resilience also connects all four stories. Alex is now successfully re-engaging in education. Sophie has achieved her life time ambition to be a teacher. James has broken away from his life of crime. For these three informants dyslexia has affected them but not paralysed them. For Rich resilience is manifest in a different way. He rejected his family to pursue a new life where he could enjoy being himself. The perpetual deficit view that he had been given was finally shaken off as he sought to re-invent a new identity for himself.

Alex's rejection of the term '*special needs*' powerfully illustrates the extent to which the terminology of special needs can pathologise individuals. The term emphasises a person's deficits, which reflects a medicalized view of disability. According to Thomas and Loxley (2007) 'there is an unspoken acceptance of need as a means of securing removal of the child' (p.54). Within this discourse the child is deemed in need to professional help from 'expert' professionals who focus their attention on locating the source of the difficulty within the child. Within a medical discourse the child is re-conceptualised as a *sufferer* and a *victim* and this reinforces a sense of powerlessness (Thomas and Loxley, 2007). Thus 'need' comes to represent deficit and disadvantage (Thomas and Loxley, 2007). There is a need to move away from such a pathologising discourse and focus on children's *rights* rather than *needs.* Such a paradigm shift has more positive connotations and emphasises the deficits in the school rather than the deficits in the child.

6. Conclusion

The narratives presented in this study evidence a united sense of resilience that emerges in all four stories. However, the resilience is demonstrated in differnet ways in each of the stories. There is evidence in these stories of low teacher expectations, for example in Rich's story, and there is evidence of marginalisation of children with dyslexia. Alex's story represents a powerful example of this. Jame's story illustrates that the costs of literacy failure can have devastating consequences and although it is not possible to make a direct link between criminal activity and literacy failure, it could be argued that James'low self-concept, could have been a significant factor in his criminal activities in later life. Parental support ranged from being supportive to over-bearing. For example, the support from Sophie's mum inevitably impacted on developing a secure sense of self which was clearly evident following her diagnosis However, Rich's mother had overly optimistic ambitions for him which resulted in his determination to rebel and dis-own his family. What emerges from these stories is a sense of success. Through determination and resilience, both Sophie and Alex have achieved their academic ambitions. James has overcome his drug addiction and is now considering re-engaging with education. Rich has made a new life for himself away from the pressures of his mother who, although over-bearing, only had what she considered to be his best interests at heart. The stories expose pain and suffering but, above all, they illumiate the discrimination experienced by all the informants in their education. Rich never had a diagnosis of dyslexia. If he had, the outcomes could have been more positive and Rich might still be in contact with his family today. Alex was denied access to a mainstream primary education. All informants believe that they have dyslexia. Some received official diagnoses, but these often came too late. Others, received no diagnosis, which left them vulnerable and unable to understand why they found reading and writing so difficult. Given the range of issues identified through these stories it is important that further narrative research is conducted and published to illustrate the effects of dyslexia on people's lives.

7. Acknowledgment

I wish to express my gratitude to all four of my informants for allowing me to write their stories of resilience.

8. References

Bochner, A.P. (2000), 'Criteria against Ourselves', *Qualitative Inquiry*, 6, (2), 266-72, in: Denzin N.K. (2003), 'Reading and writing Performance', *Qualitative Research*, 3, (2), 243-68.

Burden, R., and Burdett, J. (2005), 'Factors associated in successful learning in pupils with dyslexia: a motivational analysis', *British Journal of Special Education,* 32, (2), 100-104.

Butkowsky, I.S., and Willows, D.M. (1980), 'Cognitive motivational characteristics of children varying in reading ability: evidence for learned helplessness in poor readers', *Journal of Educational Psychology,* 72, (3), 408-422.

Clough, P. (2003), 'A Reply by Peter Clough: Things, Objects, Truths, Narratives and Fictions', *Research in Post-Compulsory Education*, 8, (3), 446- 449.

Denzin N.K.(2003), 'Reading and writing Performance', *Qualitative Research*, 3, (2), 243-68.

DES (1978), *Special Educational Needs: report of the Committee of Enquiry into the Education of handicapped Children and Young People,* London: HMSO.

DFEE (2000), *SEN Code of Practice on the Identification and Assessment of Pupils with special Educational Needs and SEN Thresholds: good practice guidance on identification and provision for pupils with special educational needs. DFEE.*

Dewhirst W (1995) 'Pushy Parents and Lazy Kids: Aspects of Dyslexia. An Investigation of the Experiences of Dyslexics and their Families in the Diagnostic Process ', Unpublished MSc in Social Research Methods, University of Teeside (in Riddick B (1996) *Living with Dyslexia* London and New York: Routledge).

Edwards J (1994) *The Scars of Dyslexia: Eight Case Studies in Emotional Reactions,* London: Cassell.

Ellis, C. (2000), 'Creating Criteria: An Ethnographic Short Story, *Qualitative* Inquiry, 6, (2), 273-77, in: Denzin N.K.(2003), 'Reading and writing Performance', *Qualitative Research*, 3, (2), 243-68.

Glazzard, J (2010), 'The impact of dyslexia on pupils' self-esteem', *Support for Learning*, 25, (2), 63-69.

Goodson, I., and Sikes, P. (2001), *Life History Research in Educational Settings: Learning fromLives*, Buckingham: Open University Press.

Greenbank, P. (2003), 'The Role of Values in Educational Research; the case for reflexivity', *British Educational Research Journal*, 29, (6), 791-799.

Gurney P.W. (1988) *Self-Esteem in Children with Special Educational Needs* Routledge: London and New York.

Hitchcock, G. and Hughes, D., (2003), Research *and the Teacher: A Qualitative Introduction to School-Based Research*, (2nd Ed), London: RoutledgeFalmer.

Humphrey, N (2001), *Self-concept and self-esteem in developmental dyslexia: implications for teaching and learning*, Unpublished PhD Thesis, Liverpool John Moores University.

Humphrey N (2002) 'Teacher and Pupil Ratings of Self-Esteem in Developmental Dyslexia', *British Journal of Special Education*,29 (1) 29-36.

Humphrey N (2003) 'Facilitating a Positive sense of self in pupils with Dyslexia: The role of Teachers and Peers' ,*Support for Learning*, 18 (3) 130-136.

Humphrey N and Mullins P.M. (2002) 'Self Concept and Self-Esteem in Developmental Dyslexia', *Journal of Research in Special Educational Needs* 2 (2) http://www.nasen.uk.com/e-journal.

Kirchner P and Vondraek, S (1975) Perceived Sources of Self-Esteem in Early Childhood, Journal of Genetic Psychology, 126 169-176, (in Humphrey N (2003) 'Facilitating a Positive sense of self in pupils with Dyslexia: The role of Teachers and Peers', *Support for Learning*, 18 (3) 130-136).

Lawrence, D (1987) Enhancing Self-Esteem in the Classroom London: Paul Chapman Publishers (in Riddick B (1996) *Living with Dyslexia* London and New York: Routledge).

Lawrence, D (1996) *Enhancing Self-Esteem in the Classroom* London: Paul Chapman.

Osmond, J (1996) *The Reality of Dyslexia: A Channel 4 Book* Cassell in association with Channel 4 television.

Peterson, C., Maier, S., and Seligman, M. (1993), *Learned Helplessness: a theory for the age of personal control*, Oxford: Oxford University Press.

Richardson, L. (2000a), 'Evaluating Ethnography', *Qualitative Inquiry*, 6, (2), 253-55, in: Denzin N.K. (2003), 'Reading and writing Performance', *Qualitative Research*, 3, (2), 243-68.

Richardson, L. (2000b), 'Writing: A Method of Inquiry' in: N. K. Denzin and Y. S. Lincoln, (eds),*Handbook of Qualitative Research*, in: Denzin N.K. (2003), 'Reading and writing Performance', *Qualitative Research*, 3, (2), 243-68.

Richmond M.J (1984) The Self-Concept of Academically Able and Less Able Children in a Comprehensive School: A Comparative Study Remedial Education 19 (2) 57-58 (in Humphrey N (2002) 'Teacher and Pupil Ratings of Self-Esteem in Developmental Dyslexia' *British Journal of Special Education* 29 (1) 29-36).

Riddick, B. (1995), 'Dyslexia: dispelling the myths', *Disability and Society*, 10, (4), 457-473.

Riddick B (1996) *Living With Dyslexia* London and New York: Routledge.

Thomas, G., and Loxley, A (2007), *Deconstructing Special Education and Constructing Inclusion*, (2nd edn), Berkshire: Open University Press.

Tooley, J. (1998), *Educational Research - A Critique: A Survey of Published Educational Research*, London: Ofsted.